Becoming a Reflective Practitioner

Fourth edition

Christopher Johns

With contributions from Sally Burnie, Simon Lee, Susan Brooks, Jill Jarvis and others.

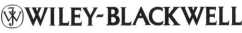

WILEY-BLACKWELL

A John Wiley & Sons, Ltd., Publication

This edition first published 2013, © 2013 by John Wiley & Sons, Ltd.
First edition © 2000 Christopher Johns
Second edition © 2005 Christopher Johns
Third edition © 2009 Christopher Johns

Wiley-Blackwell is an imprint of John Wiley & Sons, formed by the merger of Wiley's global Scientific, Technical and Medical business with Blackwell Publishing.

Registered office: John Wiley & Sons, Ltd, The Atrium, Southern Gate, Chichester, West Sussex, PO19 8SQ, UK

Editorial offices: 9600 Garsington Road, Oxford, OX4 2DQ, UK
　　　　　　　　The Atrium, Southern Gate, Chichester, West Sussex, PO19 8SQ, UK
　　　　　　　　111 River Street, Hoboken, NJ 07030-5774, USA

For details of our global editorial offices, for customer services and for information about how to apply for permission to reuse the copyright material in this book please see our website at www.wiley.com/wiley-blackwell.

Library of Congress Cataloging-in-Publication Data

Johns, Christopher.
　　Becoming a reflective practitioner / Christopher Johns ; with contributions from Sally Burnie . . . [et al.]. – 4th ed.
　　　　p. ; cm.
　　Includes bibliographical references and index.
　　ISBN 978-0-470-67426-0 (pbk.)
　　I. Burnie, Sally.　II. Title.
　　[DNLM: 1. Philosophy, Nursing.　2. Models, Nursing.　3. Thinking. WY 86]

　　610.73–dc23
2012051375

A catalogue record for this book is available from the British Library.

Wiley also publishes its books in a variety of electronic formats. Some content that appears in print may not be available in electronic books.

Cover image: Courtesy of C Johns.
Cover design by His and Hers Design, www.hisandhersdesign.co.uk.

Set in 10/12 pt Sabon by Toppan Best-set Premedia Limited
Printed and bound in Malaysia by Vivar Printing Sdn Bhd

1　2013

Contents

Preface

Welcome to the fourth edition of this book. It has been 3 years since the third edition was published. Hardly any time and yet the world is ever changing. Writing a new book is always an exciting blank canvas. Writing a new edition, the canvas is already filled with words from the previous edition. I try to approach each new edition from a reflexive perspective – how have new ideas emerged from old ones? As such, each subsequent edition of this book is like new skin on an old animal. I have not completely discarded the old skin; its remnants can clearly be seen by the reader moving between editions, like an historian plotting the emergence of reflective practice from my own particular perspective. I am less a commentator on others' ideas but a constructor of my own, juxtaposing as appropriate with the ideas of others.

I ask myself what has changed with regard to reflective practice in 3 years. Reading through professional journals, I suspect not much. There seems to be an inertia in theorising about reflection as if the dust has settled down. I get emails from around the world inquiring into facets of reflection that suggest reflection is widely accommodated into curriculum yet in a technical way. The triumph of technical rationality. This is no surprise. Teachers will accommodate reflection into the curriculum from this perspective because that is the way they know. At my own university, we missed a trick to be innovative with reflective practice with the new nursing degree programme. The result is that we will get more of the same wrapped in different paper. Perhaps they should listen to the students who generally find reflective practice a chore without much meaning. Perhaps the validating bodies should listen and ask for more, but then, would they know what more looked like? It is difficult to break out of the box and embrace reflection from a reflective perspective.

I imagine Plato's cave, the way the people only see what they see and cannot imagine another world. Technical rationality is the modern Plato's cave. Despite the heat of the licking flames and the hardness of the rock floor, it is a relatively comfortable place to be. I imagine the occupant's cry – 'I've found my place and I ain't moving!' I offer the occupant an opportunity to step outside, but it is rejected. The old cliché – better the devil you know . . .' Perhaps my failure to influence curriculum at the university has made me more cynical. Reflective practice is being open to new possibilities. It is in my bones and spurs into life whether I am in the classroom, at home writing or working as a therapist at the hospice. Reflective practice makes the world exciting. Everything becomes alive. I am like a new puppy, sniffing at everything, curious, questioning, turning things over, in my effort to realise my human potential. It is so easy to take things for granted, such as the nature of hospice or nursing. Yet these are immensely complex ideas. My image of hospice and nursing are radically different from what exists. Reflective practice opens the can and plays with the worms!

My approach to this fourth edition was to rip up the third edition and start again. Indeed, writing the book has felt much like that. Much is different, and yet I have kept many of the narratives. Reading them again I feel an attachment to them. They are such good narratives! I have edited them so they read better and have written new reflective commentaries around them. Reflective practice is like this, of revisiting narrative in light of new experience and finding different things in it. Narrative is always alive. Published papers are not covered in layers of dust but continue to inform what's happening now. It is reflection's reflexive nature. Such is the nature of this fourth edition. An invitation to step out of the cave and see reflection through new eyes.

> *Out beyond*
> *the shadows of our thinking*
> *a wholly different world appears;*
> *a world of infinite possibility.*

My cynicism melts in the hope of a new dawn. A renaissance given that I have been actively developing reflective practices these past 23 years. When the masters and doctoral students of the programmes I direct at the university construct their reflexive narratives of being and becoming, they are required to write a background chapter to inform the reader where they are coming from, given the subjective nature of narrative.

Perhaps the reader would like my own resumé to make the historical connection with my roots. My interest in reflective practice commenced in 1987 inspired by Margaret Clarke's paper, 'Action and Reflection'. The idea of learning through experience. I have always been a pragmatic person, not an intellectual. Shortly afterwards I was appointed as general manager of Burford Community Hospital, head of Burford Nursing Development Unit, and lecturer-practitioner with Oxford Polytechnic. Needless to say, I had much to do. I was also newly married with a young child. A veritable balancing act. At Burford, I developed the clinical model for reflective practice and guided reflection. This included designing the model for structured reflection (MSR), the framing perspectives, including the being available template (BAT), now widely used to enable practitioners frame learning through reflection with regard to desirable and effective nursing practice. In 1991 I moved into the university world and began exploring reflective practices on a wider canvas. I worked with numerous National Health Service (NHS) trusts to help them implement clinical supervision. I returned to clinical practice in 1998 to ensure my clinical credibility to teach palliative care. Since then, I have kept my own reflective journal and experimented with narrative form and construction. The plot of my own narrative is to ease suffering and enable growth as reflected in my personal narratives included in the book. Reflection is like opening the cover to the book of your own life, which up to now has been carefully closed (Jones and Jones 1996, p. 22).

In 2002 I commenced teaching the MSc leadership programme and in 2004 recruited my first doctoral student. I have supervised more than 80 masters dissertations all using my reflexive narrative approach (Johns 2010a,b). I currently have six PhD students, again all using reflexive narrative. All learning is guided within the community of inquiry. The plot is to liberate students to learn and to become who they desire to be.

I have become a performer, writing narrative as performance and performing widely at workshops, conferences and the public stage. Everything I do is an experiment, an opportunity to reflect and learn more about it.

I can't show performance in the book, but I would welcome approaches to perform as a means to dialogue about performance and reflexive narrative research. I would like to see performance within curriculum as a meaningful and exciting learning milieu. In 2012 I performed with Otter, my partner, in Hiroshoma, Japan and in Boulder, Colorado.

The audience response was very positive. We were approached to visit universities, hospitals and conferences as a result. Everybody is excited about performance narrative because it's learning potential is huge.

I have been experimenting with the idea of the 'reflective practice' conference. I say this in light of having convened the International Reflective Practice Conference since 1993. The last conference was at the University of Bedfordshire in 2010 where Ben Okri was the principal keynote speaker. The conference was exhilarating as always, and yet I was left with a sense of disquiet. What is the ideal format of a 'reflective practice' conference? I sensed it was not about keynotes and a succession of concurrent papers. It had to be about dialogue. In 2011 I convened the first 'reflective practice' gathering in Zakynthos. Just 17 people from around the globe spent 4 days in intense dialogue. No formal keynotes or presentation of papers. If readers are interested in this format, please contact me to arrange local gatherings around the world. In 2013, the University of Swansea hosts the 17th International Reflective Practice, returning to its conventional conference format.

This fourth edition is constructed through 22 chapters. More than I had imagined setting out. I have tried to write the text in a more reflective conversational style that invites the reader to dialogue with the text. A reflective text cannot be prescriptive. It can inform, suggest, provoke. I assume the reader is a reflective reader and, as such, is open to the possibilities of what the text has to say. It is a trigger for your own reflections. In this way I try to *show* people rather than *tell* people about reflective practice. Of course, that is more demanding of you, the reader, who would like to be told, but let me reassure you now, it is a more fruitful and satisfying path.

Reflective practice is about becoming aware of our own assumptions, how these assumptions govern our practice, how these assumptions must shift to embrace change, understanding resistance to assumption shift, and finally to change assumptions to support a better state of affairs. Without doubt, much of what passes as reflection is 'surface' work that does not address the deeper structures that govern the way the world is. This is not to say that surface work is not important. Just dig a little deeper each time.

The central focus of the book is the idea of the 'reflective practitioner' as someone who lives reflection in everyday practice. For me this is the whole point. Reflective education and research are means to this end. Becoming a reflective practitioner takes time, commitment, responsibility, discipline, and, as Ben Okri (1997, p. 22) writes, 'the biggest tasks are best approached tangentially, with a smile in the soul.' Everyone should read his book, *A Way of Being Free*, to inspire their reflective endeavour. Okri writes as a poet, and I think this is a good place to imagine.

I wanted the book to be more free flowing. As such, I have not split it into parts as previous editions. Chapter 1 is an introduction to reflective practice. It provides a background to ideas developed in subsequent chapters. I set out my description of reflective practice, that despite my tinkering around the edges, I find hard to improve upon, although my commentary on this definition is hopefully clearer. The learning potential of reflective practice is the contradiction or creative tension between the practitioner's vision of desirable practice and the practitioner's understanding of his or her actual practice. The reflective effort is to resolve any contradiction towards realising desirable practice, which is itself a movable feast. What does desirable mean as lived? Who governs what is desirable? Think differently, and the images shift.

I have always been concerned to balance what I saw as a dominant western approach to reflective theories with more esoteric or non-rational influences inspired by my interest in native American and Buddhist philosophy. This balance culminated in my paper,

'Balancing the Winds' (Johns 2005). I sense the growth of interest of mindfulness in health care stemming from Buddhist influences, for example, mindfulness-based stress reduction (Kabat-Zinn 1990). Words like reflection and mindfulness pass into general use as if everyone knows what they mean. My own approach has developed in continuous dialogue with extant theories of reflection and more diverse ideas. Most practice disciplines like nursing are concerned with 'doing' and give little thought to the underlying ideas. I know from my own university that nurse teachers (in their wisdom) consider the MST too technical for first year nursing students, and yet this is a degree programme!

Through Chapters 2–7 I set out the six dialogical movements of narrative construction. This is the 'basic scheme', moving from writing description of experiences in a journal to narrative dialogue with an audience. It does not matter whether you are a student writing a first year reflective assignment or a doctoral student constructing a thesis of being and becoming; the approach is the same. Perhaps the degree of depth is different!

It is worth noting a few significant issues. The first issue is the distinction between description and reflection. Description is the raw data of experience and the quality of the description sets up the possibility for gaining insight. In general, I sense teachers do not make this distinction clear. The second issue is the way the MSR is taken out of context of the six dialogical movements. People often say to me from across the globe, 'Oh we use your model'. I ask what model? They say the MSR and that's it. The representation of reflective practice as narrative and its presentation through performance are vital to appreciate. The third issue is the way teachers design reflective assignments around the reflective process rather than around insights gained. The MSR is a means to an end, not an end in itself. The MSR is offered in its 16th edition. I have divided it into five learning phases and have drawn attention to the idea of assumptions. As before, I emphasise its practical value in facilitating clinical skills. In Chapter 4 I explore the idea of framing insight gained from reflection. Insights change us as people. As a consequence, we see and respond to the world differently. I have downplayed the BAT in my increasing shift of emphasis on the reflective process rather than on the nature of clinical practice. If I want to know if I am more effective in person-centred practice, how would I know that? Clearly such issues are core to reflective practice. In Chapter 5, I address the mythological theory–practice gap in considering the idea of dialogue between insights and a relevant literature. Experience gives students a 'hook to hang their hats on' – and thus makes more sense than abstract immersion. I illustrate this with two narratives – Michael's wife and Sylvia. All the narratives within the book are offered as examples of reflective writing and are used to illustrate the application of theoretical ideas and evidence of learning. In Chapter 6, I explore guided reflection as the co-creation of meaning, acknowledging that the learning potential of reflection is enhanced through skilled guidance.

Many of the ideas expressed in Chapter 8 – the reflective curriculum – have been addressed in previous chapters. My exploration of the reflective curriculum in the third edition was a reflective meander without any real structure, and yet reflective learning is often like that – we follow our curious noses and see where it takes us! I have taken a more factual approach of 'how to do it' than previously. One reason for this approach is the radical nature of the reflective curriculum or what I term the truly reflective curriculum; that is, a curriculum that doesn't contradict itself. It is influenced by critical reflection and Brookfield's (1995) ideas of the critical reflective teacher (i.e. essential supplementary reading). The core of the reflective curriculum is the tension between clinical practice and theoretical ideas mediated through guided reflection. It is a simply yet radically profound movement, opening the door to art and performance-based learning. Whilst reflective-minded teachers can create bubbles of reflective activity within their spheres of influence, how can the whole curriculum become reflective?

Chapters 9–12 are edited narratives written by students I have guided within formal post-registration curriculum. They reveal the potential of learning through reflection and their authors' different writing styles. What engages you as you read these narratives? Do they trigger your own reflections? How might they influence your own reflection and writing? Would you use these narratives as a referential source in your own reflective writing, or do you dismiss them as mere anecdotes? The book is not meant to be a passive reader but a dialogue.

In Chapter 13 I set out a reflective framework for clinical practice. I have always felt that one overlooked aspect of my work in developing reflective practice is the construction of the Burford model. It has a simple logic – if we want to have reflective practitioners, then we need to structure clinical practice around reflective structures. The idea that there should be resonance and no contradiction between processes and systems. The model is built around a collective valid vision of practice and four reflective systems designed to enable the vision to be lived (Johns 1994). I rework my narrative of working with Tony to illustrate my use of the Burford reflective cues. The cues offer another approach to a reflective model in relation to appreciating and responding to the patient's life pattern as an evolving narrative of working with the patient, family and other healthcare practitioners.

In Chapter 14 I consider the idea of reflective leadership. Leadership is complex in its relationship with the transactional culture of NHS organisations with its management decree of 'command and control'. A reflective leadership seeks to work collaboratively with staff. Leaders become servants to support the front-line work, investing in staff for maximum performance and shared success. Since 2002 I have directed the MSc leadership programme at the university. In that time I have come to understand the creative tension between the idea of leadership and its potential reality within the transactional organisation. It is not an easy fit. Indeed, real leadership may not be possible.

In Chapter 15 I explore chaos theory through the narrative of Lazel, a midwifery leader, written as a masters assignment concerned with leading in a chaotic world. In essence, reflection is an element of chaos theory with its focus on the hermeneutic circle and holding creative tension – rather like the creative edge between stability and instability of systems. Throughout the narrative she holds the creative tension. She shows how the reality wall of the organisation was difficult to break down.

In Chapters 16–18 I explore another vital aspect of everyday practice – ensuring quality. It seems practice everywhere lives in the shadow of quality. The Care Quality Commission (CQC) might come knocking one day without warning. I argue that practitioners must take responsibility for quality on a daily basis. In other words, to live quality. It is not good enough for practitioners to be passive about quality – that it is something they are judged against. In the 1980s and 1990s standards of care were fashionable through the Royal College of Nursing Dyssey approach (Kitson 1989). I was a strong advocate of this approach and utilised it at Burford. Clinical audit is a reflective exercise of looking back and learning through 'experiences'. Clinical supervision hit the screens in 1993. It offers a learning space within clinical practice for guided reflection. Some narratives of clinical supervision constructed through recorded dialogue are set out in Chapter 18. These have a particular focus on ethical mapping derived from the MSR cue – 'did I act for the best and in tune with my values'. The narratives help explore the depth of this cue. I utilise 'Cathy and the GPs' narrative to explore issues around patriarchy, power and assertiveness set against the hegemonic relationship between doctors and nurses.

Initially I excluded Moira Vass's journal (Chapter 19). It had, after all, been in the two previous editions. Perhaps something new was required. I remembered my promise to her to publish her journal as an exemplar of the benefits of patient journalling to help express suffering and, with particular regards to Moira, to give her voice. As reflective practitioners we are better able to engage with our patients in reflective practice. Art therapy is a similar reflective activity practitioners can engage with patients. The therapeutic benefit of writing is well known through various research, notably by Pennebaker (1989) and Pennebaker *et al* (1990, 1997).

Chapter 20 is co-written by my artist partner, Otter, in which we explore storyboard. She uses storyboard to illustrate her experience of being bullied as a nurse. Very little dialogue accompanies the storyboard, and yet it is a very powerful narrative. People tend to be either more verbal or visual in the way they see the world. As such, visual forms of reflection and narrative may benefit 'visual' practitioners. In workshops this difference has become very apparent. I am not a visual person and struggle to use this art form. I prefer prose poetry – the focus for Chapter 21. I set out seven poems that are collectively focused on patients who I encountered in one day at the hospice where I work as a complementary therapist. It raises questions about 'what is therapy' and its ability to ease suffering. Prose poetry is an exciting development of reflexive narrative that has evolved from breaking down text into single lines and building in insight. I recently shared four of these poems in a brief reading in the USA. The feedback was very positive – in the way the poems captured something about caring that really made the listener stop and think.

In Chapter 22, I offer the narrative 'through a glass darkly' that I first performed with Otter in Hiroshima in March 2012 to an international 'peace and caring' conference to an audience of 600 people. The performance was constructed around me reading the narrative together with constructed elements of voice intonation, movement, music, background powerpoint, painting and installation. Of course, these elements are not visible within the printed version.

I decided against a specific chapter on reflexive narrative as a research journey of self-inquiry and transformation towards self-realisation. This is the focus of my book, *Guided Reflection: A Narrative Approach to Advancing Practice* (Johns 2010a,b). Of course, self-inquiry and transformation is the basis for all reflective practices.

Reading through the third edition in preparation for writing this edition left me frustrated in the way I wrote. With hindsight, this is probably a current phenomenon with authors who have moved on with their ideas as I hope I have. Reading through the fourth edition ready for publication I feel more satisfied, though every time I reread a part of it, I find myself editing. Reflective practice is rather like this. There is no resting on one's laurels. It is an insistent exploration of ideas and a way to represent them in the best way to engage others.

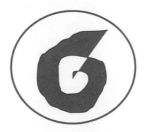

The koru is a Maori image of an uncurling fern frond. It represents peace, tranquillity, personal growth, positive change and awakening, and new life and harmony. I discovered this image when visiting New Zealand and now wear the koru, made from green stone or pounamu, as the symbol for my reflective practice. Each time I draw the koru it is different, representing how each experience is different although the basic pattern is familiar.

Throughout the book I refer to nurse/practitioner as him and her at random.

*Christopher John*s

Acknowledgements

To Otter, my partner and constant critic, for her creative genius that opens new vistas for reflective practices.

To students whose work continues to illustrate the art of reflective practice and its representation in narrative form: Sally, Simon, Lazel, Jim, Clare, Cathy, Trudy, Susan, Janet, Ted, and Jill.

To Catriona and Magenta at Wiley-Blackwell who have supported me through successive editions and have made this book possible.

Chapter 1

What is reflective practice?

Just take a moment.
Reflect and think.
Really think YOU.

Just take a moment – it needn't take very long. Just think of one situation when you were last at work. Ask yourself, 'did I respond in the most effective way?' You might wonder 'what is the most effective way'? You might reflect on factors that influenced your response. You might think about the purpose of your response. You might consider the craft of your response, the words you used. You might think about the consequences of your response. You might think about your feelings. Was it a good experience or a bad experience? How do you make these distinctions? Such questions open a path to explore and find meaning in the experience and learn through it so next time when faced with a similar situation you might just respond in a more effective way.

In this way you take responsibility for your performance. Your patients or colleagues deserve nothing less.

Reflection is a learning journey of becoming a reflective practitioner, someone who is reflective moment to moment. It is learning through our everyday experiences towards realising one's vision of desirable practice as a lived reality. It is a reflexive process of self-inquiry and transformation of being and becoming the practitioner you desire to be. Through self-inquiry we can learn to participate more fully in our own lives simply by listening 'more carefully and to trust what we hear, the messages from our own body and mind and feelings' (Kabat-Zinn 1994, p. 192). As such, reflection is always purposeful, moving towards a more reflective, effective and satisfactory life.

The *Compact Oxford English Dictionary 3e* (Soanes and Hawker 2005, p. 86) defines reflect:

- throw back heat, light, sound without absorbing it
- (of a mirror or shiny surface) show an image of
- represent in a realistic or appropriate way
- bring about a good or bad impression of someone or something (on)
- think deeply or carefully about.

Interpreting this array of definitions, reflection can be viewed as a mirror to see images or impressions of self in context of the particular situation in a careful and realistic way.

Becoming a Reflective Practitioner, Fourth Edition. Christopher Johns.
© 2013 John Wiley & Sons, Ltd. Published 2013 by John Wiley & Sons, Ltd.

It is clearly a way of thinking deeply and carefully about self within the context of one's practice. It is judgemental – to what extent was I effective within the particular situation?

The words *reflection* and *reflective practice* are used glibly, as if reflection is the most normal thing in the world requiring little skill or guidance. I recently met a district nurse at my local village fete. My partner mentioned that I was a bit of a guru in reflective practice. The district nurse recoiled and said she hated reflective practice, that she had had it shoved down her throat. I smiled. I could imagine her experience of being taught reflection in an instrumental way using a model of reflection by unreflective teachers. I know this because I see it everywhere.

Describing reflection

I currently formally describe reflection as 'being mindful of self, either within or after experience, as if a mirror in which the practitioner can view and focus self within the context of a particular experience, in order to confront, understand and move towards resolving contradiction between one's vision and actual practice. Through the conflict of contradiction, the commitment to realise one's vision, and understanding why things are as they are, the practitioner can gain new insight into self and be empowered to respond more congruently in future situations within a reflexive spiral towards developing practical wisdom and realising one's vision as praxis. The practitioner may require guidance to overcome resistance or to be empowered to act on understanding'.

I say currently because, like all things, it cannot be easily pinned down. My understanding of reflection is always evolving. It is something in motion not easily captured by words. It is more a state of being than of doing – something I am rather than something I do.

My description is full of words that need careful consideration.

Reflection on experience

Reflective practices span from *doing* reflection towards *being* reflective (Table 1.1). *Doing* reflection reflects an epistemological approach, as if reflection is a tool or device. Indeed, this is true to an extent. However, reflection is much more than that. *Being* reflective reflects an ontological approach. It is about 'who I am' rather than 'what I do'. This makes utter sense in a practice discipline such as nursing where the primary therapy is using self. The strands of reflection as an epistemological versus ontological project has been critiqued by Rolfe and Gardner (2006). My view is that the ontological subsumes the epistemological project, as if the way we think about things naturally involves us who are to think about things in the first place.

When people talk about reflection, they generally refer to reflection-on-experience. Indeed most theories of reflection are based on this idea – looking back on 'an experience'. The idea of an *experience* is difficult to grasp – where does one experience begin and another end? Is experience not the endless flow of life? Is anticipating a forthcoming event an experience in itself? I consider an experience as thinking, feeling or doing something. Each intake of breath is an experience. Each thought is an experience. Schön (1983, 1987) distinguished reflection-*on-action* with reflection-*in-action* as a way of thinking about a situation whilst engaged within it, in order to reframe and solve some breakdown

Table 1.1   Typology of reflective practices

Reflection-on-experience	The practitioner reflects on a particular situation after its event in order to learn from it to inform future practice.	Doing reflection
Reflection-in-action	The practitioner stands back and reframes the practice situation in order to proceed towards desired outcome.	
The internal supervisor	The practitioner dialogues with self whilst in conversation with another as a process of making sense and response (Casement 1985).	
Reflection-within-the-moment	The practitioner is mindful of his pattern of thinking, feeling, and responding within the unfolding moment whilst holding the intent to realise desirable practice.	
Mindfulness	Seeing things for what they really are without distortion.	Being reflective

in the smooth running of experience. The practitioner naturally adjusts to minor interruptions within the smooth flow of experience because the body has embodied knowing. Sometimes, the practitioner is faced with situations that do not go smoothly, requiring the practitioner to pause and stand back to consider how best to proceed. This requires a shift in thinking and contemplating new ways of responding. Schön (1987) drew on exemplars from music and architecture – situations of engagement with inanimate forms. His example of counselling is taken from the classroom not from clinical practice. The classroom is a much easier place to freeze and reframe situations in contrast with clinical practice grounded within the unfolding human encounter. It is easy to misunderstand reflection-in-action as merely thinking about something whilst doing it.

Mindfulness

Through writing and reflecting on practice, practitioners learn to pay increasing attention to self within practice. They become more aware of patterns of thinking, feeling and responding to situations. They become more curious and intentional. In time, with discipline, reflection becomes a natural attribute. The ultimate expression of this awareness is mindfulness; seeing self clearly at all times without distortion.

Goldstein (2002, p. 89) considers that 'Mindfulness is the quality of mind that notices what is present without judgment, without interference. It is like a mirror that clearly reflects what comes before it.' The idea of being without judgement, without interference, is very significant, as if being mindful is a precursor for making good judgements based on clear understanding. Goldstein writes from a Buddhist perspective. As a Buddhist, I too draw on Buddhist psychology to explore the nature of mindfulness or *smrti*, which implies being aware moment to moment

- of things and the world around us
- of self; our body, our feelings and thoughts
- of self in relationship with others
- of ultimate reality.

Ultimate reality can be viewed on two levels: the mundane level being concerned with holding and intending to realise a right vision of practice however this might be expressed; the transcendental level concerned with spiritual growth. Realising the mundane is inevitably a movement towards the transcendental. Being mindful, I know what I am doing and why I am doing it, and to see that what I am doing right now fits with my intention. Awareness is liberating. As Wheatley and Kellner-Rogers (1996, p. 26) write, 'The more present and aware we are as individuals and as organisations, the more choices we create. As awareness increases, we can engage with more possibilities. We are no longer held prisoner by habits, unexamined thoughts, or information we effuse to look at.'

Being mindful I am vigilant against unskilful actions and negative mental events that constantly try to distract the mind, for example anger, arrogance, resentment, envy, greed and the suchlike (Sangharakshita 1998). In Buddhism, this quality of mind is called *apramada* – the guard at the gate of the senses ever watchful for those negative mental events that cloud the mind.

Prerequisites of reflection

Fay (1987) identifies certain qualities of mind that are prerequisite to reflection: curiosity, commitment and intelligence. These qualities of mind are significant to counter the more negative qualities of mind associated with defensiveness, habit, resistance and ignorance.

Commitment is type of energy that sparks life. Yet, for many practitioners, commitment to their practice has become numb or blunted through working in non-challenging, non-supportive and generally stressful environments, where work satisfaction is making it through the shift with minimal hassle. These practitioners do not enjoy reflection. They turn their heads away from the reflective mirror because the reflected images are not positive. They do not want to face themselves and accept responsibility for their practice. Things wither and die if not cared for. When those things are people, then the significance of commitment is only too apparent. Commitment harmonises or balances conflict of contradiction – it is the energy that helps us to face up to unacceptable situations. As Carl Rogers (1969) notes, the small child is ambivalent about learning to walk; he stumbles and falls, he hurts himself. It is a painful process. Yet the satisfaction of developing his potential far outweighs the bumps and bruises. Van Manen (1990, p. 58) writes,

> Retrieving or recalling the essence of caring is not a simple matter of simple etymological analysis or explication of the usage of the word. Rather, it is the construction of a way of life to live the language of our lives more deeply, to become more truly who we are when we refer to ourselves [as nurses, doctors, therapists].

Curiosity is fundamental to the creative life, and yet many practitioners are locked into habitual patterns of practice. Often, when things get overly familiar, we take them for granted and get into a habitual groove. O'Donohue (1997, p. 122–3) writes, 'People have difficulty awakening to their inner world, especially when their lives become familiar to them. They find it hard to discover something new, interesting or adventurous in their numbed lives.'

Curiosity – why do I feel that way? Why do I think that way? Why do I respond that way? How else could I respond? Why are the walls green? Does music help patients relax? Why is Jim unhappy? Why do I feel angry each time I see my manager? Why doesn't my manager listen? Everything enters into the gaze of the curious practitioner intent on realising desirable and effective practice. Gadamer (1975, p. 266) writes, 'The opening up and keeping open of possibilities is only possible because we find ourselves deeply interested in that which makes the question possible in the first place. To truly question something is to interrogate something from the threat of our existence, from the centre of our being.'

Being curious, the practitioner is not defensive, but open to new possibilities. Every situation becomes an opportunity for learning. Being intelligent, the practitioner sees things for their merit rather than dismiss ideas out of hand because they don't fit within his or her scheme of things. The practitioner is not resistant or dismissive of new ideas but keen to explore his or her value for practice.

Reflexivity

Reflexivity is 'looking back' to make sense of self emerging through a sequence of experiences towards self-realisation however that might be expressed. Dewey (1933) describes this as links within a chain where one link leaves a trace that is picked up by the next link. If we replace the idea of a 'link' with insights, we can see that each subsequent experience is infused with insights gained from previous experiences. In practice, it is not as linear as that. We may reflect randomly for a year or more and make little connection between one experience and another. Reflexivity demands an active analysis of experiences to draw out the developmental threads that link them reflexively.

I am aware of deeper intellectual meanings to reflexivity in research (e.g. see contributions in Steier 1991) that I have steer clear of simply because I don't want to muddy the water.

Practical wisdom and praxis

Practical wisdom is the ability to mindfully weigh up any situation and consider how best to respond given the likely consequences. It draws on the praxis (or personal knowing) the practitioner uses in everyday practice; the knowing grasped at through reflection on experience. This knowing is fluid, ever changing in light of the particular experience the practitioner engages. It acknowledges that no situation is exactly like any other although it may be similar. This makes sense because every experience has never been experienced before. It is a unique encounter as if a mystery drama unfolding yet clearly influenced by past experiences and our personal knowing. Praxis is best described as informed action – breaking down any duality between theory and practice (Fay 1987). Aristotle drew a distinction between practical wisdom and theoretical wisdom. Practical wisdom does not result in knowledge which is determinate and universal; indeed, it does not result in propositional knowledge at all but in discriminations and actions.

Contradiction

Contradiction is the learning potential of reflective practice. It is the creative tension that exists between what the practitioner desires to achieve (vision) and an understanding of the practitioner's current reality (Senge 1990) as appreciated through reflection. Reflection involves understanding the nature of this contradiction and working towards resolving it so more desirable practice is realised. Contradiction is usually felt as an uncomfortable feeling, perhaps a sense that things are unsatisfactory in some way. It is this feeling that often triggers reflection, at least initially (Boyd and Fales 1983). No one likes to lead a contradictory life where there exists dissonance between our values and our actions. Practitioners might put their heads in the sand and pretend that contradictions do not exist. However, this can lead to a loss of integrity, stress and eventual burnout.

Senge (1990) notes that to hold creative tension it is first necessary to work through emotional tension. This suggests that creative tension is a rational thing and the mind requires clarity untainted by emotion. This is a moot point. I sense that working with emotions is creative tension and that resolving creative tension is more intuitive than rational.

Reflection is always action-oriented towards realising vision as a lived reality (rather than any sort of introverted navel gazing). In other words reflection is not a neutral thing but a political and cultural movement towards creating a better, more caring and humane world. As such, the ideals of a critical social science are enshrined – notably that reflection is firstly a process of enlightenment or understanding as to why things are as they are (self in context); secondly a process of empowerment to take action as necessary based on understanding; and thirdly a process of emancipation whereby action actually transforms situations for a vision to be realised (in the understanding that visions actually shift in the process of realisation) (Fay 1987). Understanding is the basis for making good judgement and taking action congruent with realising desirable practice. It is only when practitioners understand themselves and the conditions of their practice that they can begin to realistically change and respond differently. Yet, we do not live in a rational world. There are barriers that limit the practitioner's ability to respond differently to practice situations even when they know there is a better way of responding to situations in tune with desirable practice. Fay (1987) identified these barriers to rational change as tradition, force and embodiment (Box 1.1). These barriers blind and bind people to see and respond to the world as they do. To understand, the reflective practitioner creeps 'underneath his habitual explanations of his actions, outside his regularized statements of his objectives' Pinar (1981, p. 177).

These barriers are powerful resistors to transformation that govern the very fabric of our social world. They lie thick within any experience. As such, reflections are stories of resistance and possibility; chipping away resistance and opening up possibility; confronting and shifting these barriers to become who we desire to be as nurses, doctors, therapists. They are usually evident in patterns of talk when the normal talk pattern is disturbed in some way. Such patterns of talk are not easily shifted simply because they are normal

Box 1.1   Barriers to rational change

Tradition	– a pre-reflective state reflected in the customs, norms, prejudices and habitual practices that people hold about the way things should be
Force	– the way normal relationships are constructed and maintained through the use of power/force
Embodiment	– the way people normally think, feel and respond to the world in a normative and largely pre-reflective way

and reflect deeply embodied and embedded relationships that serve the status quo (Kopp 2000).

If people were rational they would change their practice on the basis of evidence that supports the best way of doing something. But even then two people may rationally disagree! Until practitioners become aware of these factors that constrain them they are unlikely to be able to change them. However, because things are normative, they are often not perceived.

Understanding requires a critical analysis of those factors that constrain self-realisation.

Fay (1987, p. 75) writes,

> The goal of a critical social science is not only to facilitate methodical self-reflection necessary to produce rational clarity, but to dissolve those barriers which prevent people from living in accordance with their genuine will. Put in another way, its aim is to help people not only to be transparent to themselves but also to cease being mere objects in the world, passive victims dominated by forces external to them.

The language of a critical social science may be intimidating with its rhetoric of oppression and misery, yet it can be argued that nursing, as a largely female workforce, has been oppressed by patriarchal attitudes that render it docile and politically passive, and thus limit its ability to fulfil its therapeutic potential. If so, then realising desirable practice may require an overthrow of oppressive political and cultural systems. The link between oppression and patriarchy is obvious, considering nursing as women's work, and the suppression of women's voices in 'knowing their place' within the patriarchal order of things. Images of 'behind the screens' where women conceal their work, themselves and their significance (Lawler 1991), and images of emotional labour being no more than women's natural work, therefore unskilled and unvalued within the heroic stance of medicine (James 1989), are powerful signs of this oppression.

Maxine Greene (1988, p. 58) writes,

> Concealment does not simply mean hiding; it means dissembling, presenting something as other than it is. To "unconceal" is to create clearings, spaces in the midst of things where decisions can be made. It is to break through the masked and the falsified, to reach toward what is also half-hidden or concealed. When a woman, when any human being, tried to tell the truth and act on it, there is no predicting what will happen. The "not yet" is always to a degree concealed. When one chooses to act on one's freedom, there are no guarantees.

I tingle with excitement as I write these words. Reflection opens up a clearing where desirable practice and the barriers that constrain its realisation can be unconcealed and where action can be planned to overcome the barriers whatever their source. No easy task, for these barriers are embodied, they structure practice and patterns of relating. Fear is a powerful deterrent for being different. Reflection enables practitioners to speak and know their truth, ripping away illusions.

The commitment to the truth is vital in Greene's words. Yet how comfortable are people in their illusions of truth? Is it better to conform than rock the boat? Is it better to sacrifice the ideal for a quiet life and patronage of more powerful others? Better to keep your head down than have it shot off above the parapet for daring to reveal the truth?

Empowerment

Reflection intends to be empowering, enabling the practitioner to act on insights towards realising desirable practice. Kieffer (1984, p. 27) noted that the process of empowerment involved 'reconstructing and re-orientating deeply engrained personal systems of social relations. Moreover, they confront these tasks in an environment which historically has enforced their political oppression and which continues its active and implicit attempts at subversion and constructive change.'

Kieffer's words may not rest comfortably with many readers. Yet the truth of the situation is stark – if practitioners truly wish to realise their caring ideals then they have no choice but become political in working towards establishing the conditions of practice where that is possible.

Practitioners, like nurses, have been socialised to be powerless and subordinate. As such, they are unable to respond to liberating opportunities when they present themselves. The emphasis must be on the practitioner coming to realise a new reality for herself, rather than have this reality explained to her. For example all shared experiences concerned with conflict have a fundamental power inequality at their root that manifests itself through different attitudes, beliefs and behaviours. This is not difficult to see or understand providing it is sought, and not just taken for granted as part of the 'natural' background of the experience.

Empowerment is the practitioner having the commitment and courage to take action towards realising more effective practice or a better state of affairs. This requires an assertive and political voice that is heard and listened to within the corridors of power. And yet so many nurses' voices are silent or suppressed for fear of sanction. Such practitioners are not so much lost for words but have no words to say. Perhaps you can remember being silenced, not so much by others but by yourself. Practitioners often say, 'I wish I had said something but. . . .'

Reflection, by its very nature, facilitates empowerment of practitioners towards self-realisation. I am drawn to theories of empowerment because I sense the way practitioners have little control over the circumstances of their practice working in transactional organisations, often leading to a feeling of resignation or a victim of the system mentality. In such worlds practitioners often feel like objects or bits within systems that impose control over their lives and stifle their professional aspirations.

They lack agency to formulate and attain their goals. They depict their lives as out of their control, shaped by events beyond their control. Others' actions and chance determine life outcomes, and the accomplishment or failure to achieve life goals depends on factors they are unable to change. To view self as a victim is to experience a loss of personhood and to project the blame for this loss onto others rather than take responsibility for self.

Bruner (1994, p. 41) notes that persons construct a victimic self by 'reference to memories of how they responded to the agency of somebody else who had the power to impose his or her will upon them, directly or indirectly by controlling the circumstances in which they are compelled to live.' Bruner's words highlight that the construction of life plots is always in relation to others. They are oriented towards avoiding negative possibilities than to actualising positive possibilities.

In theory, reflection would enhance the core ingredients of personal agency; self-determination; self-legislation; meaningfulness; purposefulness; confidence; active-striving; planfulness; and responsibility (Cochran and Laub 1994 cited in Polkingthorne 1996).

The person's work is to create a plot out of a succession of actions, as if to direct the actor in the midst of action. Locating ourselves within an intelligible story is essential to our sense that life is meaningful. Being an actor at all means trying to make certain things happen, to bring about desirable endings, to search for possibilities that lead in hopeful directions. As actors, we require our actions to be not only intelligible but to get us somewhere. We act because we intend to get something done, to begin something which we hope will lead us along a desirable route: we act with what Kermode 1966 calls the 'sense of an ending'. He writes, 'Because we act with the sense of an ending, we try to direct our actions and the actions of other relevant actors in ways that will bring the ending about' (p. 813).

However, the idea that reflection can help the individual practitioner turn this scenario around is fraught with difficulty. The transactional world is resistant to change. Reflection can so easily be like swimming in the shallow end of a deep swimming pool, literally splashing about with surface issues rather than tackling the deeper political and systems issues necessary to support best practice. However, that is not to say that tackling surface issues is not important, as indeed is developing reflective skills, and understanding of the deeper issues even if they are not amenable to change on an individual level. The need for collective reflection and action becomes vital for organisational change. If practitioners are to realise desirable practice with integrity they need to take such action. Yet is that possible against the transactional machine that will crush them? Becoming empowered will certainly need a guiding hand. The words of C.S. Lewis spoken by Anthony Hopkins in the film *Shadowlands* ring loud: 'I've just come up against a bit of experience. Experience is a brutal teacher but by God you learn . . . you learn'.

As a guide I say, 'here take my hand across the metaphoric swamp lands or hard walls of reality'. Hope springs eternal.

Development of voice

The work of Belenky *et al* (1986), *Women's Ways of Knowing*, is a useful text to reflect on the emergence of voice as a metaphor for empowerment. They describe five levels of voice: silence, received voice, subjective voice, procedural voice and constructed voice.

Silence

'Good nurses are seen but not heard'. Is this because of a fear of repercussion or humiliation? Either way it is a reflection of being put in your place. Think of a recent experience when you would have liked to have said something and didn't. Write it down and ask yourself why you were silent. What would you have liked to have said? How did you feel? What do you imagine the response of others? Perhaps you did say something – what were the consequences?

Julia Cumberlege (DHSS 1986) observed at meetings concerned with the discussion of her report on community nursing that doctors sat in the front rows and asked all the questions, whilst nurses sat in the back rows and kept silent. She commented how nurses needed to find a voice so they could be heard, otherwise they would have no future in planning healthcare services. Her comment reflected the way nurses had traditionally been socialised into a subordinate and powerless workforce through educational processes and dominant patterns of relationships with more powerful groups (Buckenham and McGrath

1983). The idea that reflection is empowering for marginal or culturally disadvantaged groups such as women in health care is a political issue. Gilligan (1982, p. 18) writes, 'The very traits that have traditionally defined the goodness of women, their care for and sensitivity to the needs of others, are those that mark them as deficient in moral development.'

Gilligan argues that women and men had different standards for moral development, yet in a patriarchal society with its higher moral claim to justice, women can be easily discounted. Do you sit in the back rows and are silent? If so, move forward a few rows next time and speak your truth.

Received voice

I remember as a student nurse sitting passively in the classroom (usually by the window where I could gaze out) being filled with facts to regurgitate when appropriate in clinical practice. Belenky *et al* (1986) describe this as received knowing – the way practitioners speak with the voices of authoritative others. Such practitioners conceive themselves as capable of receiving, even reproducing, knowledge from the all-knowing external authorities but not capable of creating knowledge of their own. I have no sense of being enabled to develop critical thinking skills, and even if I had, I suspect the all-knowing authorities within clinical practice would have soon put me in my place. Despite the rhetoric of developing the practitioner as a reflective and critical thinker, the weight of tradition and authority continues to suppress its emergence.

So when I ask a nurse – *why do you do it like that*? – she is likely to reproduce knowledge from an external authority that has been unquestioned. If I ask her how else she might do it she may struggle to think laterally simply because she has never been enabled to think. Perhaps this scenario is marginally shifting with university education.

The subjective voice

The subjective voice is finding the inner voice, listening to, valuing and accepting one's own voice as a source of knowing. This may mean confronting and rejecting the authoritative voice that has dominated the way the practitioner views, perceives, thinks about and responds to the world.

Reflective practice encourages practitioners to voice their opinions and views about their practice. As suggested above, this may not be easy to do for whatever reason. As such it cannot be taken for granted that if you give people space to express themselves they will do so, or if coerced, they might feel uncomfortable about it. Belenky *et al* (1986, p. 85) write,

> During the period of subjective knowing, women lay down procedures for systematically learning and analysing experience. But what seems distinctive in these women is that their strategies for knowing grow out of their very embeddedness in human relationships and the alertness of everyday life. Subjectivist women value what they see and hear around them and begin to feel a need to understand the people with whom they live and who impinge on their lives. Though they maybe emotionally isolated from others at this point in their histories, they begin to actively analyse their past and current interactions with others.

The focus on human relationships and alertness to everyday life is the very stuff of professions such as nursing, although it might be argued that nursing has moved away from human relationships in its desire to become more technical. If so, reflection facilitates a reconnection to such core values. Perhaps too, nurses have become emotionally blunted and detached, yet given the significance of emotion in caring work and decision making, reflection facilitates the growth of emotional intelligence.

The subjective voice is tentative, vulnerable in its uncertainty, and hence may need to be nurtured in a community of like-minded people. It may be confusing because it is competing with received voices. As such, it is easy to discount one's own subjective voice as being unsubstantiated, even ridiculed by more 'knowing' others. Listening to self, the self may see an uncanny stranger on display; a self that has been censored (Cixous 1996).

The procedural voice

The procedural voice has two complimentary ways of knowing: connected and separate knowing. Both are vital to effective practice. Connected knowing is informed by understanding the experiences of others through empathy. In contrast, the separate voice is dispassionate in its ability to critique and reason. It is the rational voice that seeks to understand things in terms of logic and procedures. It is the antithesis of received knowledge – no longer is knowledge accepted at face value but is now challenged for its validity and appropriateness to inform the particular situation. Perhaps the reader can sense Schön's (1987) metaphoric swampy lowland as the world of the connected voice and the high hard ground as the world of the separate voice.

The connected voice is the yin voice, feminine, perceived, intuited, whereas the separate voice is the yang voice, masculine, rational, logical, reasoned. Both voices are significant in health care. However, Belenky *et al* (1986, p. 106) speaks of the loss of voice when 'separate knowing has been the only voice allowed and when that voice is suppressed faced with perceived displays of brilliance or superior intellect.'

The constructed voice

The constructed voice is woven from the procedural voices into an informed, passionate and assertive voice. Belenky *et al* (1986, p. 134) note that to learn to speak in a unique and authentic voice, women must 'jump outside' the frames, and systems authorities provide and create their own frame. It is this leap of thought that enables practitioners to stand back and see things for what they really are that takes reflection into its creative and political mode. In doing so, the practitioner weaves together the strands of rational and emotional thought and of integrating objective and subjective knowing. However, having a voice is one thing, having it heard and listened to is quite another. Even practitioners who have constructed voice may be silenced. Belenky *et al* (1986, p. 146) write,

> Even among women who feel they have found voice, problems with voice abound. Some women told us, in anger and frustration, how frequently they felt unheard and unheeded – both at home and work. In our society which values male authority, constructivist women are no more immune to the experience of feeling silenced than any other group of women.

Belenky *et al*'s typology of voice offers a reflective framework for empowerment (Fordham 2008, 2012, Johns and Hardy 2005). To be an effective practitioner requires a constructed voice. At times practitioners will notice the way they use different voices dependent on the particular situation they find themselves; voices mediated by power relationships.

Whole brain stuff

The constructed voice is whole brain stuff. It is the balance of yin and yang, the left and right brain, the masculine and feminine, however way you would like to put it. The key is balance. Perhaps unity is a better word, given the whole brain rather than its parts. Virginia Woolf (1945) considered that the great mind is androgynous. She writes, 'It is when this fusion takes place that the mind is fully fertilised and uses all its faculties' (p. 97). The unbalanced mind leans too heavily towards the masculine, favouring reason over intuition, justice over care, outcomes over process, science over art. Perhaps the feminine has to be privileged to find balance. I wonder, do normal patterns of practice privilege masculine values and demean feminine values? I have often heard that to succeed in a man's world women must become more manly then men. Look about your practice – is there a grain of truth in this idea? Pink (2005, p. 22) considers 'the left hemisphere analyses the details; the right hemisphere synthesises the big picture.' How does he know that? I assume that the right side of the brain is the centre for certain qualities of mind; creativity imagination, perception, intuition, synthesis, wonder and spirit. It counterbalances the more dominant left side of the brain that is traditionally concerned with qualities of mind associated with analysis, reason, rationality and logic (Table 1.2).

Imagine the neglected right side of the brain is like the dark side of the hill tucked away out of view, out of touch. The left side whirs away in its rational cognitive way, imposing logic over intuition, reason over imagination, observation over perception, technique over creativity.

Writing story opens and nurtures the right brain that, for many practitioners, has been neglected. In the meantime the left brain has been constantly fed through education and practice processes. Paramananda (2001) writes, 'the imagination has become trimmed'. Play has become a lost art. This is why story is so important, simply because clinical practice is a playful, creative and imaginative practice. Left brain domination takes us down a rational analytical path that stifles such qualities of mind and impoverishes the practitioner. Instead of humans they see objects to be analysed. This is why it is vital to favour the right brain so it can play again and tease the left brain for its contribution

Table 1.2   Qualities of mind

Left brain	Right brain
	Creativity
	Imagination
	Perception
	Curiosity and wonder
Reason	Intuition
Logic	Spirit
Rationality	Synthesis
Analysis	Wholeness

towards the whole. Reflection is life giving, paying attention to one's being, one's spirit. This is vital to appreciate amongst the sterility of reason when the human factor is often lost amongst the facts.

Knowing reflection

My interest in reflective practice was initially stimulated by Margaret Clarke's (1986) paper, 'Action and Reflection: Practice and Theory in Nursing'. I was intrigued with the idea of learning through practice. This made sense for a practice discipline such as nursing. However, it wasn't the type of paper I could easily implement as a practical idea. However, it inspired me to begin a dialogue with key texts on reflective practice that continues today. Susuki (1999), writing from a Zen Buddhist perspective on zazen, described written teaching as *brain food*. He writes, 'Written teaching is a kind of food for your brain. Of course it is necessary to take some food for your brain, but it is more important to be by yourself by practicing' (p. 28). Such words of wisdom.

Much has been written about reflective practice. In the early days I explored the theories and ideas of Boud *et al* (1985), Boyd and Fales (1983), Brookfield (1995), Gibbs (1988), Jones and Jones (1996), Mezirow (1981), and Schön (1983, 1987). As you will discern, these references are dated and yet they remain the key theorists, as if nothing new of any significance has emerged. The reader is directed to the primary sources to explore these author's ideas.

However, a few words.

Boud *et al* (1985) posit reflection as moving through three key stages:

- returning to experience
- attending to feelings
  - utilising positive feelings
  - removing obstructing feelings
- re-evaluating experience
  - re-examining experience in the light of the learner's intent
  - associating new knowledge with that which is already possessed
  - integrating this new knowledge into the learner's conceptual framework
  - appropriation of this knowledge into the learner's repertoire of behaviour

This work resonates with the format of the model for structured reflection (MSR) and the six dialogical movements. Gibbs (1988) offers a reflective circle spanning six movements: description (what happened?), feelings (what were you thinking and feeling?), evaluation (what was good and bad about the experience?), analysis (what sense can you make of the situation?), conclusion (what else could you have done?), and action plan (if it arose again what would you do?). The circle represents the reflexivity that insights gained naturally inform future practice.

Mezirow (1981) viewed reflection as emancipatory action, influenced by a critical perspective. He posited a depth of reflection through seven levels of reflectivity spanning from consciousness, the way we might think about something, to critical consciousness where we pay attention and scrutinise our thinking processes. His work is influential because of the way he conceptualised *perspective transformation* inspired by Freire (1972) and the idea of an emancipatory approach to education, and the idea that thinking is problematic. Hence our thinking is a focus for reflection. How do I need to think differently to perceive the situation differently, and unearthing those assumptions that govern thinking. If reflection is viewed merely as a problem solving, and we used the same thinking to solve the problem that caused the problem, then we wouldn't get very far. Our solutions would quickly break down.

These theories enable practitioners to frame their reflective approach, often as a linear progression through a number of stages with the aim of developing insights into self and practice that can be applied to future experiences. These ideas about reflection reflect a generally Western technological approach to learning that can be contrasted with more esoteric approaches reflected in ancient wisdom traditions (Johns 2005). As I studied the more esoteric influences, notably Native American lore and Buddhism, I sought to balance the prevailing dominant rational approach to reflection.

Bimadisiwin

Rational approaches to reflection are prosaic couched in an intellectual language that do not easily excite the imagination. Consider *Bimadisiwin*.

Jones and Jones (1996, p. 47) write,

> Bimadisiwin is a conscious decision to become. It is time to think about what you want to be. The dance cannot be danced until you envision the dance, rehearse its movements and understand your part. It is demanding for every step needs an effort in becoming one with the vision. It takes discipline, hard work and time. Decide to be an active participant in your life journey. It is rewarding. Embrace the joy your vision brings you, it is yours to hold forever. It is freeing, for its frees the spirit. It releases you to become as you believe you must.

Jones and Jones offer a timeless wisdom. Such words stir the imagination. The idea of reflection (and clinical practice) as a dance is compelling. It suggests grace and movement, purpose and imagination. Yet to be a skilful dancer requires effort, discipline, commitment, patience, compassion and wisdom.

> Believe in the vision of you.
> Practice the vision.
> Become the vision.
>
> Jones and Jones (1996, p. 47)

Critical reflection

Practitioners and teachers who read about reflection will note a distinction in the literature between reflection and critical reflection. It is not a distinction I subscribe to. All reflection has the capacity to move into a consideration of the nature and consequence of power and hegemony within everyday practice.

Critical reflection pays attention to two particular types of assumptions – those that mask the ways in which the variable of power affects and distorts relationships, and secondly, hegemonic assumptions that establish norms that serve the best interests of the dominant group who naturally have an invested interest in maintaining such power relations and hegemonic structures (Brookfield 1995). Brookfield's work is essential reading notably in considering the reflective curriculum (see Chapter 8, where I draw on his work more explicitly).

Brookfield classifies assumptions as paradigmatic, prescriptive and causal. I do not find it easy to distinguish between them. Paradigmatic assumptions are those mostly embedded in normal cultural practice, for example, that nursing is caring and holistic. Prescriptive assumptions are closer to the surface, for example, that nurses should be compassionate or that patient's spiritual needs should be met. Causal assumptions are on the surface and hence easier to access, for example, allowing patients to choose their breakfast time would lead to chaos or that nurses should introduce themselves to patients. These assumptions might also be described as values we have grown up with and taken for granted as normal.

To ask the question 'what assumptions govern my practice within this particular experience?' is valuable. Assumptions are rather like social norms. Reflection is then the movement from one set of assumptions to another set of assumptions congruent with desired practice. As most assumptions are embedded within normal practice, this often requires collective action.

Critical reflection takes us deeper into the fabric of society, seeking to expose hegemonic structures and revealing the way these structures support the interests of the 'ruling' class. For example why is nursing curriculum governed the way it is and policed by a government body to ensure it stays that way? Yet equally, why does the same regulatory body espouse reflective practice and yet demand as a radical re-conceptualisation of the curriculum? The contradiction is stark. Critical reflection is political and fraught with danger for the naïve practitioner.

Transgression

My approach to reflection has been inspired by diverse sources. One inspiration is Ben Okri (1997). He suggests that all storytelling is *transgressive* in challenging the taken for granted and unexamined aspects of practice. Okri argues that there is no point to story otherwise.

Okri (1997, p. 63) writes,

> in storytelling there is always transgression, and in all art. Without transgression there is no danger, no risk, no frisson, no experiment, no discovery, and no creativity. Without extending some hidden or visible frontier of the possible, without disturbing something of the incomplete order of things, there is no challenge, and no pleasure and certainly no joy.

A few lines further down the page, Okri captures the critical reflection agenda: 'quietly, or dramatically, storytellers are reorganisers of accepted reality, dreamers of alternative histories, disturbers of deceitful sleep' (p. 63).

As a guide I encourage the quiet approach . . . rock the boat but do it gently, almost imperceptibly, so it is barely noticed. Narrative is a breach of the commonplace (Bruner 1986, 1996).

Being in place

The reflective journey can be viewed as a movement from *knowing your place* – the place you are placed in, determined and controlled by more powerful others, towards *being in*

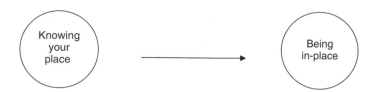

Figure 1.1   The reflective journey.

place – the place where you need to be to in order to realise desirable and effective practice (Mayeroff 1971).

I shall assume that not *being in place* is a deeply disturbing idea that creates a strong sense of internal conflict. Reflective practice opens a door to examine if we are in the right place to achieve most effective practice and if not, why not, and what must be done to move to a better place more congruent with realising desirable practice (see Figure 1.1).

Try this exercise:

- In relation to a specific experience, reflect on the tension between 'knowing your place' and 'being in place' to achieve desirable and effective practice.
- Identify what factors constrain you from being in place.
- Identify positive action you can take to being in place.
- Reflect each day on the difference such positive action enables you to move to being in place.
- Constantly review what factors continue to constrain you being in place and what help you need to overcome these constraints.
- Repeat the exercise at least weekly and mark along the line your progress towards being in place.

Whilst this exercise can be undertaken by individual reflective practitioners, it is best done in guided group reflection. However, the movement to being in place is not easy. As suggested within the exercise cues, embodied forces remind me to know my place. But that is ok. At least I am aware of this. It is my reality. It is a beginning. Perhaps all I can do is chip away at the edges, but if so, I can imagine being a sculptor chipping away slowly but purposefully at the granite slab towards creating a beautiful thing. For without doubt my image of desirable practice is a beautiful thing.

The significance of reflective practices for professional practice

Schön's (1983, 1987) critique of an epistemology of professional practice is vital to appreciate. He opens Chapter 1 of his book, *Educating the Reflective Practitioner* (1987, p. 1), with these words:

> In the varied topography of professional practice, there is the high, hard ground overlooking the swamp. On the high ground, manageable problems lend themselves to solution through the application of research-based theory and technique. In the swampy lowland, messy, confusing problems defy technical solution. The irony of this situation is that the problems of the high ground tend to be relatively unimportant to individuals or society at large, however great

their technical interest may be, while in the swamp lie the problems of greatest human concern. The practitioner must choose. Shall he remain on the high ground where he can solve relatively unimportant problems according to prevailing standards or rigor, or shall he descend into the swamp of important problems and non-rigorous inquiry?

Schön turns upside down the *normal* relationship between technical rationality and professional artistry. He suggests that reflection is the gateway to knowing and responding to the issues of everyday practice. Technical rationality provides few answers to these issues. Indeed, it might seem almost irrelevant and yet curriculum is dominated by a technical rational approach.

Technical rationality is a left brain model steeped in prescription and control. It is like wearing a coat of many theories but does not affect the person inside, whereas professional artistry is about the person inside and the way that person perceives, makes sense of and responds to the uncertain human drama of practice. Technical rationality has its place to inform this process.

Schön's notion of the hard high ground and the swampy lowlands reflect two types of knowing. The metaphor of *swampy lowlands* draws attention to the type of knowing that practitioners need in order to respond to the problems of everyday practice that defy technical solution, where the practitioner faces issues of distress and conflict within the unique human–human encounter on a daily basis. This resonates strongly with a profession like nursing where each clinical moment is a unique human–human encounter grounded in suffering. There are no easy answers to the life problems that face patients and nurses who strive to care. When we think we know the solutions to complex situations we endeavour to apply such knowledge, yet when we seek to impose control of events through applying such knowledge we somehow miss the point. Practice is a mystery drama unfolding. We may have had similar experiences but not this one. We draw parallels but it is not the same. We have to be mindful to read the particular signs or we may get it wrong. These signs are often subtle, requiring perception, imagination and intuition. Subtle differences between this experience and previous experiences demand subtle shifts of response that cannot be known outside the unfolding moment. There are no prescriptive solutions.

I take issue that the practitioner must choose which land to inhabit. Both are essential grounds to inhabit. The practitioner must dwell in the swampy lowlands, and yet be comfortable with visiting the high hard ground in order to appropriately assimilate relevant theory and research into practice (the constructed voice). Professional artistry is subjective and contextual, yet is often denigrated as a lesser form of knowing, even dismissed as 'anecdote' by those who inhabit the hard high ground of technical rationality. People got locked into a paradigmatic view of knowledge and become intolerant of other claims because such claims fail the technical rationality rules for what counts as truth.

Researchers through the past decades (Armitage 1990, Hunt 1981) have endeavoured to understand why practitioners do not use research in practice. These authors suggest that blame lies with the practitioners because of their failure to access and apply research. Is it any different today? Schön (1987) argued that little research had been done to address the real problems of everyday practice and that research always needs to be interpreted by the practitioner for its significance to inform the specific situation. The decontextualised nature of most research with its claims for generalisability makes this problematic. Any claim for generalisability *must* be treated with extreme caution to inform unique human–human encounters. Such encounter is essentially unpredictable. The insensitive application of technical rationality is likely to lead to stereotyping; fitting the patient to the theory rather than using the theory to inform the situation. Schön exposes the illusion that research can simply be applied.

Technical rationality (or evidence-based practice) has been claimed as necessary for nursing's disciplinary knowledge base because it can be observed and verified (Kikuchi 1992). Historically, professions such as nursing have accepted the superiority of technical rationality over tacit or intuitive knowing (Schön 1983, 1987). Visinstainer (1986, p. 37) writes, 'Even when nurses govern their own practice, they succumb to the belief that the "soft stuff" such as feelings and beliefs and support, are not quite as substantive as the hard data from laboratory reports and sophisticated monitoring.' Has anything changed?

Since the Briggs Report (DHSS 1972) emphasised that nursing should be a research-based profession, nursing has endeavoured to respond to this challenge. However, the general understanding of what 'research-based' means, has followed an empirical pathway reflecting a dominant agenda to explain and predict phenomena. This agenda has been pursued by nurse academics seeking academic recognition that nursing is a valid science within university settings. Whilst such knowledge has an important role in informing practice it certainly cannot predict and control, at least not without reducing the patient and nurses to the status of objects to be manipulated like pawns in a chess game. The consequence of this position in nursing has been the repression of other forms of knowing that has perpetuated the oppression of nurses of their clinical nursing knowledge (Street 1992). Has it improved in the past 20 years? I see no evidence to support that. We who plough the left field reap poor reward in academic acclaim.

Expertise

Dreyfus and Dreyfus (1986) note that for the expert practitioner clinical judgement is largely intuitive learnt through pattern appreciation and past experiences. For this reason, models and theories of reflection have limited value. They may offer the novice reflective practitioner a way to access the breadth and depth of reflection, yet it is folly to think that they can 'know' reflection in this way. These models threaten to impose an understanding of reflection that skims the surface of its potential depth and subtlety.

Benner (1984) and Benner *et al* (1996) draw heavily on Dreyfus and Dreyfus's (1986) model of skill acquisition in determining the pathway from novice to expert (Box 1.2). In contrast with novices, experts intuit and respond appropriately to a situation as a whole without any obvious linear or reductionist thinking. The novice simply does not have this tacit knowledge accumulated from past experience. Reflection as a learning process enables the practitioner to surface, scrutinise and develop her intuitive processes

Box 1.2   Dreyfus and Dreyfus's model for skill acquisition

Novice--	→ Expert
• Linear thinking and acting	→ Intuitive
• View parts in isolation from whole	→ Holistic or gestalt vision
• Reliance on external authorities	→ Reliance on internal authority
• See self as separate from situation	→ Self as integral to the situation
• Application of knowledge	→ Wisdom

and, ipso facto, to develop her tacit knowing. Hansen (2008) has developed the Dreyfus and Dreyfus model in relation to developing phronesis.

Holly (1989, pp. 71, 75) writes,

> It [keeping a reflective journal] makes possible new ways of theorizing, reflecting on and coming to know one's self. Capturing certain words while the action is fresh, the author is often provoked to question why . . . writing taps tacit knowledge; it brings into awareness that which we sense but could not explain. This is subliminal learning, revealed in the light of reflection.

Cioffi (1997) draws on the work of Tversky and Kahneman (1974) to suggest that judgements made in uncertain conditions are most commonly heuristic in nature. Such processes are servants to intuition. The heuristics intend to improve the probability of getting intuition right by linking the current situation to past experience, being able to see the salient points within any situation and having a baseline position to judge against. Without doubt, the majority of decisions practitioners make are intuitive. King and Appleton (1997) and Cioffi (1997) endorse the significance of intuition within decision making and action following their reviews of the literature and rhetoric on intuition. They note that reflection accesses, values and develops intuitive processes. The measured intuitive response is wisdom.

The six dialogical movements

To reiterate, reflection is learning through everyday lived experiences towards gaining insight that transform the practitioner towards becoming the practitioner she desires to be. This is the reflective turn. Yet how can such journeys of becoming be adequately represented in narrative form? This is the narrative turn. How can narrative be written as performance to engage audience towards social action. This is the performance turn.

Reflection commences with stories. The movement from writing stories about everyday lived experiences to performance narrative can be viewed through six dialogical movements within the hermeneutic circle (Figure 1.2).

The hermeneutic circle

The hermeneutic circle refers to the idea that one's understanding of the text as a whole is established by reference to the individual parts and one's understanding of each individual part by reference to the whole. Neither the whole text nor any individual part can be understood without reference to one another, and hence, it is a circle (Wikipedia[1]). In other words the part given attention is always viewed against the background of the whole which constantly changes in response, ever deepening and unfolding the level of understanding. It is a perpetual dialogue between the whole of our understanding and the insights emerging from reflection on a new experience. Each new experience challenges, informs and ultimately transforms the existing practitioner's personal knowing or the knowing the practitioner draws on to practice, knowing that is largely tacit. Within the hermeneutic circle the six dialogical movements flow as a dynamic whole. They offer a sequential route to constructing *reflexive narrative* as a formal research methodology (Johns 2010a).[2]

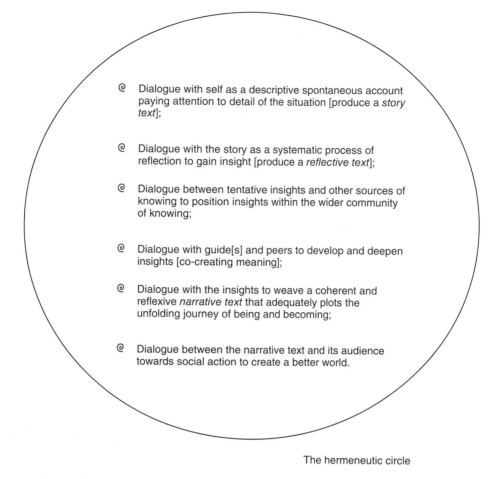

@   Dialogue with self as a descriptive spontaneous account paying attention to detail of the situation [produce a *story text*];

@   Dialogue with the story as a systematic process of reflection to gain insight [produce a *reflective text*];

@   Dialogue between tentative insights and other sources of knowing to position insights within the wider community of knowing;

@   Dialogue with guide[s] and peers to develop and deepen insights [co-creating meaning];

@   Dialogue with the insights to weave a coherent and reflexive *narrative text* that adequately plots the unfolding journey of being and becoming;

@   Dialogue between the narrative text and its audience towards social action to create a better world.

The hermeneutic circle

Figure 1.2   The six dialogical movements of narrative construction.

Dialogue

Dialogue is a specific form of conversation between practitioners (Bohm 1996, Isaacs 1993). Isaacs (1993, p. 25) describes dialogue as a discipline of *collective* thinking and inquiry. Based on Bohm's work I identify six *rules* of dialogue:

- commitment to work with others towards consensus for a better world
- awareness and suspension of one's own assumptions and prejudices
- proprioception of thinking
- to be open to possibility and free from attachment to ideas
- to listen with engagement and respect
- to have a mutual appreciation of dialogue.

Dialogue can be with oneself as if self is both object and subject, or with groups of people. It is always *moving towards* consensus for a better world. The emphasis on *moving towards* acknowledges a *letting go of attachment* to old ideas. The idea of a better world suggests all action is moral social action towards this end. To dialogue people must not only know and suspend their assumptions and opinions, but also be aware of the thinking that gave rise to these assumptions in the first place. Where do they arise from, how tenacious do we cling to them? Why do we cling to them? This requires a *proprioception of thinking*, an awareness of where the mind is at the moment. Within the dialogical process there is a shift from problem solving towards acknowledging and resolving paradox that requires thinking about the way people think about things. If we use the same thinking that caused the problem to try and solve the problem we fail. Hence we need to change the way we think to view the problem differently.

Bohm (1996, p. 25) writes,

> We could say that practically all the problems of the human race are due to the fact that thought is not proprioceptive. Thought is constantly creating problems that way and then trying to solve them. But as it tries to solve them it makes it worse because it doesn't notice that it's creating them, and the more it thinks, the more problems it creates – because it's not proprioceptive of what it's doing.

Only then can people transform their perspectives to see things differently. Dialogue is *listening*. Only when people *really* listen can they hear what is being said or not being said. Yet listening seems a rare quality in the patterns of talk that dominate practice and education. Do we listen to what we want to hear, or distorting what we hear in order to fit into our own scheme, to confirm our own assumptions? Listening opens the gateway to creativity. The six dialogical movements are unfolded through the following chapters.

Evaluating reflection

One student practitioner writes,

> Reflection is transforming my practice in so many meaningful and profound ways. . . . I have never felt so free to care and to be true to what I consider to be ideal practice. . . . Reflection had enabled me to contextually refocus on the individual. My interactive skills are being sharpened and I am rediscovering the therapeutic value of establishing a close relationship with clients. Until now I have never been able to find an approach to nursing which recognises the true potential of this unique relationship. . . . My first few reflections were triggered by a feeling that I had failed to achieve my goals in some way . . . guided reflection had enabled me to make use of the creative energy of conflict. I have been challenged to stoke up a far more challenging style of practice. I have become empowered to provoke and maintain the contradictions I feel between my goals of desirable practice and actual practice. Just as there are no limits to my expanding consciousness. . . .

Reflective practice has been criticised for its lack of definition, modes of implementation and for its unproven benefit (Mackintosh 1998, p. 556). Mackintosh singles out the Burford reflective model for criticism. She writes,

> The benefits of reflection are largely unaddressed by the literature [*that* is *beyond unsubstanti-ated claims*], and instead the underlying assumption appears to be that reflection will improve nursing care or the nursing profession in some intangible way. This is demonstrated by Bailey (1995) who, although describing the introduction of reflection into a critical area and claiming that an improvement in problem-solving skills occurred, gives no evidence that the quality of care was improved in any way. These failings can also be found in much of the literature

describing the Burford reflection in nursing model (Johns 1996a,b,c), which attempts to integrate reflective practice into a clinically grounded nursing model through use of a series of 'cues'. Much of the published evidence regarding the model's impact on clinical practice appears to be based on personal anecdote, and again, evidence in support of its impact on patient care is of a mainly qualitative and descriptive nature. [italics mine]

I continue to use this quote because it so pointedly addresses the tension of knowing the impact of reflective practice on practitioner performance. The accounts within *The Burford NDU Model: Caring in Practice* (Johns 1994) was not cited in the above references. Yet in this book there are four collaborating accounts from Burford practitioners and accounts from four other nursing units besides Burford – accounts that testify to the impact of the Burford model on clinical practice. In other words, Mackintosh reviews the literature with her own partial eye, seeing or interpreting what she wants to read to support her prejudice against reflective accounts and qualitative methodologies. Without doubt, there is a strong prejudice within healthcare research and education against what Mackintosh pejoratively describes as anecdotal accounts. Stories, by their nature, are one person's perspective, and that perspective is partial and distorted. It is the canvass for reflection and movement towards gaining insight expressed as narratives of being and becoming. Attempts to evaluate the impact of reflective practice on patient outcomes is fraught with difficulty given the variables of health care. However, practitioner reflective accounts do shed considerable light on the practitioner experience, just as personal narratives shed a compelling light on patient experience of receiving health care (Frank 2002b). Indeed, the nuances of care can only be revealed by such accounts.

Reflection is self-inquiry. As such, reflective accounts are subjective and particular to the situation. Such knowing is always evolving and deepening in light of new experiences. It is the dynamic interplay with the movements within the six dialogical movements and the hermeneutic circle. Its claim for truth is *authenticity* (Wilber 1998). Authenticity is revealed in two fundamental ways. Firstly, in the practitioner's reflexive account of being and becoming guided through the six dialogical movements (each movement with its own criteria for coherence), and secondly, in the reader's identification of the experience as real. I have had published numerous narratives that are used by teachers worldwide in their teaching both in terms of its clinical focus and narrative construction. It is only such accounts that offer any genuine evaluation of the impact of reflective practice on practitioner development and patient outcome as reflected through the narrative.

The limitations of reflection as a mode of learning has been highlighted by (amongst others) Platzer *et al* (2000). They noted that students may be resistant to revealing self, a point also highlighted by Cotton (2001), that reflection becomes a type of surveillance, assessment and control. Yet education has always been a socialisation process. Where teachers use reflection from a teacher-centred perspective, then it may be resisted. They further noted that the socialisation of nurses and their previous educational experience made the self-directed approach associated with the adult-learning process difficult, as nurses had not been encouraged to think for themselves. Without doubt there are barriers, but the barriers are a focus for learning and shifting, both within self and within the organisational culture. Real education isn't necessarily easy. Students may prefer to be fed what they need to know, but is that an adequate preparation for developing critical thinkers?

The MSR is widely utilised in university nursing departments across the globe. Why? Because it has been tested and found to be beneficial in enabling students to develop self-awareness and caring potential (Novelestsky-Rosenthal and Solomon 2001).

A study involved 50 students from one cohort in their final year degree course in community healthcare nursing to ascertain whether the students found reflection to be a meaningful activity, whether there are perceived benefits associated with reflective practice, and whether it is a valid process on which to access the outcomes of the course relating to the competencies of specialist practice (Smith and Jack 2005). The findings neither fully supported or refuted the usefulness of reflective practice. It became apparent that the student's learning style was pertinent to his or her perception of the usefulness of reflection. The data collected a web-based discussion board and focus group interview.

The study's description pays no attention to the quality of the student's reflective experience. The idea of diverse learning styles is widely known. However, the reflective curriculum maintains diverse learning approaches. At the end of the day, are practitioners better practitioners because they are reflective? The risk is a soft edge to pander to individual needs under the name of 'student-centred learning' that is psychologically demoralising for the teacher (Brookfield 1996).

Such studies offer very limited perspectives. Burton (2000) challenges why the UKCC and ENB insist that nurses, at all levels of experience, reflect, when the evidence to support its benefits is unsubstantial. Perhaps she should ask why do people think in the first place and read research findings? Yet Burton's words, again like Mackintosh, reveal the way people who inhabit a behavioural paradigm view reflection. They impose their own rules of injunction without appreciating the nature of reflection.

Reflection is *not* primarily a technology to produce better patient outcomes, and yet it follows that if reflection does enable practitioners to realise desirable practice, this realisation is best illuminated through reflexive narratives as compellingly illuminated through completed doctoral work (Jarrett 2009), and ongoing doctoral work by Foster, Fordham and others.[3] Examples of reflexive narratives have been published in my other books (Johns 2006, 2010a, Johns and Freshwater 2005) that demonstrate the impact of guided reflection on knowing and realising desirable practice. Reflection is essentially about personal growth, and its impact on personal growth can only be known through the stories these people tell. As narratives exquisitely illuminate, the impact on patient care shines through yet not in any reductionist sense.

Journal entry

Email from Marcia Ring (University of Vermont, August 2008):

> I can't believe this is the first time I am writing to you since June when you graced us with your presence and wisdom. Some of the Masters in Expanded Psychiatric Nursing [MEPN] students found your work and conference life altering. I even changed the final assignment for the MEPN students in psych to allow them to do their final Interpersonal Process Recording utilizing your method. Only one took advantage of that but it was truly stunning. If you like, I can find out if I can send it to you. You'd love it. I think she should publish it.

Conclusion

Reviewing what I have written, I am mindful that very little new literature contributes to knowing reflection. Reflection has been largely adopted within healthcare education from a technical rational approach, an ironic position considering Schön's idea that reflection tunes the hierarchy of professional on its head. Radical ideas like reflection are accommodated into normal structures despite their rhetoric of brave new worlds and becomes an awkward fit with the educational machine, reduced no more to an educational technology (see Chapter 8). Still, I remain positive because I know through my own work that reflection makes a significant difference to the lives of practitioners and the patients they serve.

Notes

1 http://www.Wikepedia.org
2 The development of reflexive narrative is the focus of my book, *Guided Reflection: A Narrative Approach to Advancing Professional Practice.*
3 School of Reflective Practice, Narrative Inquiry and Performance, University of Bedfordshire.

Chapter 2

Writing self: the first dialogical movement

Before we can reflect we need stories to reflect on. Stories are the raw data of our experience. We pay attention to a particular experience in order to write a story about it – a rich descriptive account as the prelude to reflecting on it and learning through it. As Wheatley (1999, p. 143) writes, 'we paint a portrait of the whole, surfacing as much detail as possible.'

I write in a journal. In fact I write two journals: a reflective work journal related to my clinical work and a personal journal. Writing takes me deep into myself and opens the doors of perception and possibility.

Mimesis

In writing self, the practitioners write to capture something of the past experience through rich description, paying attention to detail and drawing on all the senses in order to capture the reality of their experience as best they can. It is our senses that can lead us to appreciate self in relation to practice in new ways.

The attention to reality, what actually took place, is the mimetic nature of reflective writing. Boud *et al* (1985, p. 27) suggest the value of mimetic writing as

> one of the most useful activities that can initiate a period of reflection is recollecting what has taken place and replaying the experience in the mind's eye, to observe the event as it had happened and to notice exactly what occurred and one's reaction to it in all its elements, it may be helpful to commit this description to paper, or to describe it to others. By whatever means this occurs the description should involve a close attention to detail and should refrain from making judgments.

However, mimetic writing should not be naïve (Mattingly 1998). There is a distinction to be made between the actual lived experience and telling the story. The remembering of the story becomes distorted through perception and memory even when written shortly after the event. The reflective practitioner is aware that capturing the exact nature of the

Becoming a Reflective Practitioner, Fourth Edition. Christopher Johns.
© 2013 John Wiley & Sons, Ltd. Published 2013 by John Wiley & Sons, Ltd.

experience is elusive because of her subjective partial view. This is natural and is not a problem, not least because the practitioner's subjective partial view becomes a focus for scrutiny through the subsequent dialogical movements.

For some people it may be easier to capture the reality of the experience by writing about it soon after it happened. My own edict is to write the story approximately 24 hours of the experience. Whilst I have no hard evidence to support this, practitioners say this is useful advice. It is often enough time for the emotional mud to settle and for things to become clearer and yet detail not to be forgotten. However, it might suit others to write at a later time when the immediacy of the experience has settled.

At work, I carry my journal with me, so it is available for making notes I later develop into story if I feel it is significant. The notes are usually facts about the situation or actual dialogue. In developing the story I usually write directly onto a computer screen. From a reflexive perspective, writing is significant, motivated by a plot. It isn't simply a recollection of any event. My own writing, in the broadest perspective, is focused on realising my vision to ease suffering as both a therapist and nurse, in collaboration with others. Within this plot, a plethora of sub-plots emerge that are significant in easing suffering. These sub-plots are like threads, that when woven together, create the bigger picture of my effectiveness. Reflective writing always has this purpose. It is not something in itself. I also write about personal experiences not directly linked to my professional practice, some of which have been developed into published papers and performance. These include visiting my mother in a nursing home the day before she died (My mother's death), accompanying my partner for a cardiac catheterisation (Three blind mice and the movie star), and killing a deer in Ashridge Forest (Flowers for your grave). These stories were my attempt to work through my feelings. My intention was not so much to learn through these experiences, although these experiences have proved valuable to inform my understanding of suffering from a more personal perspective. I describe this writing as auto-ethnographic (Bochner and Ellis 2002) where I explore the cultural conditions that govern my experience.

Creative writing

The one text I recommend people study with regard to writing is Manjusvara's (2005) 'writing your way'. It is full of practical ideas and it won't convert you to Buddhism. The key is to write *spontaneously*. By spontaneous I mean not to overly think about what you are going to write about the situation but write what comes to mind. To aid spontaneity, I suggest 'do not take your pen off the page', as if taking the pen off the page leads to thinking. Let the mind go and the imagination take over. Imagination is the gateway to creative writing. When practitioners think about an experience, they tend to see what the mind has taught them to see. It is a very partial view. When people can let go of thinking and dwell within their experience then more becomes manifest. Thinking is a kind of self-talk with built-in censors that limit the natural flow of mind.

Reading letters home by Sylvia Plath (1975, p. 147), she writes in one letter to her mother (25 October 25 1954):

> the thing about writing is not to talk, but to do it; no matter how bad or even mediocre it is, the process and production is the thing, not the sitting and theorizing about how one should write ideally, or how one could write if one really wanted to or had the time.

Plath's words are a reminder about not getting caught up in technique. I advise practitioners to write spontaneously for say 15–20 minutes in the first instance to get people absorbed into the writing, to facilitate the art and discipline of paying attention. Writing can take any time at all.

Afterwards, practitioners are often surprised by what they have written. Often the writing has gone off on tangents to the extent that people did not write what they had intended to or hadn't yet come around to the specific point. They seem to enjoy this creative form of writing even though it may at first seem alien and difficult to start.

'How do I write,' one student asks.
'Just do it,' is my response, 'let it come and flow as naturally as water flowing in a stream.'

Stemming from socialised patterns of learning based on technical rationality, practitioners are overly sensitive about doing it right – as if they will be judged. Hence, there is no way of doing it right. Like the poet, the practitioner finds her own way. The guide teaches them to find their own way, knowing that this way will ultimately be the most productive way. To show them the way reinforces an instrumental approach.

'Give me a clue,' the student asks.
'Were you at work yesterday?' I respond.
'Yes.'
Think of one patient you nursed –now write a story. For example, Mr Smith is 46. He sits in his chair by the bed. 'I am frustrated that I do not have enough time to spend with him as Mr Brown demands my attention. . . .'

The pen writes furiously for 20 minutes. A flush of excitement.

Creativity may be aided by making the journal an art form. For example, explore *Artists' Journals and Sketchbooks: Exploring and Creating Personal Pages* by Lynne Perrella (2004) to inspire the imagination. My journal format undoubtedly lacks imagination. They are words on a page, but words that come alive with imagination as I explore my world of being and becoming in relation to particular experiences.

Bringing the mind home

To write self, I need to be in the right state of mind, what Susuki (1999) terms the 'right posture'. I describe this posture as *bringing the mind home* inspired by Sogyal Rinpoche (1992). He writes,

> We are fragmented into so many different parts. We don't know who we really are, or what aspects of ourselves we should identify with or believe in. So many contradictory voices, dictates, and feelings fight for control over our inner lives that we find ourselves scattered everywhere, in all directions leaving no one at home. *Reflection then helps to bring the mind home* (p. 59).[1] Yet how hard it can be to turn our attention within! How easily we allow our old habits and set patterns to dominate us! Even though they bring us suffering, we accept them with almost fatalistic resignation, for we are so used to giving into them. (p. 31)

Bringing the mind home shifts the balance from viewing reflection as a cognitive activity to a more meditative activity – a time of quiet contemplation to pay attention to self. Be patient with self. Jones and Jones (1996) write,

We must slow down or we will miss all that has meaning. Meaning is revealed only when you pause, when you stop, when you pay attention. Learn the lesson of the tribal people. Put your busyness on pause, eliminate distractions, and allow the meaning of life and living to return to you. Slow down in order to connect to the meaning of life. (p. 90)

Can we create this space within ourselves to bring the mind home? Do you have the patience to wait till your mud settles and the water is clear? (Lao Tzu 571 BC[2]). Taking time out from practice or any other daily activity to reflect sounds easy, but when our lives are addicted to being busy, it may be hard to focus one's thoughts within rather than be scattered outside.

Writing a journal is not natural for most people.

Susan Brooks (2004) writes:

One of the most priceless skills learnt over the last two years of study on the MSc leadership programme, is 'bringing home my mind' – slipping out of the noose of anxiety, releasing all grasping and relaxing into my true nature (Rinpoche 1992). Rinpoche (1992) records that by relaxing in this uncontrived, open and natural state we obtain the blessing of aimless self-liberation of whatever arises. This has certainly been my experience and the joy of feeling able to distance myself from the daily pressures of work by bringing my mind home is immense and a practice that, I believe, will stay with me indefinitely. Hatha yoga has become an element of my daily practice as a means to bring my mind home and to promote my own physical and mental well being in a meditative context. Such practice has revealed to me that I do matter as a person and am not simply a faceless cog in the healthcare organisation. How many times have I said or heard the comment, 'I am just a nurse'? Nurses generally have not trusted their own sense of self-importance enough and yet the fact that nurses do matter is a fundamental truth (Tschudin 1993). Bringing my mind home focuses me on me, underpins my own sense of self-importance but also emphasises my crucial need, as a transformative leader, to recognise and encourage the development of the personhood and thoughts of others. Reflective thought has become a pleasure rather than a threat and as I sit to review the period of this study and my journey so far, I am contentedly aware that my mind is unshackled by the contradictory voices, dictates and feelings that usually fight for control over our inner lives (Rinpoche 1992). Being available to self in this way has implications for my leadership, support and development of others since I would argue that unless I am truly available and knowing to self, transference of such availability would be problematic.

Susan notes hatha yoga had become a daily practice to help bring her mind home. My own practice is meditation linked to my Buddhist practice. I use my breath in a moment to bring the mind home, for example before I journal, before I teach, at the door to a patient's room at the hospice where I practice, or when I feel angry and my instinct is to retaliate. The breath helps see the anger for what it is and may stop me from reacting to it. Gardening or walking up Carn Brea in Cornwall where I live also works to clear the mind.

I most often write my reflections in the evening when I can dwell with my thoughts and consider the events of the past few days with less distraction than at a desk at work. Even the most ordinary events have great significance for the reflective practitioner. Everyday experiences are a source of rich learning.

Dividing the page

One technique that may be useful to novice writers is to divide the page into three columns (Figure 2.1).

Rich description	Reflection (using reflective cues)	Anticipating what I might do differently given the situation again

Figure 2.1   Dividing the journal page in three columns.

In writing, I get glimpses of myself through the reflections of others within the particular experience. I get glimpses of the relationship between my thinking and my action, between the relationship of my practice with knowledge, between my values and the assumptions I find myself holding, and perceiving signs that point to deeper social, political and cultural assumptions that are not obvious on the surface of the experience.

Susan Brooks (2004) reflects on being invited to keep a journal with the intent of constructing her leadership narrative:

Having never attempted to keep a reflective journal before, the journey ahead seemed a little daunting as evidenced by the first recorded entry.

Today I start my journal. What shall I write? I'm really worried about this whole thing –will I get time to do it – will I want to do it – will I do it right? If I'm honest in it will it matter if others read it? Reflective practice, reflective practice – what is it really? I think I know but I don't think I've ever really done it properly. I feel so uncertain about everything at the moment and a bit scared and threatened. I don't feel I know anything about myself really and I suppose I just do what I do to fit in. I need to get over this and get on with it – pull yourself together Sue – you know you can do it.

This first journal entry reveals my initial uncomfortable reactions to the prospect of journal writing. I had doubts about my capacity to write, felt threatened by having to face myself on paper, questioned my ability to manage my internal censors that may inhibit complete honesty and held the naïve assumption that there is a correct way to keep a journal – all classic reactions to journaling (Street 1995). My initial fears were quickly dispelled as the value of my journal soon became evident. After I while, it seemed to become a powerful emancipatory tool in giving my innermost thoughts voice. I was the only person with access to the journal and, possibly because of this, it became a very cathartic experience to write. As the process continued, I soon recognised that I did not need to confront all the chaos of my personal or professional life at any one time and became more discriminatory about the events that I considered worthy of deeper reflection and subsequent action (Street 1995). The journal became, in a sense, my autobiography containing both positive and less than positive experiences – a non-hagiographic record of my daily life. My journal had, after just a few months on the course, become a silent but very powerful and challenging teacher – perhaps more persuasive and influential than any human embodiment that I had met. The following entry signifies just how my attitude had changed since that first entry at the start of the course.

July 2002 – I read of a teacher today who got very excited about writing his journal. He wrote that he felt especially good about writing for himself instead of someone else. His written thoughts were entirely his own regardless of lack of style, format or academic expression. He had never written like this before and felt that he was really communicating with and understanding himself. That's just how I feel now and I wish I had started writing like this ages ago. To be unrestricted by structural rigour, academic expectations and the approval of others is so liberating!

From the practical aspect, a double entry technique was used with the factual account (data collection) of the experience written on the left of the page and the reflective thought (the analysis) on the right (Moon 2002). Both the ordinary and extraordinary events of every day practice were included to prevent selective inattention, particularly to the seemingly mundane, where habitual routinised practice is thought most likely to occur (Heath and Freshwater 2000). I considered myself to be the primary research tool here. If the journal was to accurately and consistently record my own experiential world I needed to maintain a strong sense of commitment to the task and demonstrate the skills necessary to the reflective cycle – self-awareness, description, critical analysis, synthesis and evaluation (Atkins and Murphy 1993). Keeping a journal enabled me to enter into a dialogue between my objective and subjective self and it transformed my feeling self into a spectator and analyst of my own personal professional drama (Street 1995). Street (1995) writes that 'journaling provides the reflector with a process for meta-theorising, that is thinking about the processes of thinking. This significantly developed not only my skills of reflection but also my skills as a learner in general, moving me away from my previously held attitude that knowledge (and not necessarily enhanced learning skills) was the goal to be achieved.

Commentary

Susan extols the virtues of keeping a journal. And yet, at the beginning she felt daunted. It is a serious matter for the practitioner to enter into reflective practice. It requires commitment and responsibility. Perhaps this is why so many practitioners struggle to keep a reflective journal. They are tired at the end of the day, they want to switch off, they don't see the value, they do not have the discipline, they don't find it meaningful, they don't know how to write, or they don't see the point.

Writing rather than telling

Some people like to tell their stories whilst others prefer to write them. I always advocate writing because writing is creative and imaginative and stimulates the reflective process. Many practitioners get stuck between telling their story and writing it. It is as if they hit a mental block. Perhaps the oral telling is more spontaneous whilst writing is more considered, more cognitive, more self-conscious. I sense the presence of an internal censor at work in writing that tries to fit the description into learnt ways of writing that dismisses or denigrates feelings and imagination. Whatever, some people struggle to write. Perhaps telling stories is essentially a creative right brain activity whilst writing is essentially a left brain activity and between the two sides of the brain the connections are fuzzy and censored. If so, I might say to the struggling writer – tell me about an experience you might like to write about – and then when the words flow – I say – that's what you need to write to hit the spontaneous vein.

Reflection is most often triggered by negative feelings such as anger, guilt, sadness, frustration, resentment or even hatred (Boyd and Fales 1983). It is these feelings that create a sense of drama significant enough to reflect on. It is as if practitioners do not pay attention to the little, more subtle aspects of their practice that have become taken for granted, and yet, these are rich with story, and yet, are significant triggers for reflection.

Negative feelings create anxiety within the person and bring the situation that caused these feelings into the conscious mind. As such, the practitioner may *naturally* reflect either consciously or subconsciously to try and defend against this anxiety. They may distort, rationalise, project or even deny the situation that caused these feelings.

Writing self is initially often triggered by negative feelings. This is significant because our feelings give access to our inner world, often a negative feeling or sense of discomfort about something that has happened during the day. So write the feeling in your journal (large letters can help!)

Whilst it may be natural to pay attention to negative feelings because they disturb us, practitioners can also be encouraged to reflect on positive feelings such as satisfaction, joy and love. In my experience, this is less likely because such feelings are not viewed as problematic or dramatic enough. Experiences that arouse no strong feelings are simply taken for granted, that is, until the practitioner becomes aware enough to pay attention to every aspect of their practice.

Think of one recent experience when you felt angry.

Write angry on the page.

Now let the pen or keyboard flow with this feeling of anger and see where it takes you. (Dog sounds optional!)

ANGRY!

> I'm angry at Jane, the junior nurse, because I asked her to help a patient wash, but she ignored me and went to help someone else. I am puzzled why she did this. It made me angry but I couldn't challenge her. I didn't want to make a fuss. I'm still angry, angry at myself for letting her get away with it. Maybe I should have confronted her later. Grrghhh

For novice reflective practitioners, it is more natural to pay attention to things that haven't gone well than things that go well. As a consequence the practitioner may get into a pattern of negative thinking about self and practice. She may despair about her organisation and her colleagues. Not much fun.

To help balance this I suggest that practitioners focus on one experience that was good, and one experience that was less than good. As practitioners become more experienced with reflection, they often shift their focus from negative to affirming experiences, when guided to balance the focus of their reflections from the outset.

Having said that, the practitioners learn by being where they are and experiencing their life as it is right now. It is significant to experience our anger, our sorrow, our failure, our apprehension; for these feelings are all our teachers when practitioners do not try and defend against them. Then learning is not possible. That's not hard to understand, just hard to do (Becker 1997).

Tapping the tacit

Writing may be difficult for practitioners because, as Schön (1983) suggests, much of our knowing is tacit and not easily explainable. In other words, they may struggle to write what they know. This can be frustrating.

Schön writes,

> When we go about the spontaneous intuitive performance of the actions of everyday life, we show ourselves to be knowledgeable in a certain way. Often we cannot say what it is we know. When we try to describe it we find ourselves at loss, or we produce descriptions that are obviously inappropriate. Our knowing is ordinarily tacit, implicit in our action and in our feel for the stuff with which we are dealing. It seems so right to say that our knowing is in our doing. (p. 49)

Spontaneous writing taps the tacit; it brings it to the surface like a bubbling underground brook. Holly (1989, p. 71) notes that 'writing taps the unconscious; it can make the implicit explicit, and therefore open to analysis.' It is bringing feelings and thoughts to the surface where they can be looked at. Ferruci (1982, p. 41) says 'writing can be much more powerful that we may think at first. We should not be surprised that unconscious material surfaces so readily in our writing.' Perhaps that is one reason to keep writing superficial. Yet it is these deeper reaches of the mind where old stuff lies buried, stuff that is fundamental to the assumptions we hold and which govern our practice. If we are to gain insight, then it is necessary to access and shake up these assumptions. No easy task. Assumptions by their nature are resistant to recognition, understanding and change (see Chapter 1). Otherwise we scratch at the surface of our experience and it doesn't seem meaningful.

Writing is creative. Pay attention to everything no matter how tangential it is. Do not discard anything. Let the imagination run riot! Writing should be approached with a playful and creative spirit. IT is YOU! In writing, you are writing yourself, your body, nurturing your precious and unique self. In writing you change yourself on a subliminal level. As Ferruci (1982, p. 42) says, 'it is like cutting a new pathway in a jungle.'

Opening the reflective space through the humanities

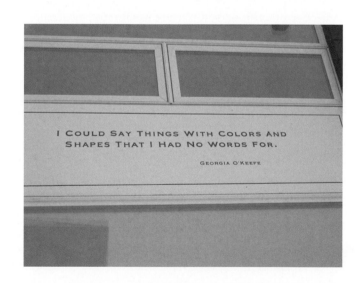

I photographed these words from the outside of a building in Boulder, Colorado. It suggests that words may limit our ability to express our experience. Art, especially if you are a visual sort of person, can be a short cut to the right brain, bypassing the potentially constraining use of learnt language and cognitive structures, especially for those practitioners who are more visually oriented. This resonates with the realm of art therapy, whereby patients are helped to express difficult feelings and trauma through art.

A number of studies use art and poetry to help practitioners find meaning in their experiences of being with suffering patients (Begley 1996, Brodersen 2001, Eifried *et al* 2000, Parker 2002, Vaught-Alexander 1994). These studies reflect the way humanities can open a space where practitioners can dwell with their own vulnerability within a safe space – where expressions of vulnerability can be expressed in whatever form and learnt through. As McNiff 1992 (cited by Picard *et al* 1999) puts it, 'whenever illness is associated with a loss of soul, the arts emerge spontaneously as remedies.' Put another way, whenever activity is related to the soul, the arts emerge spontaneously as soul food.

A particular use of reflective art is a storyboard that constructs story through a number of visual scenes with or without commentary (see Chapter 20).

The therapeutic benefit of writing

The subtitle of Rachel Remen's (1996) book *Kitchen Table Wisdom* is *Stories That Heal*, that in telling our stories we can connect to something vital within us, something healing.

She writes, 'Whatever we have denied may stop us and dam the creative flow of our lives . . . avoiding pain, we may linger in the vicinity of our wounds . . . without reclaiming that which we have denied, we cannot know our wholeness or have our healing' (p. 70).

The reclaiming is in telling or writing the story. I consider writing better because it creates the space to identify and work through the dam. Writing is the creative flow of our lives. If we do this consistently then it washes away traumatic debris before it can accumulate into a dam. Then we have crisis. Jourard (1971) argues that self-disclosure of upsetting experiences serves as a basic human motive. As such, people naturally discuss daily and significant experiences with others. Talking through a trauma with others can strengthen social bonds, provide coping information and emotional support, and hasten an understanding of the event. The inability to talk with others can be unhealthy.

Pennebaker (1989, p. 213) writes,

> When given the opportunity, people readily divulge their deepest and darkest secrets. Even though people report they have lived with these thoughts and feelings virtually every day, most note that they have actively held back from telling others about these fundamental parts of themselves. Over the past several years, my colleagues and I have learned that confronting traumatic experiences can have meaningful physiological and psychological benefit. Conversely, not confiding significant experiences is associated with increased disease rates, ruminations and other difficulties.

Pennebaker and his various colleagues (Pennebaker *et al* 1990, 1997) demonstrated the therapeutic benefit of therapeutic journalling in well-being, notably the benefit of connecting strong feelings to past traumatic events. Smyth *et al*'s (1999) review of the literature suggested that emotional expression has a salutary health effect, whereas emotional inhibition has a detrimental health effect.

Without doubt, healthcare work is stressful, embracing suffering on a daily basis and working under conditions that do mot necessarily facilitate caring work. As such, it seems imperative that practitioners have a mode for expressing and sharing their feelings, for example in clinical supervision (see Chapter 17). Smyth cites Pennebaker *et al*'s (1997, p. 175) claim that 'Written emotional expression leads to a transduction of the traumatic experience into a linguistic structure that promotes assimilation and understanding of the event, and reduces negative affect associated with thoughts of the event.'

Smyth's review highlighted that the 10 review studies demonstrated significant superior health outcomes in health participants; psychological well-being, physiological functioning, general functioning, reported health outcomes, but not for health behaviours. Smyth noted that these studies demonstrated that short-term distress was increased but is thought to be related to long-term improvement.

Pennebaker *et al* (1990, p. 536) write,

> The present experiment, as well as others that we have conducted, found that writing about transition to college resulted in more negative moods and poorer psychological adjustment by the end of the first semester. Our experiment may have effectively stripped the normal defences away from the experimental subjects. With lowered defences, our subjects were forced to deal with many of their basic conflicts and fears about leaving home, changing roles, entering college.

Indications from this study suggest that the power of confronting upsetting experiences reflects insight rather than cathartic processes. In follow-up questionnaires, for example, the overwhelming majority of the subjects spontaneously wrote that the value of the experimental condition derived from their achieving a better understanding of their own thoughts, behaviours and moods. The stripping away of defence mechanisms means that practitioners may benefit from guidance to support them through the consequences of the writing experience. Perhaps one way practitioners deal with negative experience is to avoid it, to bury it deeper into the subconscious. Writing opens the door to the subconscious with the threat of lifting these buried experiences into the conscious mind. Whilst this may be upsetting, burying experiences has a psychological impact that is not conducive for well-being and effective practice. In other words, healthcare practitioners have a responsibility to be fit for practice. However, writing about experience and disclosing these experiences are two different issues. Writing is an introvert activity whereas disclosure is a more extrovert activity perhaps more suited to different personalities. Having written the story the practitioner now stands back to reflect on it – the focus for the following chapter.

Reflective activity

> Think of the last time you were at work. Now think about one particular situation. It needn't be dramatic. It can simply be something mundane or ordinary, something you wouldn't normally give a second thought.
>
> First relax and bring your mind home. Now write a description of this situation for 15–20 minutes. Do not to take your pen off the paper. Do not stop and think about the why's of the situation. Just let the pen or keyboard flow spontaneously, in rich graphic description, paying attention to detail, drawing on all your senses. Just write.
>
> After 20 minutes, pause and stand back. Read what you have written with an open and curious mind. Ask yourself, 'what is significant in what I have written towards becoming a more effective practitioner, towards realising my vision of clinical practice as a lived reality?'
>
> As you do, you enter the reflective spiral. This is the focus for the following chapter.

Notes

1   Italics are my emphasis. I substituted 'meditation' with 'reflection'.
2   Quote reflections.blogspot.co.uk

Chapter 3

Engaging the reflective spiral: the second dialogical movement

Having written my story text, I stand back from the text to reflect on it. Reflection guides practitioners to access, understand and work towards resolving any contradiction between their vision and their perceived reality. The point of this activity is towards gaining insight.

Standing back, I intentionally move into a dialogue with the text to see it more clearly. Easier said than done when the text reflects who I am. It reflects my mental models, those deeply ingrained assumptions, patterns, attitudes and values that influence how I am in my practice and, more generally, in life itself.

Standing back is a playful posture. Wheatley and Kellner-Rogers (1996, p. 69) write, 'life is playful and life plays with us. The future cannot be determined. It can only be experienced as it is occurring. Life doesn't know what it will be until it notices what it has just become.'

How does it notice? Through reflection, and yet what it notices is inevitably a partial view. Others would see the experience differently. The reflective practitioner naturally challenges her partial views and works to clean the *smudges on the mirror* that distort seeing self clearly.

At first, it may be difficult to discern the objective–subjective tension simply because the practitioner is wrapped up in her experiences, especially if it has a strong emotional impact. Over time, with experience, this becomes easier as she becomes more mindful and discerning. Imagine my self-dialogue – 'Now Chris – what were you up to here? What were you thinking? What made you respond in that way?'

Dialogue is both a creative and rational activity. Tuffnell and Crickmay (2004) use the word conversation. They write, 'Creating becomes a conversation when we enter into a dialogue with whatever we are doing. In this conversation we are drawn along in the moment by moment flow of sensation, interchange and choice, rather than following a predetermined intention or idea' (p. 41). One thing evolves or unfolds into another. Pattern finds itself.

As I noted in Chapter 2, reflection might be facilitated by dividing the journal page into three columns (Figure 3.1).

Becoming a Reflective Practitioner, Fourth Edition. Christopher Johns.
© 2013 John Wiley & Sons, Ltd. Published 2013 by John Wiley & Sons, Ltd.

Rich description	Reflection (using reflective cues)	Anticipating what I might do differently given the situation again

Figure 3.1   Dividing the journal page in three columns.

Models of reflection

The practitioner will utilise a model of reflection to help her to explore the breadth and depth of experience. There are many on the market to review (see Chapter 1). The practitioner should be guided to review all models for their value, rather than accepting the authority of any model on face value. Rather like the skilled craftsman, the practitioner will choose the tool that is most helpful. I am wary of cyclical or stage models of reflection because they suggest that reflection is an orderly step-by-step progression. Reflection is not a neat movement between different stages or cycles. To view it in this way suggests a mechanical flow through discrete stages. Reflection is complex and holistic, whereby the mind engages all the cues or stages. There may be some value for stage models for novice practitioners in helping them grasp the essence of reflection.

It is natural for someone approaching reflection for the first time to ask certain 'technical' questions:

- What is reflection?
- How do I do it?
- How do I know if I am doing it properly?
- How do I learn through reflection?

Guarding against a prescriptive legacy

These are important questions that face the practitioner experiencing reflection for the first time.

I must emphasise that all models of reflection are merely devices to help the practitioner to access reflection; they are not a prescription of what reflection is. Put another way, models are heuristic – a means towards an end, not an end in itself.

Rinpoche (1992, pp. 64–5) writes, 'Largely because of our Western technological culture people tend to be absorbed by what I would call 'the technology of meditation (reflection). The modern world, after all, is fascinated by mechanisms and machines, and addicted to purely practical formulae. But by far the most important feature of meditation (reflection) is not the technique, but the spirit: the skilful, inspired, and creative way in which we practice (reflect), which could also be called the "posture".'

It is easy to get wrapped up in the technology of reflection, especially in a learning culture dominated by technical rationality.

My caution is that stage models immediately present reflection as some technical linear task. In a technologically driven society the risk exists that reflective models will be grasped as a technology and used in concrete ways. From a technological perspective (as opposed to a reflective perspective), the risk is that practitioners will fit their experience to the model of reflection rather than use the model creatively to guide them to see self within the context of the particular experience. Whilst alternative frameworks are available, it is vital that the practitioner views reflection as a path towards gaining insights that do not show themselves easily.

The model for structured reflection (MSR)

I designed the model for structured reflection (MSR) to enable practitioners to access the depth and breadth of reflection to facilitate learning through experience. The first edition of the MSR was constructed in 1991 through analysing the pattern of conversation between myself as a guide, and practitioners in guided reflection relationships. I then framed this pattern within Strauss and Corbin's grounded theory paradigm model (Johns 1998a). Since then, the MSR design has been reflexively developed, culminating in the 16th edition (Box 3.1). I have now delineated five phases:

- Preparatory
- Descriptive
- Reflective
- Anticipatory
- Insight.

Box 3.1   The model for structured reflection (MSR) (Edition 16).

Preparatory phase
- Bring the mind home

Descriptive phase
- Focus on a description of an experience that seems significant in some way (balance between experiences that were affirming and experiences that were problematic)

Reflective phase
- What issues are significant to pay attention to?
- How were others feeling and why did they feel that way?
- How was I feeling and what made me feel that way?
- What was I trying to achieve and did I respond effectively?
- What were the consequences of my actions on the patient, others and myself?
- To what extent did I act for the best and in tune with my values?
- What knowledge did or might have informed me?
- How does this situation connect with previous experiences?
- What assumptions govern my practice and what factors influence the way I feel, think and respond to the particular situation?

Anticipatory phase
- How might I reframe the situation in order to respond more effectively?
- What would be the consequences of responding differently for the patient, others and myself?
- What factors might constrain me responding in new ways?
- How do I NOW feel about this experience?

Insight phase
- What insights have I gained? (framing perspectives)

The cues are arranged in a sequential order through the five phases, enabling a movement of thought through each cue and phase, although they do not have to be used sequentially. The cues reflect a dynamic movement towards gaining insight. With repeated use, the reflective cues become embodied and shape the clinical gaze in mindful attention. In this way practitioners become reflective practitioners. They also have considerable value in developing clinical skills as I indicate in relation to each cue.

Moving into dialogue with the story text the practitioner is drawn into a reflective spiral – moving from an initial perception of what is considered significant towards gaining insight enfolded within the spiral. These insights are rarely obvious and are often realised with a sense of ah-ha at some random moment.

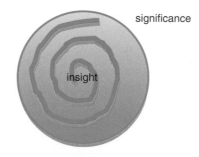

The reflective spiral is a journey into oneself to find meaning. Van Manen (1990, p. 58) writes,

> It is not a simple matter of etymological analysis or explication of the usage of the word. Rather, it is the construction of a way of life to live the language of our lives more deeply, to become more truly who we are when we refer to ourselves as doctors, nurses, therapists.

The more frequently practitioners use the MSR, the more the cues are internalised and used naturally in all aspects of her practice, not just reflection. The reflective practitioner will begin to use the cues within her spontaneous writing, breaking down the separation between the first and second dialogical movements. Besides their value in gaining insight, the cues have considerable value in developing clinical skills as I highlight through my exploration of each cue in turn.

The first two cues – *Bringing the mind home* and *Focus on a description of an experience that seems significant in some way* – have already been explored in Chapter 2. They are included in the MSR as the descriptive phase. To reiterate, description is the data for reflection. However, as the practitioner becomes adept at reflection the first and second movements become increasingly integrated. Indeed, all the movements exist in a dynamic integrated flow.

First a story.

Tom.[1]

I go with Marie, a healthcare assistant (HCA) to wash Mr Sturch. 'Hello Mr Sturch. . . .' I introduce myself as Chris, a visiting nurse. He says, 'Call me Tom.' I sense his need to be recognised for who he is and a need for familiarity.

At the shift report we had been informed how miserable Tom was being in hospital and being shut in a single room because of the risk of cross infection due to his diarrhoea. We were waiting for results of a bowel culture. If Tom's stools were clear he could be moved back into the main ward.

As I was scheduled to work with Marie, I paid attention to her. She is in her 50s and very committed to caring. She loves it and would love to be a nurse. She is experiencing strain in her personal life with her mother very ill. She and her husband moved here some years ago. Now she travels every weekend driving about 3 hours each way to care for her mother. I listen and help her talk through her feelings and options, even though we are little more than passing strangers.

Marie's approach to Tom is familiar and caring, but task focused. I immediately notice the characteristic pattern of parent–child communication. Tom is a little boy, upset but trying hard to be good. Marie is mother, protective, kind, although her tolerance is limited to the extent that there is work to be done.

I ask Tom 'How are you feeling this morning?' I say it with intent holding his gaze. He easily expresses his distress at being in hospital and shut up in this room. His tears are close to the surface. He is lonely inside the side room and embarrassed that these poor girls have to clean him up.

Marie kindly informs Tom that we are going to wash him. This is not negotiated with him. He needs considerable physical help as he has Parkinson's disease. His left hand in particular continues to tremor and his right side has been weakened by a previous stroke. I want to say to her 'stop, let's talk to Mr Sturch and see what's best for him. Treat him with respect rather than an object to be processed.' I want to say this because this task approach is the antithesis of person-centred nursing. I have met so many Maries who practice in this way. But I say nothing. It isn't the time.

We begin to wash him as he lay on the bed, when he asks for the commode. I note the impact of his Menière's disease characterised by his nausea on standing. The symptom is poorly controlled. Ensuring he felt safe, we left him to use the commode. Afterwards, we help him complete his wash whilst sitting on the commode. I help him stand whilst Marie washes his bottom. On seeing Tom like that I am struck by Mary Madrid's (1990) account about the nurse imagining who the patient is in terms of his past. Tom tells me he had been a staff sergeant in the army during the Second World War, working in recruitment training. I can imagine him like that. How straight and proud he must have been and now, what a different way to parade. And yet I can say that to him with humour, acknowledging his past while being empathic with this moment. I realise the significance of this approach in respecting people. After the war, Tom had been an engineer in microwaves, work that reflected his intelligence. I resist a sense of pity at his current state. I have learnt from previous experience about acknowledging self-discomfort towards patients and families and confronting this through enabling the other to talk through their experience.

After his wash, Tom cleans his own teeth. He appreciates the wet shave I give him. He is normally shaven by the nurses using an electric razor because the nurses feel clumsy with wet shaves even though Tom prefers a wet shave. I am mindful how this 'little thing' (Macleod 1994) of shaving Tom makes a difference to caring. I know this informs Tom of my concern for him. By paying him attention, my concern is fed and grows. I am also compensating for the task approach. Although we had only just met, I had been involved with him in intimate physical care – washing him, being here while he was on the toilet, wiping his bottom, shaving him – and seeing and responding to him as a suffering human being. My personal vision and that espoused by the ward, but the contradiction between the vision and reality hits home.

Tom easily discloses other aspects of his life. He has been married for 59 years to 'wifie', his endearing term for his wife. Indeed, his diamond anniversary was in February. He becomes alive talking about his wife and their life together. She visits in the afternoons.

He desperately wants to go home but is anxious about the future. He is so dependent physically and even though they had a support package, he fears he will be too much of a burden for 'wifie'. I wonder if he would be happier with television, some music, or a paper? No, he just wants 'wifie' and to go home. I sense my need to 'fix it' for him, a need to take his distress away from him. But of course, I am becoming anxious on his behalf, beginning to absorb his distress, which I recognise and repattern to be available to him.

Rubbing his smooth face, he thanks me. It feels good. His offers me a 'Murray mint – too good to hurry mint' (for those who remember the TV advert) – his gift in return for my attention, my respect and kindness. In seeking to connect with me, he needs to give something back. By accepting, I honour this need and he can honour himself. We begin to tune into a reciprocal relationship, where I can respond with an appropriate level of involvement with Tom. In this way I synchronise our rhythms of relating with each other at this moment (Newman 1999). In tune with him, I am most available to him.

I am mindful of the ways I paid attention to him in response to his feelings and needs, which had made him so happy this morning when he had been so miserable. Nurses are focused on the tasks of the morning and don't necessarily see him from his perspective. They may see him as a person but that's not their frame for responding. Marie noticed the difference in him this morning and passed this off as 'male company being good for him'.

I inform the doctor that Tom's stool is now semi-formed and to assert Tom's desire to move back into the main ward. This request was granted. I could also challenge the adequacy of the medical treatment for Tom's Menière's disease, to prompt a review of the medical response. The doctor welcomed my feedback. I felt good advocating for Tom and being genuinely listened to by doctors. This has not always been the case. Collaboration between the nurse and doctor is precarious depending on the doctor's attitude. Playing the doctor–nurse game I have been socialised into (Stein 1978, 1988). The game alive and kicking! However, a niggling doubt – did advocating for Tom take away his autonomy? How easy to render people like Tom silent despite our good intent.

Joan

At lunchtime I move over to the dinner trolley. Cook–chill. The domestics say the quality is quite good. They are serving the dinners. I express my surprise at the absence of a nurse. 'That's alright, the nurses are often busy so we get on.' Default pattern but is it therapeutic? I feel uneasy but hold my tongue. It's not the time.

Joan has severe arthritis. She struggles to eat one-handed with an adapted fork, chasing the food around the plate. She has neither plate guard nor slip mat. The adapted fork is not effective as she holds the handle below the padded stem. I fix a plate guard. These things are so obvious – why can't others see them?

After lunch I sit with her considering whether I might offer her some therapeutic touch. My agenda – yet I am sensitive not to impose this on her, mindful of Hall's (1964) challenge to nurses of 'strutting their new skills'. These people are so passive, it would be so easy to impose a parental, 'we know best' stance. We talk. I need to know this woman, who she is, to understand her experience of being here in hospital, and her perceptions of the future. Joan is only 78 although she looks older, small and wrinkled but always with a smile on her suffering face. She is stoic and courageous, and would never make a fuss. Her twisted wrists give visual evidence to her advanced arthritis. She is in hospital for respite care. Her stay has been extended following a new mild stroke she experienced 5 days earlier. She is extremely anxious and distressed. She is afraid she won't go home because her husband can no longer manage to care for her. He is 80 and not in good health. She cries. Clearly it was deeply in her mind. Behind this brave and cheerful face she presents to the world she doesn't want to be a burden to anyone. She needs to be the co-operative, uncomplaining patient. Perhaps she has learnt this way of being through her chronic illness career. To be the proverbial 'good' patient.

I help her explore her home possibilities, how we need to sit down with her and her husband and see what can be done. For example, her major fear is getting to the toilet, but she has not considered the possibility of a commode. She has not walked for 5 days since the stroke but has not been seen by a physiotherapist. I offer to help her take a few steps. She is happy with this idea. She stands by herself. She struggles to grip the zimmer frame, her normal walking aide, but refuses my help, murmuring through gritted her teeth 'I will do it'. She walks six steps before losing her right-hand grip.

Her notes are scanty. They tell me nothing about her and are associated with activities of living; Joan has difficulty washing, going to the toilet, with obvious goals of assistance. I write a commentary in her care plan about her needs amending her care plan. I emphasise her need for physiotherapy and her anxiety about going home. In writing the notes I remind myself of the Burford cue questions (Johns 2009a): 'How does this person see the future for self and others? and 'what support does this person have in life?' I write these two questions together with a brief summary of our work together within the 'progress' notes to help others see her as I have done.

I am reminded of Hall's (1964) words: 'it is impossible to nurse anymore of a person than that person allows us to see.' I thought 'how blind we have been'. Perhaps there is a taken for grantedness by staff because Joan is a respite patient despite her stroke. The staff seemed well disposed to her, although I sense they unwittingly contribute to her suffering by not seeing and responding to her and her husband in terms of their concerns. Her husband did not seem to be in the nurses' gaze at all. Perhaps his needs were met by providing respite care? Even in this ward dedicated to elderly people with chronic illness, the nurses essentially view practice through a medical/physical-oriented lens. The inappropriateness of this lens is stark, and yet no one can see it despite their claim to holistic practice.

Considering the paucity of the notes, I realise that notes are not an effective way to communicate these concerns. I decide to reinforce my notes by tentatively talking it through with the nurse in charge. She is receptive to my feedback, although I'm wary about overstepping my welcome as some critical interfering academic. Better to avoid potential conflict? Yet if so I would compromise my integrity. In failing to assert my concern I fail Tom and Joan. Without doubt, we need to create environments of care whereby we can express ourselves assertively without fear of upsetting the apple cart.

I share with Joan what I have written and urge her to express her fears with the staff, that the staff will be receptive. But I doubt whether she will be able to do this. Later I see her husband and go to talk with them. He is small like Joan and he is very deaf. She is pleased to be with him and thankful for my intervention. I never did my therapeutic touch but as with Tom, I felt good. I had quickly established a connected relationship with Joan and later with her husband. I felt certain that she, like Tom, connected with my concern.

Later, reflecting, I begin to doubt myself – did I enable the staff to see Tom and Joan in their humanness enough? I realise that practice culture is deeply embodied and not easily shifted, but I can chip away at it through role modelling – food for thought for my visit next week.

Maybe then it will be time to be critical.

What issues are significant to pay attention to?

Standing back from the text I ask myself: what is significant within the text? The story points to many issues. In Chapter 2 I quoted Wheatley (1999, p. 143): 'we paint a portrait of the whole, surfacing as much detail as possible.' She adds, 'we inquire into a few pivotal events or decisions, and search for great detail there also.' If I have written the story well enough, significance lies thick on its surface. What may seem significant on the story's surface may shift as the practitioner dwells more deeply within the reflective spiral.

So, what emerges for you as significant within this story?

Start with the most obvious and then scratch deeper at the surface to reveal less obvious significant issues.

The story text feels like an exposé of nursing culture, as if I have lifted the edge of the curtain to reveal what goes on inside. One significant issue is listening to the voices of Tom and Joan and appreciating the meanings they give to their illness experience. It is not just listening but creating a space where their voices might be heard and respected amidst the din of task-focused practice. The story text is also about my voice and the tensions with asserting my voice. The idea of advocating becomes significant. Does my advocating for these patients disempower them? By advocating I sense I also wanted to open the eyes of the staff to see these people in their suffering. The unwitting carelessness of the staff is significant as are my values that might judge such carelessness. I was frustrated with Marie. She was not mindful of her impact on him – like so much of care, it had become routine, as if these patients had become objects of care rather than engaged in care. What time would Tom liked to wash? Probably, given the choice, he would say whatever time is convenient to you. I know from previous experience that patients like Tom endeavour to fit in with nursing patterns, they want to be co-operative, they do not want to be a nuisance despite their suffering. Perhaps they have learnt from previous experience it pays to fit in rather than be viewed as some difficult, dirty, demanding, old man. Perhaps Tom knows he will get more kindly attention if he fits in. So the list goes on. I am certain that you can tease out many more issues that are significant for you.

Practical skills

- Paying attention and recognising significance within the unfolding situation
- Developing perception
- Becoming aware of the person and self within the context of the practice environment

How were others feeling and what made them feel that way?

Without doubt, illness and admission to hospital create significant anxiety for people. How did Tom, Joan and Marie and others involved in my reflection feel? And why did they feel that way? Was Marie wrapped up in her own concerns with her mother and hence less available to give herself to Tom? I sense this was true but I did not know Marie. Such ideas are speculative. I mustn't jump to hasty conclusions and label her as uncaring even though the signs point me to that conclusion. Within the context of normal ward practice I imagine her practice is caring. What *is* caring?

Tom and Joan's feelings are worn on their sleeves for anyone to see if they paid attention. They were close to despair, fearful of uncertain futures. I was aware that Tom's needs (and his wife's needs) were not being met. Understanding how others are feeling strengthens my empathic inquiry – my ability to know and connect with the experience of the other person. Practitioners often greet people, 'How are you feeling today?' Said with caring intent, such questions can open a cathartic space. However, as I illuminate in Chapter 18 with Michelle's story, it can open a can of worms. Said, as a routine greeting, it is meaningless.

This cue prompts the practitioner to connect with the other person, to sense what the other person is experiencing and to appreciate the meanings the other gives to their experience. The cue – what made them feel that way? – challenges the practitioner to check out their interpretation of the other's feelings and surface the assumptions that led them to interpret it that way.

Practical skills

- Developing empathic inquiry
- Catharsis

How was I feeling and what made me feel that way?

I felt a mixture of satisfaction and frustration. Satisfying because caring is vital for patients and myself. It is why I chose to nurse. Frustrating, because it is not easy to witness uncaring practice. Perhaps my frustration lies with attitudes based on ignorance. Marie was kind, but her attitude was not appropriate and yet she did not realise that. No one had pointed it out and so I had a more general feeling of frustration with the hospital.

Paramananda (2001, p. 58) writes, 'Whenever we begin to feel frustrated in what we are doing, we should slow down and pay closer attention to it. Frustration takes us away from ourselves; we become alienated from our experience. When we feel this beginning to happen we need to pay more attention to our experience.'

Reflection is often triggered by negative or uncomfortable feelings (Boyd and Fales 1983). As such, models of reflection draw the user's attention to feelings (Boud *et al* 1985, Gibbs 1988). It seems natural to focus on negative experiences because it is these situations that present themselves to consciousness. Much of experience is not reflected on simply because it is unproblematic. In other words, much of practice is taken for granted. Negative feelings disturb us and are played out as anxiety. People are strongly motivated to resolve anxiety through the use of defence mechanisms. As such, people may naturally reflect to defend against anxiety rather than to learn through it. I use the word reflect loosely because in this sense it does not lead to insight. It is an effort to deal with the consequence of a situation rather than its causes.

Some practitioners may find writing helps them work through their feelings, but for other writers, reflecting on events, especially traumatic events, may be distressing.

Gray and Forsstrom (1991, p. 360) write,

The process of 'journalling' may sound simple and easy to execute, but at times it was extremely difficult. Mostly the incidents recorded were identified because there was an affective component. This may be related to feelings of personal inadequacy to cope with the demands of the situation. Alone, it was emotionally painful to journal events that were largely self-critical.

Through writing I work out and convert negative feelings such as pity, frustration, anger and hatred into to positive energy for taking action. Thomas Moore (1992, p. 235) writes,

> Day by day we live emotions and themes that have deep roots, but our reflections on these experiences tend to be superficial . . . not only are our reflections often insufficient to account for intense feelings, but we may have been living from a place that is too rational and dispassionate. Rainer Maria Rilke advises the young poet to 'go deep into yourself and see how deep the place is from which your life flows.' We could all take note of this advice, go deep into ourselves and discover how deep is the source of our everyday lives.

The difficulty with going deeper is what will it reveal? Better to swim in the shallow end? I imagine the guide saying, 'let's keep this light and comfortable'. Exploration of feelings leads to deep insights into self and the development of therapeutic poise or equanimity. C Yoko Beck (1997, pp. 42–3) writes,

> For a time our life may feel worse than before, as what we have concealed becomes clear. But even as this occurs, we have a sense of growing sanity and understanding, of basic satisfaction. To continue practice through severe difficulties we must have patience, persistence and courage . . . we learn in our guts not just in our brains.

Reflection is about coming to know 'who I am' so I can better use my self for therapeutic work. As George Elliot (1876/1996) wrote in *Daniel Deronda*: 'There is a great deal of unmapped country within us which would have to be taken into account in an explanation of our gusts and storms.' Reflection is mapping, charting the unknown self, to better recognise, understand and control these gusts and storms in order to be more effective in our practice – what I term as poise. It may not be easy to understand our emotions. They may stem back to earlier unresolved issues in our lives. In his book, *Awakenings*, Sacks (1976, p. 15) writes,

> In our study of our most complex sufferings and disorder of being, we are compelled to scrutinise the deepest, darkest, and most fearful parts of ourselves, the parts we strive to deny or not to see. The thoughts which are most difficult to grasp or express are those which awaken our strongest denials and our most profound intuitions.

Reading these words may give an impression that reflection is more like therapy. Paying attention to feelings is undoubtedly significant in decision making (Callahan 1988). This understanding challenges the idea that decision making is a rational process where emotions are morally suspect and distort reason. As such, paying attention to feelings develops emotional intelligence, notably the idea of knowing and managing our emotions and fears (Salovey and Mayer 1990).

Through reflection we become aware of our fear and see the way it constrains our practice. Perhaps we see the fear as huge and immovable as if it were a boulder. As we reflect, we can begin to accept the fear as our own rather than something that will destroy us. As we do, the boulder seems to dissolve, loosens and falls away. We can learn to shift our images of fear and see fear as a cloud obscuring the blue sky. We can see that it is not permanent and will float away. Slowly our attachment to fear weakens and, as Rosenberg (1998) notes, 'little by little, we're not so enslaved to things' (p. 145). At every point, reflection is freedom to become who we desire to be.

Practical skills

> • Developing emotional intelligence and poise – knowing your emotional self and learning to manage this
>   therapeutically, thus becoming more available to the patient and less anxious
> • Developing sympathetic resonance and balance with empathic inquiry
> • Learning to focus the emotions in decision making
> • Nurturing compassion

What was I trying to achieve and did I respond effectively?

At every turn with Tom and Joan, I appreciate the unfolding situation, making decisions, being deliberative, acting intuitively, responding to their perceived needs, weighing up the impact of my response in terms of meeting their needs. But was I most effective? How could I judge that? I might think I am but am I? The reflective posture takes nothing for granted. Hence, reflecting on situations that went well always has this element: 'so that went well, could it have gone better?'

The idea of effective action can be viewed as four movements (Figure 3.2) .

Reflection on outcome informs future situations within a spiral of increasing effectiveness. The cue gets to the very core of clinical practice. Collectively, I describe these four movements as the aesthetic response. My use of the word aesthetic was inspired by Carper's fundamental ways of knowing in nursing (Johns 1995). Carper identified *aesthetics* as one of four fundamental ways of knowing in nursing. The other ways are *the empirical*, *the ethical*, and *the personal patterns of knowing*.[2] Carper's understanding of aesthetics is having an awareness of the immediate situation, seated in immediate practical action, including awareness of the patient and their circumstances as uniquely individual, and of the combined wholeness of the situation. More broadly, aesthetics is a branch of philosophy dealing with the nature of beauty, art and taste, and with the creation and appreciation of beauty.[3] Here, I would include performance. Watch a nurse go about her practice and you witness a performance that integrates all aspects of her practice. Perhaps

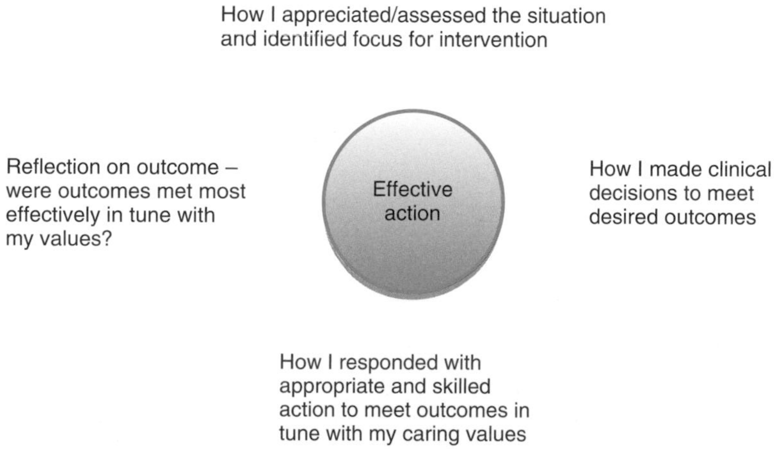

How I appreciated/assessed the situation
and identified focus for intervention

Reflection on outcome –
were outcomes met most
effectively in tune with
my values?

Effective
action

How I made clinical
decisions to meet
desired outcomes

How I responded with
appropriate and skilled
action to meet outcomes in
tune with my caring values

Figure 3.2　Effective action through four movements.

it flows with grace and perhaps it stutters awkwardly. Like a dancer I move about the patient. Like a sculptor I shape my practice. Like an actor I play out the drama. Like a poet I sense the poignancy within the unfolding moment.

The cue challenges the practitioner's pattern of decision making, lifting it from a non-reflective to a reflective mode. In terms of response I know that practitioners tend to respond based on three inadequate criteria:

- Responses they have used before
- Responses that have worked before
- Responses they are comfortable using.

These criteria reflect a habitual and unreflective practice that certainly does not lead to effective practice. Through reflection the practitioner constantly seeks to expand her repertoire of available responses in response to the patient's and family's needs.

Practical skills

- Developing appreciation and assessment skills
- Developing clinical judgement
- Developing effective action
- Evaluating efficacy in terms of meeting patient need

What are the broader consequences of my actions on the patient, others and myself?

In the previous cue, the practitioner has considered whether his or her actions were effective in meeting the patient's needs. In this cue, the practitioner is challenged to contemplate the broader consequences of her actions on both others and herself. The cue is deceptively deep. All actions have consequences. On the surface of things, the consequences of actions may be quite obvious, yet when the practitioner begins to pay attention, she can see that often her actions have far more reaching consequences, some of which could not be anticipated or even known about. It is like throwing a pebble into a pond and seeing the ripples spread out.

The cues enable the practitioner to develop foresight – to weigh up the likely consequences of actions as part of the decision-making process. It leads to the development of what Aristotle termed phronesis or practical wisdom – being mindful of the best way to respond within a particular situation considering the ethical consequences of such response (Delmar and Johns 2008).[4] Foresight is intuitive, for how can consequences be known given the uncertainty of life. Intuition in this sense suggests deeper embodied way of knowing. It is significant considering the impact of our actions not just for the patients we work with but more broadly towards creating better worlds for generations to come.

Practical skills

- Recognising the impact of actions, both intended and not-intended
- Developing practical wisdom

What knowledge did or might have informed me?

Without doubt, the effective practitioner is an informed practitioner. This cue guides the practitioner to access and critique all forms of knowledge for its value to inform the particular experience. In this way, knowledge is assimilated within personal knowing to inform future practice, enabling the development of *praxis*. Keeping informed is a mighty onus on the practitioner, given the vast amount of knowledge out there. As such, an organisational response is required, for example, developing standards of care and protocols that have systematically and periodically reviewed knowledge with ensuing clear guidelines to inform practice. Obvious examples are responses to wound care pressure relief. Yet, care does not lend itself easily to formulaic responses. It is important to caution about using such guidelines as prescriptions simply because all clinical situations are unique, they have never happened before. In medicine, National Institute for Health and Clinical Excellence (NICE) guidelines do prescribe specific responses to specific situations. However, this does risk turning practitioners into technicians to apply the prescription and patients into objects to be manipulated. Much of practice is complex and indeterminate with no easy solutions to simply apply (Schön 1987). Hence applying theory must always be viewed through a sceptical eye (Dewey 1933).

Consider my experience with Tom and Joan. What theory might inform my decisions and actions? One example, enabling patients control of their environment whilst in hospital has been shown to be significant for self-esteem and maintenance of competence (Charmaz 1983).

Practical skills

- Accessing, critiquing and assimilating relevant theory with practice (developing praxis)

To what extent did I act for the best and in tune with my values and beliefs?

Healthcare professionals are expected to practice within a code of professional ethics that set out their responsibility to act ethically at all times. As such the practitioner is always mindful of always acting for the best or good. Every story is a moral story concerning the practitioner's intent to act for the good. It was certainly my intention with Tom and Joan. My person-centred values can be discerned within the story, as are the factors that constrain me.

The cue has two interrelated issues: firstly, an ethical reflection on the 'best', and secondly, a review of the practitioner's values and beliefs that constitute desirable practice. I added beliefs to the MSR because people may view values and beliefs as different.

The healthcare world is always changing. The consumer movement demands the right for people to be involved in decision making about their health care. People are no longer passive recipients of health care. They are more informed: 'Google' any health condition to reveal an overload of information, challenging the idea of professional knowledge being known only to the initiated.

Applying ethical principles in practice is complex. Often they contradict each other. As such, *acting for the best* always needs to be interpreted within each moment (Cooper

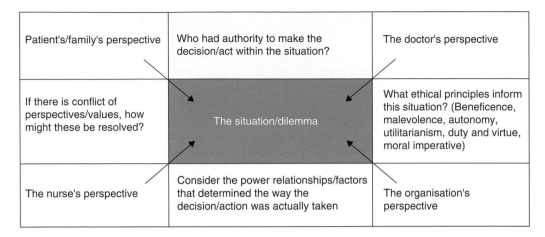

Figure 3.3   Ethical mapping (Johns 1998b).

1991, Parker 1990). This may be challenging if practitioners have different values, agendas and levels of authority to make decisions.

To guide the practitioner to explore acting for the best, I developed ethical mapping (Figure 3.3).

The ethical map trail

1 *Frame the dilemma*

Most ethical issues can be reduced into a dilemma.

For example, should I confront Marie's approach to Tom or not? Should I walk Joan or not?

2 *Consider the perspective of different actors, commencing with the nurse(s) own perspectives*

By considering the perspectives of people involved within the experience, the practitioner is challenged to see and understand their perspectives alongside their own perspective. These different perspectives are all partial and not necessarily motivated by what's best but by personal, professional or organisational interests. In this way the practitioner can gain a global or helicopter view of the whole.

3 *Consider which ethical principles apply in terms of the best decision*

Having gained an understanding of partial perspectives, the practitioner can consider the way ethical principles might inform the situation. The major ethical principles to consider are

- Autonomy
- Beneficence and non-malevolence
- Justice or utilitarianism.

Autonomy is the possession or right of self-government (Compact Oxford English Dictionary 2005, p. 58). Seedhouse (1988) views autonomy as the highest ethical principle. It has two aspects: firstly, the practitioner respects the patient's right for self-determination and secondly, the practitioner creates the space for the patient to exercise their autonomy. Hence Tom and Joan might not assert their right for autonomy for many reasons, such as learnt passivity, fear of reprisal and the suchlike. They may be happy for professionals to make decisions for them although, as the story reveals, this is not necessarily in their best interests.

By contrast, professional autonomy is concerned with the practitioner's right for self-government safeguarded with the ethics of beneficence and non-malevolence enshrined within the Hippocratic oath that doctors should do good (beneficence) and not do harm (non-malevolence). In past days, professional autonomy was universally accepted in a capitalist construction of health care whereby the person gave up his or her rights in return for health care (Talcott Parsons 1952). However, the world has changed with an ever-increasing recognition of patient's rights to be involved in decisions about their health care. This creates a natural tension between professional and patient autonomy within which the practitioner must position herself.

professional autonomy ⟷ patient autonomy

From a person-centred perspective, the practitioner naturally leans towards patient autonomy although this perspective may not be shared with other professionals and hence the ground for contestation and conflict.

Another key ethical principle is utilitarianism – the idea of greatest good whereby the needs of the individual are in tension with the needs of society as a whole due to finite resources available.

Needs of the individual ⟷ needs of society

Professional codes of ethics are constructed around the ethics of virtue or duty; the way the practitioner should conduct herself as befitting a nurse. An obvious example of this is that a nurse should always act in caring manner. This also means not causing suffering through careless action, for example, failure to provide Joan with a plate guard when she is unable to use a knife and fork. A further ethical principle is Kant's moral imperative – 'do as you would be done for'. In other words imposing your own values into the situation – 'if that was my mother'. The problem with this principle is that the patient is not your mother and that imposing such values may be misguided.

With Tom and Joan, I was faced with the dilemma of whether to advocate in their best interests or empower them to act for themselves. Certainly, I should have negotiated my advocacy role. Acting on behalf of others is described as paternalism by Benjamin and Curtis (1986) who set out three criteria to legitimate such action:
- Harm – would Tom and Joan come to some harm if I hadn't acted for them?
- Autonomy – are Tom and Joan able to act for themselves?
- Ratification – would Tom and Joan thank me for my actions at a later date?

According to these criteria, I was ethically wrong to talk about them without their knowledge to other health professionals. And yet how easy it is to respond like this and treat patients as objects of care rather than respect their autonomy.

4 *Consider what conflict exists between perspectives/values and how these might be resolved*

Having considered the different perspectives of people involved and diverse ethical principles, the practitioner can consider the best decision to make or if there is conflict between professionals, how such conflict can be resolved in the patient's best interests.

5 *Consider who had the authority for making the decision/taking action*

This part of ethical mapping challenges the practitioner to consider her autonomy, authority and accountability for making and acting on decisions. According to Batey and Lewis (1982), autonomy has two dimensions: legitimate autonomy as set out in the person's job description and discriminant authority – the autonomy the person believes she has. However, job descriptions are often vague, and working in bureaucratic organisations may diminish discriminant autonomy, especially for professionals such as nurses who may perceive themselves or be perceived by other professionals as a subordinate workforce. In this sense, reflection empowers practitioners to expand their field of autonomy and counter any sense of oppression.

6 *Consider the power relationships/factors that determined the way the decision/action was actually taken*

In the real world, decisions are not necessarily made in terms of what's best for the patient or family, but in terms of power and fear of sanction.[5] These patterns of power are implicit within normal patterns of relating between professionals. However, they can be made explicit and ethically challenged for their legitimacy in terms of the patient's best interests.

A number of questions are useful to inform stages 5 and 6:
- Who defines the problem?
- Whose terms are used?
- Who controls the domain or territory?
- Who decides on what resources are needed and how they are allocated?
- Who holds whom accountable?
- Who prescribes the activity of others?
- Who can influence policy makers?

Ethical mapping is a very practical tool and widely used in guided reflection.[6]

Practical skills

- Ethical decision making
- Integrity
- Empathy and therapeutic relationships
- Resource management
- Conflict management

How does this situation connect with previous experiences?

An experience is not an isolated moment in time. It is part of a continuous stream of unfolding experiences. How the practitioner responds today is influenced by how she responded yesterday and beyond. As Jones and Jones (1996, p. 78) write, 'If we don't stay connected and remember the lessons from the past, are we not doomed to repeat them?'

Patterns of thinking and behaviours become embodied as normal, often leading to habitual and unreflective practice. Practitioners carve out comfort grooves and then get stuck in them. We are creatures of habit and quickly become complacent. O'Donohue (1997, pp. 163–4) writes,

Many people remain trapped at the one window, looking out every day at the same scene in the same way. Real growth is experienced when you draw back from that one window, turn and walk around the inner tower of the soul and see all the different windows that await your gaze. Through these different windows, you can see new vistas of possibility, presence and creativity. Complacency, habit and blindness often prevent you from feeling your life. So much depends on the frame of vision – the window through which we look.

Imagine going round your mind opening shutters to see your practice from different vistas. It is a powerful metaphor for seeing my experience with Tom and Joan from new angles – challenging the normal and taken-for-granted aspects of my practice. It links to the qualities of openness and curiosity I noted as prerequisites of reflection in Chapter 1.

Reflection helps me appreciate links between my practice with Tom and Joan and others involved in the experiences and see patterns of my behaviour grooved out over 30 years as a nurse. I see my intolerance to uncaring and my hesitant response to such behaviour because I am anxious about conflict. I have never been assertive yet strive to be so. I have worked with many old people like Tom and Joan who are dependent on others for help. I know it is easier to take over and do to them rather than enable them, especially when busy in a practice culture dominated by a task approach to doing work.

This is a disturbing cue for at least two reasons. Firstly, it pulls you out of autopilot and now you have to think about what you do. Secondly, you may realise that learnt patterns are not the best patterns and feel a deep sense of guilt. The good news is that guilt is energising if we are committed to best practice.

Practical skills

> • Being mindful of how patterns of thinking and behaviour influence the current situation

What assumptions govern my practice and what factors influence the way I feel, think and respond within the particular experience?

In the sequential order of the MSR, this cue doesn't quite know its place. Factors such as ethics, knowledge and past experiences are all influencing factors on how the practitioner thinks, feels and responds within practice. The idea of assumptions is helpful. As Bohm (1996, p. 69) writes

> Normally, we don't see that our assumptions are affecting the nature of our observations. But the assumptions affect the way we see things, the way we experience them, and consequently the things we want to do. In a way we are looking through our assumptions; the assumptions could be said to be an observer in a sense.

Assumptions govern our way of looking at our practice. As such the practitioner needs to appreciate these assumptions and shift them as necessary towards realising more desirable practice. As I explored in the last cue, assumptions are deeply embodied and not easily perceived. Think of the last time you said 'I assume. . . .' It is the way someone interprets the world.

This cue is a gateway to knowing self – what makes me tick, what factors pull my strings? It is deceptively difficult to respond to because the self tends to view itself normatively.

This cue can feel scary because it is introspective, unearthing and revealing influences that stem from social and cultural practices or past experiences that have left a trace. These influencing factors can be threatening. Perhaps this is one reason why some practitioners turn away from the reflective mirror or actually *smudge the mirror* to distort the image of self being reflected back to give a better impression. Lather (1986a,b) describes this distortion as 'false consciousness'. This distortion is not done consciously; it is a defence mechanism at work protecting the threatened ego. As such, it is not easy for the practitioner to recognise distortion. A guide is necessary to challenge the practitioner and pull away the masks of false consciousness and help the practitioner reveal and accept their true self (see Chapter 6 for exploration of guidance).

Through analysing practitioners' reflections, I have identified a number of common influencing factors (Figure 3.4). The grid is reorganised around the 'expectations tension'.

Expectations from self how I should respond

Expectations from others how I should respond

Conforming to 'normal practice/habit? *The weight of tradition*	Expectations from others how I should act?	Negative attitudes and prejudice?
Limited skills/discomfort/ confidence to act in other, or appropriate ways?		Fear of sanction? *The weight of authority*
Emotional entanglement/over identification? Deeper psyche factors?	What factors influence my decision making and actions?	Misplaced concern – loyalty to colleagues versus loyalty to patient? Anxious about ensuing conflict?
Assumptions that seemingly govern my practice?		Knowledge to act in specific ways? *The weight of theory*
Wrapped up in self-concern? Pity? Guilt? Frustration? Need to be valued? Dependency?		Doing the right thing? (ethical mapping) Time/priorities?
Need to be in control	Expectations from self about 'how I should act'	Stress

Figure 3.4   The 'influences grid'.

Other factors identified in the 'influence grid' influence this tension. I could write a supplementary book on the nature of these influences. These factors are grounded in issues of tradition, authority (force/power) and embodiment; issues that Fay (1987) identified as barriers to rational change. The weight of embodiment is heavy indeed. It reflects how I have come to be who I am through socialisation. To change who I am requires awareness and understanding of these influences so I can begin to let go of them and learn new patterns of being more congruent with desirable practice. As the motto goes 'old habits die hard'. They need active and prolonged confrontation. It can be like hitting your head on a brick wall – what I term the hard wall of reality (see framing perspectives). Issues of force and tradition are evident within normal patterns of relating and again tend to be embodied. These too are hard to shift because they are grounded in patterns of relationship that require changing others besides self.

Many of these factors are debilitating, such as stress and fear of sanction. Fear of sanction from more powerful others reflects how expectations from others can dominate the expectations tension when practitioners feel powerless to assert themselves and practice with integrity. People can become victims of the system. I reflect on stress as a subheading. The deeper psyche factors are fear, dependency, insecurity; factors that may have left emotional scars. Identifying these old patterns is a significant step in healing them with the help of a guide or therapist. Jones and Jones (1996) describe these factors as crooked arrows that continue to hurt us. They advocate a focus on straight arrows that develop a strong sense of self-acceptance and love. Too often we get wrapped up in our negative parts of self and neglect strengthening the positive aspects. It is about the 'self' being fit for practice. Some of the influencing factors can have dramatic impact on the quality of the practitioner's relationship with patients.

Warshield

One exercise I use with reflective practitioners is to construct a warshield and decorate it to remind the person of their crooked and straight arrows. Using the warshield is an imaginative approach to dealing with stress and developing poise. Learning becomes playful as the practitioners bend over tables or lie on the floor with their imagination, paints and crayons.

The grid is always expanding and is adaptable to suit your own design. For example, issues surrounding racism continue to surface (Blackford 2003, Puzan 2003). Puzan writes,

> There is so much familiarity in talking about the alleged racial differences of non-white people in public discourse and so little familiarity in talking about those racial properties attached to being white, that the concept of whiteness (or a recognition of racial formation) has little resonance within nursing. While issues related to cultural difference are not ignored, they rarely include the difference specifically engendered by 'whiteness', which is structured to avoid and deflect interrogation or critical reflection. (p. 194)

Reflection opens a space for such discourse. So, what factors were influencing me at the community hospital that cold day in spring? I felt the tension between my expectation to be person-centred and expectations from others to get through the work. I sense the tension between my expectations of self to speak out (integrity) versus (unspoken) expectations from others not to be critical. Linked to that I sense the tension between speaking out for others (paternalism) and enabling others to speak for themselves (empowerment). I found myself to some extent absorbing the suffering of both Tom and Joan, identifying with them, pitying them to some extent. I can imagine the strain on staff to find time to prioritise being with them in the demand to get through the work. I could feel this cultural strain ripple through the unit.

The influences grid gives the practitioner a structure to view both their own and others' perspectives within ethical mapping – this is illustrated in Chapter 18.

This cue inevitably explores the boundaries with therapy and highlights the vital need for self-development in human–human encounter work that espouses the intention to work with people from spiritual, psychological and emotional frames of reference.

Practical skills

- Knowing self and developing the therapeutic self and self's impact on practice

Stress, anxiety, and coping with work

Stress accumulates without realising it. Neck and shoulder muscles ache giving headaches and sapping energy to balance the body. So many practitioners' shoulders are knotted and aching. Stress leaves us feeling heavy and drained. With our energy depleted we are not available to our patients. Anxiety kills, and in the survival effort we sacrifice the patient to save ourselves. The reality of today's National Health Service (NHS) is that nurse shortages are reportedly reaching crisis point, establishment shortfall is nationally 20%, one-third of all nurses are allocated no study time, and bed occupancy is running at 98% (Hall 2003). In such an environment, Wall *et al* (1997) note that NHS staff suffer considerably more stress than any other workforce with 28% recording levels above the symptom threshold.

Feeling fluffy–feeling drained scale

We can be stressed for many reasons. The first remedy for dealing with stress is to recognise its aetiology. One reflective approach is to use the 'feeling fluffy–feeling drained' scale (Figure 3.5). The scale consists of a visual analogue scale (VAS) 10 cm long. It asks the practitioner to mark along the scale the extent they feel either fluffy or drained at the end of their work shift.

The scale then poses three questions:

- What factors contribute to your sense of feeling drained?
- What factors contribute to your sense of feeling light and fluffy?
- What can you do to go home feeling more fluffy and less drained?

Feeling fluffy is a feeling of lightness at the end of the day where one's energy remains full, whereas feeling drained is having no energy at the end of the workday. I am sure every reader has experienced both feelings at the end of the day.

At the end of the workday, the practitioner scores the extent they feel either fluffy or drained and explore contributing factors and what they can realistically do to improve

Week commencing......20 May 2002
Day – Wednesday
Please score on the scale the extent you feel light and fluffy or drained at the end of the workday:

I go home feeling light and fluffy	⬅——————————➡	*I go home feeling totally drained*
What factors contribute to your sense of feeling drained?	*Arrived in the morning to a horrible phone call from a patient's relative who held me personally responsible for his wife's wait in A&E when I had already advised him that there were no beds in the hospital.*	
What factors contribute to your sense of feeling light and fluffy?	*Did teaching session – I always enjoy teaching. Also put together a bid for further training in the hospital. Didn't think I would be able to do it this quickly.*	
What can you do to go home feeling more fluffy and less drained?	*I confronted the relative and listened to his worries. He apologised to me for being rude. Whilst I felt better because he apologised I need to learn not to take relative's anger so personally. I recognise he was projecting his frustration – that I was in the firing line. Instead of defending myself I need to be more mindful and see the anger for what it was – this will help diffuse it.*	

Figure 3.5   Feeling fluffy–feeling drained scale.

their fluffy score by acknowledging and enhancing feel-good experiences and working at neutralising energy-draining situations. As with all reflective activity, it is first necessary to become aware of and pay attention to these experiences. Only then is change possible based on a realistic appreciation of the situation, perhaps requiring guidance, given the practitioner's embodied responses to stressful stimuli within 'normal' patterns of relationships.

The practitioner can use the scale daily over a period of time (giving structure to a reflective journal) to monitor the (intended) improvement in 'fluffiness'.

In Figure 3.5, I give an example of one practitioner's score. Her normal score was around 7, suggesting a relatively high residual level of stress. On a very good day, this might drop to 5. In the example, her score is 10 – due entirely to an altercation with a patient's relative despite its successful resolution. Such was the stressful nature of the situation it submerged her feeling fluffy factors. In clinical supervision, she was able to explore the situation in more depth, her response to it and ways of resolving it, so if she faced a similar situation her energy would not be so drained. Imagine what better shape she would be in, if her average score was 3 rather than 7?

Use the scale. Does it help you identify and reduce stress?

Practitioners seem to suffer more stress related to organisational issues and conflict than issues related to patient care (Vachon 1988). Is this observation true for you? If so, this may have ramifications for giving patient care. Taylor (1992) noted a theme within the literature of how nurses have been dispossessed 'of their essential humanness as human beings and as people, by emphasising their professional roles and responsibilities' (p. 1042). Taylor draws attention to the fact that nurses are human too and, as such, are vulnerable to the same issues that face their patients and families. The lack of recognition of humanness in nursing through a focus on roles and responsibilities has led practitioners to strive to be something they were clearly struggling to cope with. Taylor (1992) noted that practitioners didn't recognise or understand their own ordinariness as human beings. Consequently, they become alienated from themselves in their efforts to cope with and live with the contradictions in their lives. Jourard (1971) noted that such striving damages 'the self' and reinforces the need to cope in a vicious downward spiral of self-destruction towards burnout and a state of anomie.

Jade, one of the primary nurses at Burford Hospital, said, 'I don't come to work dressed in protective armour' (Johns 1993). As Dewey (1933, p. 30) observed, 'Unconscious fears also drive us into purely defensive attitudes that operate like coats of armour – not only to shut out new conceptions but even to prevent us from making new observations.' Dewey believed that anxiety limited the practitioner's ability to learn through experience. The professional is closed to protect self rather than open to possibility. 'Armour' is akin to professional detachment.

Water butt theory of stress

Lydia Hall (1964, p. 151) writes,

> Anxiety over an extended period is stressful to all the organ functions. It prepares people to fight or flight. In our culture, however, it is brutal to fight and cowardly to flee, so we stew in our own juices and cook up malfunction. This energy can be put to use in exploration of feeling through participation in the struggle to face and solve problems underlying the state of anxiety.

Stewing in our own juices is not healthy. Reflection opens a space for people to express and appreciate their anxiety and stress and work at ways of dealing with it in a similar way of expressing negative feelings. This releases energy. A guide may be a necessary catalyst for converting this energy into positive energy for taking action.

However, some people are unable to express or work out their anxiety, that is, until they are unable to contain it anymore. Then one of two things tend to happen. Either they blow up inside and have a breakdown or they blow up outside – literally they 'blow their top' similar to a water butt that spills over when full. One difficulty with 'spilling over' is that it creates a mess that others may feel uncomfortable with. No one likes overt displays of anger or despair. Such people are motivated to clear the mess up and pretend it didn't happen, characteristic of the 'harmonious team' that sweeps up and brushes emotional mess under the carpet and pretends that everything is okay on the surface.[7] In other words, the underlying issues that caused the stress are not dealt with.

Slowly, drip, drip, drip, the water butt fills up again, until the person blows again. Sometimes, a violent storm fills the water butt quickly and, like lightning, the practitioner snaps and blow her top and rage at events or people (Parker 1990, Pike 1991, Wilkinson 1988). Pike (1991, p. 351) writes, 'Moral outrage ensues when the nurse's attempts to operationalize a choice is thwarted by constraints. The outrage intensifies when these constraints not only block action, but also force a course of action that violates the nurse's moral tenets.'

Many practitioners wear this T-shirt. However, the water butt does have a drainage tap. The practitioner can learn to be aware of monitoring her stress levels, drain stress off and convert the stress into positive energy necessary to take appropriate action to resolve the sources of stress. Likewise, the gardener draws water from the water butt to water the flowers and nourish their growth. However, the tap might be blocked, requiring help to unblock it – again the value of guided reflection.

The risk of burnout

Failure to realise desirable work or manage anxiety in constructive ways leads inexorably to burnout. Cherniss (1980) describes burnout as a process in which 'the professional's attitudes and behaviours change in negative ways in response to job strain' (p. 5). Maslach 1976 suggested that the major negative change in those experiencing burnout in people-centred work was 'the loss of concern for the client and a tendency to treat clients in a detached, mechanical fashion' (p. 6).

Not good news then.

McNeely (1983) observed that when practitioners felt they had lost the intrinsic satisfaction of caring, they became focused on the conditions of work, for example, off duty rosters and workload issues, characteristic of bureaucratic models of organisation. McNeely believes that bureaucratic conditions are antithetical to human service work and strongly advocated that such organisations needed to move to collegial ways of working staff in order to offset the risks of burnout. Burnout is a descent into a black hole when the caring self has been scrapped away on the uncaring sharp edges of systems despite rhetoric to the contrary. The contradictions are no longer tenable. Benner and Wrubel (1989) believe that the answer to stress and burnout is to reconnect to caring rather than the development of personal detachment as advocated by Menzies-Lyth (1988). There is little organisational sensitivity to the profound nature of journeying with another person to help ease that person's suffering. The lack of recognition of emotional labour (James 1989, Bolton 2000), that somehow emotional work is natural women's work, and therefore is unskilled, doesn't need to be taught, and is not valued, when emotional work is the greatest gift nurses can offer patients. Yet if the organisation doesn't seem to care why should I? Quick route to burnout.

Yet burnout can be viewed as a healing space, whereby the nurse can discover herself. It may be dark, lonely and painful, but it can still be a necessary healing space. Such healing is a journey to discover rather than recover, because recovery suggests returning to what she was before, only for the hurting to start all over again.

The looking forward cues

In Chapter 2, I suggested dividing the page into three columns: the left column for the rich description, the middle column for reflection and the right column for imaging how the practitioner might respond differently given the experience again.

Janet writes

Saw V again today, still very tearful and anxious about breastfeeding. Positioning and attachment (of baby onto breast) much better, but nipples red and cracked, and strong evidence of deep breast thrush in her, and oral thrush in baby. Has seen GP as I suggested last week – he has prescribed for baby but says he does 'not believe' in deep breast thrush, and refuses to prescribe. V refused to see another GP and says she does not want to make trouble or waste their time . . . so how will things ever change? Am frustrated and annoyed . . . have prescribed a topical anti-fungal. It's not the best treatment but all I can do. Why do people pander to GPs like this?

It was after this experience that I began to experiment with the 'left-hand column'. Senge (1990) suggests as a strategy for challenging and revealing how mental models operate to distort and manipulate reality. I divide the page into two columns. I write the description of my experience in the left column, and use the right column to respond to MSR cues. In doing so, I am writing an explicit and implicit story:

1.1 The explicit story	1.2 The implicit story
Saw V again today.	V is taking up a lot of my time.
Doctor does not believe in deep breast thrush.	My diagnosis is being questioned, which makes me look and feel foolish.
V refuses to seek another opinion and does not want to make trouble.	V senses the tension between me and the doctors.
V does not want to waste the doctors' time.	V values my time less than that of the doctors.
How will things ever change?	I feel powerless to change things myself.
I prescribe a less efficacious treatment.	I feel forced to compromise my professional integrity by the doctor.
I am frustrated and annoyed.	I am not in control of the situation.
Why do people pander to doctors like this?	I want to avoid a confrontation with the doctors, and want V to do it on my behalf.

In this experience, the cue – 'what issues seem significant to pay attention to?' – raised my awareness of my need for status and recognition. The cue – 'to what extend did I act for the best?' – prompted my ethical consideration of my prescribing decision and V's right to act autonomously. The cue – 'what factors influenced the way I was feeling, thinking or responding?' and 'how do I *now* feel about this experience?' – highlight my conflict avoidance and struggle for autonomy against the background of GP dominance.

A third column could be utilised based on the cue, 'How might I respond more effectively given this situation again?' Most significantly, would my response in tune with my values of collaborating with both the mother and the GPs? At the core of this new story is my desire to confront both V and the GPs with their respective attitudes and to confront myself in order to overcome my frustrating sense of subordination and to assert my perspectives. But could I respond differently? Do I have the skills? Am I powerful enough? What will the consequences be? My fear is that it will go pear shaped and create conflict. I don't do conflict well. I want my mothers to need me and despite my frustration I need the GPs to value me. Chris (my guide) says it will work out fine – that I always look at consequences from a negative perspective. Maybe that's true, but somewhere deep within is the assumption that doctors punish nurses if they do challenge them. It is a psychological hold that isn't easily shifted. Chris says 'imagine they are toads not gods'. That's funny. Ribbit, ribbit, ribbit. The power of imagery. The fear flakes off.

Reflection helps me see things clearly and sharpen my frustration, but it doesn't hurt so much because I sense what I need to do and can convert this energy into taking action.

Over time, as I look back on this experience, I can see it was groundbreaking – the crisis so to speak that began an inexorable shift in my relationship with both mothers and GPs. I now appreciate the GP's resistance to my insistent demand to be heard, and as such, it is no longer demoralising but inspiring as I sort to 'be with women' – my vision of midwifery practice. Paradoxically, the GP now values me more because I assert my point of view rather than demand it like a petulant child even though we do not always agree. Writing that, I realise I still need to be valued. Subordination is not easy to shrug off. It is also hard to admit.

How might I respond more effectively given this situation again?

In the above scenario, the cues guided Janet to reflect back on her experience with the intention of appreciating and resolving the creative tension between desirable and actual practice. She then turned towards the future to anticipate how she might respond more effectively given the situation again.

I term this the anticipatory phase of reflection. I can't emphasise enough the significance of this cue. It opens a creative learning space to play with possibility. It challenges normal ways of perceiving and responding to practice situations and thinking patterns that govern these normal ways. For this reason, it is not necessarily an easy cue to respond to. I know from guiding many practitioners it is difficult to shift perception to think differently especially is there is an emotional impasse. Another reason why a guide may be essential for reflective learning to pull open the practitioner's shutters to view the experience from new angles.

Applying this cue to my experience with Tom and Joan,

- Linked to the tension between advocacy and enabling them to assert their own voice, I could have asked them if they would like me to speak for them.
- I could have confronted Marie with her approach to Tom or asserted a more holistic approach.
- I could have anticipated Tom's need for the commode before his wash. Butterfield (1990) describes this as 'thinking upstream' – often we pull people out of the stream who fall in when we should consider ways of preventing them falling in the first place. In other words, a focus on **prevention** rather than **rescue**.
- I could have taken Marie aside and asked her to reflect more on what made Tom so happy this morning when he had been so miserable.
- I could have asked the domestic to apply a slip mat and plate guard rather than do that myself.
- Perhaps I would not have walked Joan, but contacted the physiotherapist directly, to come and see her. Walking her may have put her at some risk.
- I could have been less frustrated. I feel certain my voice had a critical edge as I gave feedback to the senior nurse. I felt her slight recoil. Her defensive posture diluted my message.

The list is endless. Every response could be different. Contemplating new ways of responding is like planting seeds of possibility so that if I was faced with a similar situation the seeds might germinate and I respond differently (Margolis 1993).

And this is the significant thing about this cue – the fuelling of inquiry and opening to other possibilities in the quest for effectiveness and professional responsibility.

What would be the consequences of alternative actions for the patient, others and myself?

This cue challenges me to consider the possible consequences of responding in different ways within the particular situation. It helps me weigh up my judgement and develop practical wisdom. Imagine the consequences of confronting Marie with her normal approach to patients such as Tom? Would that have been in his best interests? If I did confront her, when should I have do that? Perhaps we should have a discussion about our approach before we commenced his wash? These questions reflect the way this cue opens new possibilities of response to scrutiny.

What factors might stop me from responding differently?

Weighing up the consequences of different ways of responding leads the practitioner to choose the preferred option. Yet can I actually respond as envisaged? Do I have the skills? Am I assertive enough? Can I move through my natural inclination to avoid conflict to respond more effectively? Can I move through pity to compassion?

The cue challenges any ideal response and makes me take a realistic look at myself.

Practice skills

- Challenging habitual practice
- Appreciating new ways of responding within particular situations and their consequences
- Developing skills associated with responding differently
- Creativity
- Developing foresight and practical wisdom

How do I NOW feel about this experience?

Remember, reflection is often triggered by negative feelings. The release of feelings is both cathartic and energising, enabling the practitioner to work through and learn from these feelings without defending herself. If not, unresolved negative feelings store up trouble for the body causing stress and potential ill-health, reducing the practitioner's energy for therapeutic work.

Having worked through the cues, I naturally convert any negative feelings or energy into positive energy for taking ensuing action. I feel better about the situation. I no longer feel guilty about any neglectful responses simply because I know what I need to do next time. I feel more open, more curious, more responsible. I feel as if the heavy clouds that depressed me and obscured my perspectives have lifted. I am more fluffy!

Practice skills

- Releasing negative feelings and energising self

Am I now more able to support myself and others better as a consequence?

This cue challenges the practitioner to consider if adequate support is available within the workplace to ensure she can be most available to patients. This is both an individual and collective enterprise.

Caring is a reciprocal relationship. If nurses and other healthcare practitioners are expected to care, then they need to work in caring environments. If the practitioner is suffering, it is likely that other colleagues re also suffering, sapping their energy and limiting their availability to be with patents. And yet often, nurses seem to need to cope, to not expose their vulnerability, as if it is a weakness not to cope or admit to strain. They would prefer a collusive silence. To care, we need ways to penetrate the silence to support each other and create a therapeutic team – a team whereby its members are actively and genuinely available to each other. As such, the reflective practitioner is mindful of her colleagues' well-being.

Consider the following questions:

- Are adequate support systems in place?
- Are people stressed or worse, burntout?
- If so, why do you think that is?
- Do you see seeking help as a strength rather than weakness?
- Do you explore your anxiety as a learning opportunity?
- Are you truly available to support your colleagues?

Practice skills

- Ensuring support for self and others within practice is valued and available as necessary
- Keeping self fully (emotionally) fit for practice (emotional intelligence)

Conclusion

I have set out the reflective spiral moving from significance on the surface of experience towards gaining insights folded deep within it. The final MSR cue – 'what insights do I gain?' – is the focus for the following chapter.

Notes

1 A version of this narrative was first published in *Nursing Inquiry* (Johns (1998b) Caring through a reflective lens: giving meaning to being a reflective practitioner).
2 I outline Carper's work as a way of framing insights in Chapter 4.
3 http://www.merriam-webster.com/dictionary/aesthetics
4 The 13th International Reflective Practice conference held in Aalborg was dedicated to the development of phronesis through reflective practice. Papers from this conference were collected in the book, *The Good, the Wise, and the Right Clinical Nursing Practice*, edited by Delmar and Johns (2008).
5 As I indicated in Chapter 1, power is the central tenet of critical reflection.
6 Chapter 18 comprises narratives using ethical mapping to explore dilemmas and conflict.
7 See Hank's complaint, Chapter 18.

Chapter 4
Framing insights

The point of reflection is to learn and gain insight. Insights, by their very nature, change people. In changing people, insights inevitably impact on the wider community as the practitioner responds differently, more congruently with her values. Other people feel the ripple of change and also begin to respond differently, sending further ripples of change through the community, shifting norms and weaving more therapeutic patterns of relationships to create better worlds for practitioners and those they serve. Carson (2008, p. 139) writes, 'when you change the way an individual thinks of himself, you change the way he lives in his community and thereby you change the community in some way to a greater or lesser extent.'

Insights are at the level of understanding, empowerment and transformation. They can be explosive moments of revelation, perhaps something so obvious that we simply have not seen it before. They may be subtle, their subtlety only revealed through subsequent reflection. Insights are more than thinking about things differently. Indeed, our thinking may block gaining insight simply because it is the way we have always thought, whereas insights reflect different thinking. In gaining insight we learn to think about our thinking. It is this dimension of reflection that becomes mindful and deeper.

Dwelling within the reflective spiral is intuitive, being open to its possibilities but without forcing it. The key is to stand back far enough to gain a wider perspective. Wheatley (1999, p. 118) writes, 'when we concentrate on individual moments or fragments of experience, we see only chaos. The complexity of our practice may seem like chaos – just how do I sort the wood from the trees to see clearly? But if we stand back and look at what is taking shape, we see order. Order always displays itself as patterns that develop over time.'

The idea of pattern is useful because insights are always in relation to the whole. Insights are not necessarily easy to translate into words. Subhuti (1985/2001, p. 90) writes, 'we need to make this attempt to describe the indescribable because words help us to reduce this cosmic complexity to a workable simplicity for the purposes of everyday functioning.'

Becoming a Reflective Practitioner, Fourth Edition. Christopher Johns.
© 2013 John Wiley & Sons, Ltd. Published 2013 by John Wiley & Sons, Ltd.

Single lines

One facilitative approach towards gaining insight is to break the story text into single lines and scrolling down the text. This opens up the text and enables the practitioner to literally read between the lines where meaning and insight is often found. However, insights are not simply lying in these spaces waiting to be revealed. As I scroll down text, it is like entering a new place where things are not so familiar, in search of the insight (Winterson 2001). It is helpful to keep a wide perspective rather than focus too narrowly – the art of standing back and it will come to you. It is like trying to name the ineffable, rather like the nature of tacit knowing – I know something but can't easily explain what it is I know. As Polanyi (1958) has noted, this tacit knowing is the core of professional craft and artistry, and it is the knowing accessed and developed through reflection on a tacit level. Of course, this is one reason why practitioners struggle to name their insights.

The breaking down of text into single lines leads to the development of what I term 'prose poems'. As I break down the lines, I find myself rewriting the lines as new ideas spring to mind. As I do this, insights often emerge. It is a movement towards weaving the narrative.[1] It is an evolving process as one thing leads to another, like watching a washing machine go round and round, and with each revolution something new is spun out.

Dwelling with the text, I scroll down it, seeking to find the edges of the unfamiliar so I can pull away the veneer of normal practice to sense another world altogether less familiar. The insight is more likely to be a hunch, an ah-ha moment more than a logical deduction. This is an imaginative, intuitive and creative process. Tuffnell and Crickmay (2004, p. 119) write, 'imagination is not a separate faculty, rather it engages all parts of the mind and intelligence – fusing or bringing together often surprising aspects of what we feel or know, imagination expands our seeing.'

As I have noted, much of our educational experience has trimmed our imagination. Paramananda (2001, p. 71) writes,

Of course, the sad thing, the tragic thing, is that many of us do get trimmed. We all start off with real heads full of space and imagination, but slowly, somewhere along the path that we call growing up, our heads get trimmed. We become caught up in the doings of this world, the realities of adult life, and we get down to size . . . without imagination the world loses its mystery and sense of depth in which we can find meaning.

The good news is that reflection nurtures imagination. Imaginatively, I scroll down the text in creative play. Okri (1997, p. 21) writes,

Creativity, it would appear, should be approached in the spirit of play, of foreplay, of dalliance, doodling, messing around – and then, bit by bit, you somehow get deeper into the matter. But if you go in there with a businessman's solemnity or the fanaticism of some artistic types you are likely to be rewarded with a stiff response, a joyless dribble, strained originality, ideas that come out all strapped up and strangled by too much effort.

The idea of dallying suggests giving the mind free rein to explore, allowing the imagination to wander and accept anything that comes up. Laughing at our in-built censors that constantly seek to trim us.

So, as we dwell in the text, we are curious, contemplative, compassionate and discriminating, moving within the hermeneutic cycle, letting go of attachment to ideas to allow the imagination and creativity to flow until tentative insights emerge, as if rising to the surface. But be patient, these insights are not forced. At times, I put aside the text and then, later, a new idea will dawn, perhaps as I sleep, or walk, or during meditation, or indeed at any time of the day. It is as if the insight has been germinating within my body. Insights are not necessarily new, but a deepening of things already known or sensed to some degree. In this way insights reflexively build on each other.

Dwelling within my text of Tom and Joan, what insights emerge?

The experience reinforces an overall negative perception of the failure of nurses to care from a holistic or even person-centred perspective. I recognise the folly of any claim to holistic practice as untenable due to the traditional nature of nursing practice. Can tradition be so powerful? It cannot be underestimated because it is deeply embedded in culture and grooved within psyche. I can no longer accept the tenet of holistic nursing – that the whole is more than the sum of its parts. If I accept that Joan and Tom are human beings, there are no parts – there is only Tom and Joan in their humanness. Yet I am left with a disturbing thought. To claim holism is to set up a tension that leads the practitioner to lead a contradictory and frustrating life. I felt just like this. I liberate myself from the oppression of holism. Instead I seek a person-centred care grounded in easing suffering.

Framing insights

Such is the diverse nature of insight, that practitioners may benefit from schemes to frame insights. One obvious weakness with this idea is that the frameworks set boundaries for the nature of insights. In other words, practitioners are likely to fit their insights into the box – the problem with all models or criteria.

I have experimented with two framing schemes: Carper's (1978) fundamental ways of knowing in nursing and the framing perspectives.

Carper's fundamental ways of knowing

Previous to the 12th edition of the model for structured reflection (MSR), I utilised Carper's fundamental ways of knowing in nursing to frame learning through reflection. Carper offered a ready-made and compelling approach to framing insights within the domains of nursing knowing. I was able to link each MSR cue into the different ways of knowing.

I viewed the aesthetic as the core way of knowing simply because it reflected the knowing the nurse used in practice informed by the ethical, empirical and personal ways of knowing (Figure 4.1). Other theorists had played with Carper's scheme and postulated other ways of knowing. White (1995) suggested the socio-political ways of knowing to contextualise the ways of knowing within societal norms, whilst Munhall (1993) suggested 'unknowing' as a way of knowing, which influences the clinical response. I too felt something missing from this scheme which led me to develop a fifth way of knowing that I labelled *reflexivity* to account for the dynamic personal knowing the practitioner developed through reflective practice (Johns 1995). Reflexivity is a transitional and embodied knowing that informs future practice.

As a practical scheme, Carper's approach was too abstract. I needed something more practical and meaningful to frame insights.

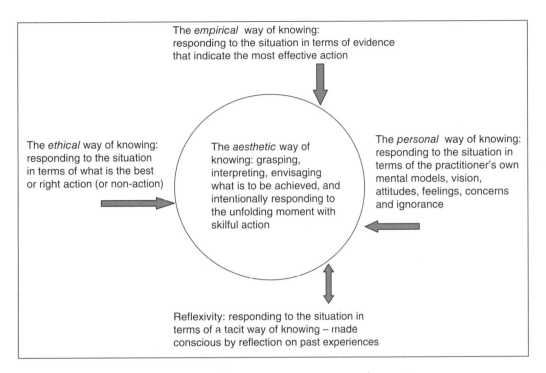

Figure 4.1   Carper's fundamental pattern of knowing in nursing (1978) (Johns 1995).

The framing perspectives

My solution was to construct 'The framing perspectives' (Figure 4.2). This was a commonsense approach of simply analysing the scope of knowing apparent within emerging insights. As such, it was a more practical and meaningful approach for practitioners. It is no surprise that the framing perspectives mirror to some extent the MSR cues. One thing leads to another. The framing perspectives are self-explanatory with the exception of parallel process framing and developmental framing.

In parallel process framing, the guide explicitly role models and rehearses specific ways of being that can be transferred to clinical situations. For example, using of Heron's six-category intervention analysis.

Developmental framing: the being available template

Developmental framing seeks to represent the whole of practice. So, for example, if my vision is to realise holistic nursing – how might that be known? Similarly, if my vision is transformational leadership – how might that be known? Clearly, there are theories of holistic nursing and transformational leadership that might be mapped as reflective frameworks. If no adequate theory exists to frame one's vision, then it can be constructed through analysing patterns of insights emerging through guided reflection.

Philosophical framing: *How has this experience enabled me to* confront and clarify my beliefs and values that constitute desirable practice?	Problem framing: *How has this experience enabled me to* focus problem identification and resolution within the experience.	Reality perspective framing: *How has this experience* barrier of reality whilst helping me to become empowered to act in more congruent ways?
Parallel process framing: *How has this experience enabled me to* make connections between learning processes within my guided reflection process and my clinical practice?	insights	Theoretical framing/mapping: *How has this experience enabled me to* draw on extant theory and research in order to help me make sense of my knowing in practice, and to juxtapose and assimilate theory/research findings with personal knowing?
Temporal framing: *How has this experience enabled me to* draw patterns with past experiences whilst anticipating how I might respond in similar situations in new ways?	Developmental framing: *How has this experience enabled me to* frame becoming a more effective practitioner within 'whole' appropriate theoretical frameworks.	Role framing: *How has this experience enabled me to* clarify my role boundaries and authority within my role, and my power relationships with others?

Figure 4.2   Framing perspectives.

The being available template (BAT)

As such, I constructed the being available template (BAT) as a reflective framework for holistic/person-centred practice. Holism is commonly understood to be more than the sum of its parts; therefore, simply reducing holistic practice to a set of attributes had to be avoided.

I delineated that the core *irreducible* quality of holistic practice was the practitioner *being available* to work with the person(s) to enable the person to find meaning in their experience as the basis for negotiated decision making about their health and to assist them as appropriate to help them meet their health needs.

The extent the practitioner can be available seems to be determined by the pattern of six interrelated *influences*: holding and intending to realise a vision, concern for the person, knowing the person, aesthetic response, poise and creating an environment where being available can be possible (Figure 4.3). The first five influences concern the therapeutic relationship. The sixth influence positions the therapeutic relationship within the wider organisational and societal environment.

Practitioners like this scheme because it relates immediately to their practice. It is easy to understand and actually helps to develop clinical skills and insight. Elements such as

The practitioner's mindful ability to be available is influenced by the following:	Brief significance of each factor:
The practitioner intends to realise a vision of practice. The practitioner knows the other.	Vision gives purpose and direction to practice. Holding intent, the practitioner is more likely to realise the vision in practice. Through empathic inquiry the practitioner appreciates the pattern of the person's wholeness and the meanings they give to health. It is tuning in and flowing with the unfolding pattern of the person's experience.
The practitioner is concerned for the other; has compassion.	Concern for the other and compassion is caring energy. Concern creates possibility within the caring relationship. The greater the practitioner's concern for the other. The more available the practitioner is.
The practitioner is effective in meeting the person's needs as best as possible (the aesthetic response).	Five abilities constitute effective performance: 1 The ability to grasp and interpret the clinical moment. 2 The ability to manage the advocacy-enablement tension. 3 The ability to make most appropriate and ethical clinical judgement. 4 The ability to respond with appropriate skilful action to assist the person to meet their health needs. 5 The ability to evaluate one's efficacy.
The practitioner has poise. (equanimity/emotional intelligence).	The practitioner knows and manages self within relationship so that their personal concerns do not interfere with being available to the person. It is the flip side of compassion; where compassion makes the practitioner vulnerable, poise manages the vulnerability. Poise is defined by the *Compact Oxford English Dictionary*, 3rd edition (2005), p. 785 as • A graceful and elegant way of holding the body • Calmness and confidence • Ready and prepared to do something
The practitioner creates and sustains an environment where being available is possible.	This includes such factors as Creating and sustaining collaborative and assertive patterns of relationships with other healthcare workers towards realising a shared vision of practice; Being political to maximise available resources to ensure availability to the patient and counter coercive patterns of management; Collaborative attitude and skill to manage conflict (Thomas and Kilmann conflict mode instrument); Having a constructed voice (Belenky *et al* 1986) that is influential.

Figure 4.3   The being available template (adapted from Johns 2009).

vision, compassion, poise and assertiveness are minimally taught within traditional nursing curriculum. As a curriculum model, BAT has much to offer in the way it frames the whole curriculum.

BAT has been continuously tested over 20 years. To reiterate, it is only a representation. It is not holistic practice itself, but it does give the intended holistic or person-centred practitioner a measure to sense the scope of holistic practice and a measure to judge self against.

Conclusion

The point of reflective practice is to gain insight. This can be facilitated through techniques such as Carper's fundamental ways of knowing in nursing and the framing perspectives. It can also be developed through using theoretical mapping, the focus for the following chapter.

Note

1   In Chapter 21, I set out a number of prose poems for the reader to contemplate insights.

Chapter 5

The dance with Sophia: the third dialogical movement

In the first dialogical movement, the practitioner writes stories that are rich descriptions of her experiences. In the second dialogical movement, the practitioner stands back from her story in order to dialogue with it in order to learn through it and gain insight. Now, in the third dialogical movement, the practitioner dialogues with a wider literature to inform and develop these insights. In doing so, she positions herself within the wider knowledge field.

Theories and ideas from literature help the practitioner see her experience from new angles, opening possibilities of understanding and ways of responding differently, challenging the practitioner's previously learnt and partial views. It confronts the practitioner's habitual ways of thinking and doing things. Juxtaposing with relevant theories and ideas helps to affirm the practitioner's interpretation and strengthens her interpretative confidence. It emits an ah-ha, an affirming sense of recognition, and yet the reflective practitioner is always mindful not to be seduced by any compelling theoretical view but to hold it loosely, until it can be metaphorically chewed over and checked out for its appropriateness to inform. As such, no theory is accepted on face value – it is always critiqued for its authority to inform the tentative insights. As Dewey (1933) cited by Tann (1993, p. 54) writes, 'Reflective action entails active and persistent consideration of any belief or supposed form of knowledge in the light of the grounds that support it and the consequences to which it leads.'

Theory helps the practitioner to frame and reframe issues of uncertainty and problems arising from practice. From a reflective perspective, all practice is uncertain because it has never been practised before. As such, every aspect of practice should be in potential dialogue with a wider field of knowledge to justify it providing the practitioner is open to the possibilities the text has to offer.

Theory leads practitioners into conversations with others – 'I have been reading this . . .' – noting its challenge, inspiration or even rejection of the ideas offered. Guiding masters and doctoral students, I take texts into the classroom and read passage in order to stimulate dialogue, always leading the students back to their own narratives. I encourage students to bring in their own texts into the community for critique and assimilation into personal knowing.

Becoming a Reflective Practitioner, Fourth Edition. Christopher Johns.
© 2013 John Wiley & Sons, Ltd. Published 2013 by John Wiley & Sons, Ltd.

Theory can help to untangle the practitioner from a web of emotions that has blurred seeing other perspectives and from seeing the bigger picture, and the way the bigger picture is framed by cultural, embodied and power forces. Brookfield (1995, p. 36) writes, 'Theory can help us name our practice by illuminating the general elements of what we think are idiosyncratic experiences. It can provide multiple perspectives on familiar situations.'

Reading a text is like travelling with a trusty companion. Writing this book, I stretch myself across dozens of books in dialogue with my ideas on reflective practice, in my quest for deeper understanding.

The dance with Sophia

The type of knowing developed through reflective practice is the knowing practitioners need to practice. It is ever shifting in response to the particular experience. Schön (1983, 1987) described this type of knowing as professional artistry. In the epistemological hierarchy, such knowledge has generally been considered of less importance than technical rationality, a universal and abstract knowledge constructed as facts about the world. Schön turned the epistemological hierarchy between technical rationality and professional artistry on its head. He believed that professional artistry was a more significant form of knowing for practice disciplines simply because it is the knowledge practitioners need to traverse the complex and indeterminate lowlands of professional practice. Professional artistry is practical wisdom or what Aristotle (2004) described as phronesis – the knowing practitioners use in making clinical decisions, considering its intended and moral consequences. He distinguished phronesis with *Sophia*, usually translated as wisdom or philosophy, as the ability to think well about the nature of the world and to discern why the world is the way it is. It involves deliberation concerning universal truths. One can learn the principles of action, but applying them in the real world, in situations one could not have foreseen, requires experience of the world. *Sophia* represents truths that are generally held as universal, reflecting the nature of life and, as such, intends to guide the way people go about things, for example, the nature of the caring relationship. At this level of dialogue, I accept I am not alone in the world but am situated within a community that shares common ideas and values as the basis for social and cultural life. At this level of dialogue, I dwell critically within these ideas, problematising both my insights and the wisdom literature for its potential to inform my insights.

Mihn-ha Trihn (1991, p. 157) says 'Experience, discourse, and self-understanding collide against larger cultural assumptions concerning race, ethnicity, nationality, gender, class, and age.'

Collide, rub against, grate . . . words of friction that scrape and open up the surface of insights: words that capture something of the tension between personal knowing and a wider universal knowing.

In my experience, healthcare practitioners rarely engage with philosophy, reflecting a curriculum that is largely devoid of history, politics, caring theory and philosophy. Why is that? Cynically, I might suggest it is because nurses are trained to apply accepted ideas, not think about those ideas, that is until you become a nurse researcher.

The non-engagement with philosophy is a form of self-oppression, reflecting an assumption that nursing is about doing, not being, or even thinking too deeply. Reflection confronts this attitude. It demands that the practitioner focuses or refocuses on a values-based foundation to clinical practice. Ask yourself: what does it mean to be a nurse or indeed any other healthcare identity? These are vital questions that this third dialogical movement grapples with.

When I first read theory, it is 'out there' in a space that my mind grapples with. Gradually, as I dialogue with the theory within the context of my particular experience, I absorb and assimilate the theory as my own. It becomes part of me and begins to influence the way I see and respond to the world.

D. Soyini Madison (1999, p. 109) captures this unity:

> Performance helps me live a truth while theory helps me name it – or maybe it is the other way around. My mind and body are locked together in a nice little divine kind of unity: the theory knows and feels, and the performance feels and unlearns. I know I am un/learning body in the process of feeling. You too.

Dialogue as creative play

Dialogue with theory and ideas is creative play. I do not look at theory just once, but again and again through a succession of experience. With each reading I make new connections.

Theory comes alive, intriguing, because it is immediately applied to practice and viewed through a sceptical eye for its value to inform, to make sense. As such, theory looses its eminence. It is cut down to size to simply inform, not to predict and control.

Indeed this whole book reflects a dialogue with all sources of knowing: theory, theology, philosophy, science, ancient wisdom and the suchlike, as I move to embody ideas and transform myself through my performance as an educator and clinician towards enabling myself and those with whom I work towards self-realisation to become more fully human, whatever that might mean for the individual and for society.

Of course, this overturning is controversial within a culture traditionally dominated by a rational scientific view. This is most apparent in the way knowledge produced through random control trials is viewed as the gold standard of research, yet one person's story is denigrated as anecdote and where forms of self-inquiry are regarded as soft research. Random control trials are valued because they offer an alleged predictable approach to control health care – and yet portrays a world where people are consequently reduced to statistics and objects that can be manipulated.

Mapping

A practical way to dialogue with theory is to map the theory. This enables the practitioner to position herself within the theory. The map can then be used over a sequence of experiences to plot any developmental shift of position. There are many examples of this through the narratives. A good example is the Thomas and Kilmann conflict mode instrument (see Cathy and The GPs, Chapter 18).

Narratives of health illness

There are many narratives written by people experiencing health care or illness to inform practitioners. Such narratives are useful because they get to the heart of meaning. When well written, they engage the reader and invite dialogue. Some examples I have used alongside my own journey are *Grace and Grit* (Wilber 1991), *Bald in the Land of Big Hair* (Rodgers 2001), *The Cancer Journals* (Lorde 1980), and *Cancer in Two Voices* (Butler and Rosenblum 1991). These autobiographical accounts reveal what are invaluable for appreciating the experiences of living and dying with illness within healthcare systems.

Michael's wife

In the following text, Michael's wife, I break the text into single lines to help me find meaning. I leave it in this form to illustrate how I might read the text as performance, giving emphasis to any turning points. Following the text, I dialogue with a relevant literature (Sophia) to inform my understanding of specific issues related to easing suffering (italicised in the text). I could pull out other significant issues to pay attention. There is only so much the practitioner can pay attention to with one experience without cluttering the narrative. This reflection, although written some years ago, remains 'live' in the sense of linking to new experiences and deepening my understanding of easing suffering.

Michael's wife

Holding my blue wooden box of essential oils
I wait in the corridor outside the door,
waiting for Linda to return from the bathroom.
I glance across the corridor and catch the eye of Michael's wife.
She sits alone by the side of Michael's bed as if in vigil.
I imagine her eyes shift anxiously not knowing quite how to be at his bedside
For sure *the waiting* is not easy.
The *loneliness of dying* for those who wait
Beyond consolation they endure.
I know, for I have journeyed many times with those who wait
I have heard their stories and shared their despair.
We had met last week when I had given Michael reflexology,
Then smiles and easy talk on the surface of things
The only time we have conversed.
Now all has changed though not unexpectedly.
Can anything really prepare you confronts me for death's final call?
I give a sad smile and truncated wave and look away.
Yet I feel her deep despair drift across the space
As if she might shatter.
I feel the pang of contradiction that, to look away, adds to her suffering when my vision is to ease it.
The *ethical demand* not to *pass her by* confronts me.
How should I respond to this demand for the best?
Should I move across the corridor and spend just a few moments with her and Michael?
But would that fulfil my need rather than hers and Michael's?
Perhaps she needs to be alone to endure her loneliness when anything else might be a distraction or intrusion, that forces her to engage, even smile when her heart is heavy and her mind buried in its thoughts.

I hesitate and then move across the corridor into the room and ask 'how are things?'
Michael is not doing so well.
She says 'It will be a sweet release when he 'goes' for both of us.
It's hard to watch him struggle'.
She looks down.
I touch her arm.
Just a light touch as if sensing the boundary between us,
Touch, is dangerous ground
I have been there before and felt its recoil.
Michael's wife looks up.
Her eyes meet mine, eyes full of suffering.
My empathic inquiry to connect with her
No words spoken
We sit alongside his broken body seeking pattern in the chaos.
Tears spill down her cheeks.
I cannot recall the few words spoken
I remember more *the silence* between the words and how words are often no more than an effort to fill the silence that brings us face to face with Michael's dying.
Perhaps words spoken help us feel less alone or less uneasy with the emotional work.
I feel her aloneness in the world as death pulls her apart
In the quietness of the fading light we dwell,
the room a sacred space infused with grace.
My head turns.
Linda waves at me from the open door.
I feel the demand and the spell is broken.
Michael's wife places her small hand over mine
She thanks me for my time
Time had ceased in that brief moment.
Without doubt practice is a mystery I tread with care.
Care *is* being mindful, being fully present in corridor moments
Caring is *lifting*, lifting us both into a lighter place
As lifted by *Avalokiteshvara's thousand arms*
Caring is liberation uncoiling in space
Caring is intuitive, for there is no prescription for how I should respond in such moments
I now know better than to look away and pass people by.

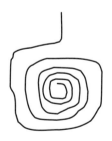

Passing people by

Perhaps the trigger for writing this reflection is the idea of *passing people by*. It is a theme developed in earlier published text (Johns 2008). In this paper I acknowledged the way I paid attention to some people at a hospice day centre and not others. This acknowledgement raised fundamental questions about ethics – how I prioritised my limited time with patients. In catching someone's eye, it is hard to pass them by – perhaps why so many practitioners avoid eye contact to avoid any demand for attention. Interestingly, it is not a topic much written about in healthcare literature. Johnson and Webb (1995) suggest reasons why some patients might be avoided because the nurse has difficulty with them for whatever reason and that the conditions for labelling are socially constructed. Am I more attracted to some patients more than others? If do, does this influence who I give attention to?

Waiting

As Michael's wife waits, she suffers, so how can the waiting be made easier for her? Or is her suffering inevitable? One constant theme of easing suffering is the idea of *waiting*. Waiting for the person to die is a common experience of many patients, families and even healthcare staff. It is a unique and significant experience that seems to be a significant marker in the idea of the 'good death' especially when the dying person defies expectations.

Lunghi (2004) recognises the need to be active in waiting. . . . I sense how difficult to passively wait. The question is, how to be active most sensitively? Lunghi suggests simple presence. Presence is being with the other with poise. It is to dwell with the other. It is more than being a witness to what is unfolding, it is being an emotional part of the drama unfolding not separate from it and yet poised within it.

Loneliness

Another constant theme is the idea of loneliness. I dialogue repeatedly with 'The loneliness of the dying' (Elias 1985) as I try and make sense of the idea whether people are lonely facing death. Is this natural? Do they need to be alone? Do I intrude? The reader will raise many other related questions. Loneliness is a complex phenomenon, and yet it is vital to appreciate in respect of easing suffering. I can read about it as a concept, but what does it mean in practice and how best to respond to it are vexing questions.

The idea of the *ethical demand* stems from Logstrup (1997).

He writes of the ethical demand:

> By our very attitude to one another we help to shape one another's world. By our attitude to the other person we help to determine the scope and the hue of his or her world; we make it large and small, bright or drab, rich or dull, threatening or secure. We help to shape his or her world, not by theories and views but by our very attitude to him or her. *Herein lies the unarticulated and one might say anonymous demand that we take care of the life which trust has placed into our hands.* (1997, p. 18) (my italics)

As a healthcare practitioner, these words get to the heart of my attitude. What does it mean to take care of the life which trust has placed into our hands? Certainly, that we create a climate of trust and accept the demand despite its unpredictable consequences. This is rather like compassion – that it is not situational but open-ended. However, being reflective practitioners, we are aware when the demand exceeds our resources and can direct as appropriate. Think about this demand when you are next with a patient.

Caring

A major focus of any narrative of suffering is the broad idea of caring. Indeed the ethical demand is itself a particular focus of caring. Frank (2002a, p. 13) writes,

> Caring is one of those activities that people know only when they are involved in it. From within, and only from within, caring makes sense. To try and explain care leads to the circularity expressed in statements such as 'caring for this person requires doing this, and I do this because I care for this person'. Philosophy teaches that, for some activities, there is only practice.

It follows that if we accept Frank's position, we can only know caring from within caring – the professional artistry perspective. Caring is therefore not a thing that can be known as an abstract idea. The practitioner knows herself as caring only within the moment. As such, caring is a mystery drama unfolding.

Buddhist influence

The reflective practitioner, mindful of self within the moment, is aware and curious of this drama unfolding, seeking to know it and shape it as it unfolds. As a Buddhist, I am influenced by Buddhist philosophy or doctrine that permeates through the text like a soft stream. Reference to Avalokiteshvara reflects this influence and conjures up imagery of the Bodhisattva who, with deep compassion and wisdom, dedicates himself to alleviating suffering wherever it is found (Sangharakshita 1999).

Lifting

The idea of 'lifting' and its therapeutic significance was inspired by the writing of Joseph Rael.
  Rael (1993, pp. 88–9) writes,

> There is an energy that comes to all of us from the sacred place, the vibrations from an ancient past, wisdom we would come to find one day. Once the sacred place is discovered, we begin to open to the wisdom. It descends upon us just as it did when the beings from the spirit of life brought spirit to the people. What is interesting about this lifting energy is that when it happened to us, it also happens to other people who are also being lifted to the next level (and) when we began to lift ourselves from where we were before to a higher place, something dramatic happens in our life.

Lifting gives healing energy a name. I guess every reader will know the way that some people lift them and other people drain them. As a practitioner I am integral to the patient's environment. Hence my energy impacts on the person creating a healing environment or sacred space (Quinn 1992, 1997). As practitioners we should actively seek to lift our patients. The idea that our presence is healing is compelling and powerful. When you pay attention to this idea and cultivate 'lifting energy', then it becomes a powerful therapeutic energy. My healing energy, like caring itself, is inchoate, always being formed, always being known through successive experiences in its subtlety.

Rael is a Native American who's wisdom may be hard to swallow for the rational western mind. I imagine the clamour – 'what is the evidence'. And yet, such wisdom is my truth. I feel it vibrate through me like a soft healing wind. As a therapist, open to the possibility, Rael speaks a universal truth that is so obvious to me.

Silence as therapeutic is very significant. Ben Okri (1997) writes,

> At best our cry for meaning, for serenity, is answered by a greater silence, the silence that makes us seek higher reconciliation. I think we need more of the wordless in our lives. We need more stillness, more of a sense of wonder, a feeling for the mystery of life. We need more love, more silence, more deep listening, more deep giving.

Okri's words draw my attention to the idea of silence. Am I comfortable with silence? I can distinguish between an awkward silence and a therapeutic silence. I sense that therapeutic silence is a gateway to being with someone, not just as they face death, but with any potentially healing encounter. Okri's words remind me to be still in the midst of apparent chaos when often we are compelled to fill the silence with words in our vain effort to fix the situation – or rather fix our own awkwardness of not knowing what words to say. The idea of silence cannot be separated with the idea of deep listening – which returns me to the idea of empathic inquiry.

As if she might shatter

The word shatter was lifted from Audre Lorde's book, *The Cancer Journals* (1980). She writes, 'I must let this pain flow through me and pass on. If I resist or try to stop it, it will detonate inside me, shatter me, splatter my pieces against every wall and person that I touch' (p. 12).

Seeing Michael's wife, I felt these words. I sense the effort to hold herself together when inside she was detonating. Such words helped me appreciate what she was experiencing.

The texts I dialogue with are not obvious caring texts. Everything I read can inform my practice simply because I read with a mind open to that possibility. Just Google *lifting energy* or *therapeutic silence* and see what emerges. However, it is time-consuming.

Sylvia

In the following reflection I dialogue with the words of Murray Cox to explore significant aspects of therapeutic work. In my view, any healthcare worker should be cognisant of such issues and work towards using self in a therapeutic way as indicated with any claim to holistic or person-centred practice. The title of Murray Cox's book is *Structuring the Therapeutic Process: Compromise with Chaos*. The recognition that practice is chaos resonated with Schön's swampy lowlands of practice where nothing is certain, and everything is complex and indeterminate.

Sylvia

Murray Cox (1988) writes.

> The therapist needs to be able to enter therapeutic space in a natural spontaneous way, although to be 'spontaneous' in such an emotionally charged and often frightening situation can take years of training. It is to be hoped that the therapist gradually develops an increasing sense of being at ease within himself, so that he may enter the orbit of his patient's experience along an appropriate trajectory. (p. 53)

Sylvia lies in bed in the single room. I enter her orbit. No family about. She stares into space.

Death hangs heavy in the air. A glimmer of a smile as I take her hand. I say who I am. It is difficult to make out her speech. Muddled? Not easy to ascertain.

'Are you sad?' I ask. She affirms. "Shall I massage your hands?" I ask with concern. She looks up at me. Is it the words or my tone of voice she responds to? I sense her aloneness, her helplessness, as if such decisions are beyond her.

Murray Cox writes,

> It is the gauging of what the client needs and not what the [therapist] wishes him to need that is the guideline to optimal structuring of the therapeutic process (p. 83). It is matter of profound importance that the personal views of the therapist must not set a limit on the person his patient is becoming. (p. 101)

Which way should I go? All decisions are personal. My assumption that massage will help her. Where does that idea stem from? Beyond the fact I am here to do such work? That she might simply be an object for my intention. That I might be blinded by the blue box I carry.

The ethics of practice. Do I think I can help ease her suffering? Or, do I just like to strut my stuff? I like to think the former, but ego is a subtle thing. No resistance to my touch. I feel her warmth. I continue to hold her hand. She looks away into another space. I sense her despair. I add oils of lavender and grapefruit. Sitting by her side, my hands embrace her own.

Her hands are small and bony. Mine are large and soft. We dwell in this embrace. It seems to comfort and relax her. Do I simply want to believe that? That I ease her suffering? Or do I merely touch its outer edge. Even irritate that which has settled. She might prefer to be left alone? What is the appropriate trajectory? I wonder her thoughts. I sense my feelings. Tinged with sadness. The human response to the other's suffering. I am at ease, easing. The relationship between my ease and my ability to ease is profound.

Murray Cox writes,

> The therapist must, at all times, be himself. He will fail his patient and become either rigidly hyper-defensive, or chaotically unbounded, if he does not remain himself as he engages with the patient in the hard work of therapy. It has something to do with a genuine ontological emotional engagement, rather than the adoption of a professional role. (p. 51)

Am I at ease? Or do I like to imagine that? Can we, who work with the dying, ever engage in genuine ontological engagement? Is there always something that triggers a defence to the ontological threat? I distance myself from the professional cloak. Only then can I be open to the moment. And yet, how open am I?

Murray Cox writes,

> Is it possible for one person, by professional training involving self-scrutiny at depth, to become sufficiently free from his own emotional 'bias' so that, relatively uncluttered by himself, he can focus concern on his current needs presented by his patient? (p. 82). The therapist's attitudes 'colour' the atmosphere of therapeutic space. He is never neutral as he thinks! (p. 100)

Cox exposes the myth of neutrality. That is the detached position I reject. I use my breath at the door to wipe away any concern that might clutter the therapeutic space. I muse the idea of 'relatively uncluttered'. No matter how hard I try there will always be ego remnants and demands, always ego threats. It is the human condition. To deny is the point of self-deception. Can I contain them so they do not clutter? Yet they persist, and perhaps, persist harder, the harder I try and push them away. Detracting from the natural posture. Ease the mind through the breath if I am mindful enough.

Murray Cox further writes,

> In response, every experience is the opportunity for growth when I pay attention to it with learning intent. Reflection opens the learning space. Ontological insecurity is the condition for learning . . . such tensions always exist, they can never be resolved within the mystery of the human–human encounter. Security would simply be an illusion. (p. 107)

I write my learning intent in dialogue with Murray Cox's words. Reflection opens the learning space. Yes! Ontological security is not the condition. It is not even the intent. Perhaps ontological mindfulness. How would I know ontological security beyond its illusion?

Murray Cox writes,

> Therefore, when the therapist also experiences ontological insecurity, it can ease the burden for his patient who does not have to 'go it alone'. The therapist can never be a merely neutral, impassive facilitator of cognitive-affective self-awareness for his patient, because he also shares the predicament of humanness. Paradoxically, it is precisely because of the ontological insecurity in the therapist, that the patient dares him to trust enough to risk the 'abandonment to therapeutic space. (p. 107)

Sylvia, did you feel less alone as I sat with you and gently stroked your hands. The air infused with oil? Did I burden you with insecure presence, with my knowing not quite how to be? With my struggle to find the appropriate response that can never be predicted in the human encounter. That is, unless I pretend it can be and then I would struggle.

Murray Cox writes,

> [the therapist's] previous encounters colour the current encounter . . . (p. 108).

Sylvia, I have met many people facing death. Who stare into space as if lost in the waiting. Betwixt and between worlds. I wonder the extent these many people colour our encounter? For sure, I have learnt through my dedicated reflective journey 'Not to know', except that nothing is for certain.

Murray Cox writes,

> The knowledge that the condition of human predicamentness is inevitably shared with the therapist, enables the patient to tolerate an ever-increasing measure of those parts of his experience found to be intolerable. (p. 114)

I think Sylvia was aware of what she and I shared in that moment. But then I might be wrong.

My assumption shatters in the reflective moment. I wonder what did she think in that moment, what would she have responded if I had asked and she had a mind to answer. She would have been silent, but she knew my presence. I wonder if any part of my manner she found intolerable. But I never gave that a thought. The unreflective mind takes self for granted. Reflection disturbs complacency, unsettles the ego confident in its practice.

Lorna

The doctor approaches and if I might help Lorna, lift her out of her flatness. She is 37. Cancer of her ovary and now, a stroke resulting in a dense left hemiplegia. Her speech is affected, and there is a question about her cognitive ability simply because she only says 'yes'. She is a scientist. She has two young children aged 4 and 6.

I enter her orbit. A blue head scarf covers her head. Does she wear it to hide her hair loss due to chemotherapy? I don't ask. She wears glasses and looks very young. Just gazing at her, I sense her tragedy. She takes my offered hand and smiles weakly. I say who I am and what I do – Murray Cox's – primary and secondary structuring. She is open to my approach. 'Would she like some therapy?' I ask expectantly. She says 'yes' but I am uncertain because, as I have been told, she always says yes. How knowledge structures the view, that if I had not known she only says 'yes', would I have responded differently? Less from my body and senses, more from my head filled as it is with knowledge? How do I read the signs? I move to touch her hand yet mindful of my touch. She does not resist my continued hold. My inclination is to give some reflexology and therapeutic touch. I sense reflexology would help stimulate and balance her body and ease her despair. I say this and she says yes. She returns my smile. Connection. Permission to move forward in mutual engagement. A relative uncluttering of my mind. Simply focused. Mindful of the appropriate trajectory but held loosely, or otherwise I would be wrapped up in my concern. Oils mixed. I guide Lorna to relax. Being at her feet feels remote. Perhaps holding her occiput would have less so. But then, for who's need?

Her husband David arrives and quietly slips into the room and sits by her side, holding her hand. Afterwards, I ask how she feels and she says 'yes', but there is a glint in her eyes and she utters a cry as David embraces her. I show David the small kitchen and offer a therapy if he should need it. He shrugs of his own despair. Acknowledges it is tough, very tough for him right now. Lorna died the following Thursday. I feel a tinge of sadness.

The fragility of ontological security.

Conclusion

Every narrative in this book engages to varying extent in the dance with Sophia. It is time-consuming. It can be intense and extensive or superficial, executed for academic purposes where such dialogue is viewed as scholarship.

Chapter 6

Guiding reflection: the fourth dialogical movement

In the fourth dialogical movement the practitioner enters the community of inquiry where reflection is guided towards developing and deepening insights. In this way, insights are co-created. Without doubt, the learning potential reflection can be facilitated by expert guidance. Boud *et al* (1985) suggest that whilst reflection was something the student could do for themselves, 'the learning process can be considerably accelerated by appropriate support' (p. 36).

Dialogue

The nature of 'guidance talk' is dialogue. It can be contrasted with debate. Debate means literally to 'beat down'. As Isaacs (1993, p. 24) writes, 'in debate one side wins and another loses; both parties maintain their certainties, and both suppress deeper inquiry.'

Dialogue comes from the Greek word *dialogos*, which can be taken to mean 'meaning flowing among and through us, out of which may emerge some new understanding' (Bohm 1996, p. 6).

Isaacs (1993, p. 25) describes dialogue as

> a discipline of collective thinking and inquiry, a process for transforming the quality of conversation and, in particular, the thinking that lies beneath it . . . a movement towards creating a field of genuine meeting and inquiry where people can allow a free flow of meaning and vigorous exploration of the collective background of their thought, their personal predispositions, the nature of their shared attention, and the rigid features of their individual and collective assumptions . . . as people learn to perceive, inquire into, and allow transformation of the nature and shape of these fields, and the patterns of individual thinking and acting that inform them, they may discover entirely new levels of insight and forge substantive and, at times, dramatic changes in behaviour. As this happens, whole new possibilities for coordinated action develop.

Dialogue cannot be assumed to exist. As such it always needs to be cultivated within the guidance relationship through the six dialogue 'rules' (chapter 1, p. 30).

Becoming a Reflective Practitioner, Fourth Edition. Christopher Johns.
© 2013 John Wiley & Sons, Ltd. Published 2013 by John Wiley & Sons, Ltd.

Why reflection needs to be guided

In previous editions of this book I established reasons why guidance is necessary (Johns 2009a, p. 86). As I review these, I am disquiet. One reason overlaps with another. To simplify matters, I suggest that the primary reason why reflection needs to be guided is to co-create and express meaning in coherent form. This can be viewed to encompass a number of processes:

- to enable the practitioner to take responsibility for her own learning and nurture the prerequisites of reflection, commitment, curiosity, openness and intelligence;
- to enable the practitioner to realise and hold creative tension;
- to explore the depth and breadth of reflection through the model for structured reflection (MSR) or similar models of reflection;
- a catalyst for releasing and conversion of anxiety/energy into positive energy for acting on insights towards realising more desirable and effective practice;
- to construct a coherent and engaging narrative;
- to build the emotional intelligence of the group (Druskat and Wolff 2001).

Co-creation of insights

The guide enables the practitioner to touch the breadth and depth, to sense the subtlety of each MSR cue, to become more aware, more proprioceptive of her thinking and being. It is all too easy to scrape along the surface of the MSR cues and miss the point. The guide points the finger. The practitioner will always have a partial view, and guidance helps the practitioner to expand her view to see things from wider perspectives, pulling away any masks that distort seeing self and reality for what it really is. Lather (1986a,b) terms this self-distortion as 'false consciousness'. The first step is for the practitioner to accept that her perceptions may indeed be distorted. Brookfield (1996, p. 33) writes,

> An intrinsic problem with private self-reflection is that when we use them, we can never completely avoid the risks of denial and distortion. We can never know just how much we're cooking the data of our memories and experience to produce images and renditions that show us off to good effect.

From its subjective nature all reflection is naturally partial and distorted. The practitioner's perspective is loaded with assumptions that govern her practice and which are taken for granted as normal. It is cleaning the reflective mirror of smudges that have accumulated over the years and which obscures and distorts the view. Not easy work, considering how the way we perceive the world and ourselves has been moulded through socialisation until we have embodied a way of being that is not easily amenable to change. We cannot learn if the basis of understanding is built on false assumptions. It has to be worked at with commitment, discipline, hard work and a sense of play to lift the load when it seems arduous. As Cox *et al* (1991, p. 285) write, 'Reflection in isolation is difficult to sustain because of the difficulty in surfacing and transcending our own distorted self understandings, asking ourselves difficult, often self-exposing questions, facing difficult answers to such questions, and, perhaps most particularly, keeping our vision directed toward new possibilities for understanding and action.' Both the practitioner and guide know this and accept that the guide's role is to help the practitioner expose these self-distortions.

The guide focuses the practitioner to dwell within the experience, slowly turning it over to see it for what it is, enabling her to open doors to see other ways of being and responding in situations. This might involve actually opening doors for the practitioner, confronting attitudes that had been partial and prejudiced, nurturing and developing personal power so the practitioners can feel empowered and take action congruent with their vision, and reinforcing integrity and self-worth. The guide proceeds with caution, mindful of what door is opening in relation to the many doors that might be opened. Why this one? The guide may tentatively offer his own interpretation but without imposing any authority onto what the experience might mean. It is holding back, not crowding the reflective space, not cramping the practitioner.

Through dialogue the practitioner and guide shape meaning, crafting insight, fusing horizons, whereby their perspectives are transcended in reaching new perspectives (Gadamer 1975). Horizon is a metaphor for our understanding. As we move forward and learn, horizons shift. Horizon also suggests the limits of our vision to see things. The guide is mindful that his own understanding has a horizon, and so through dialogue works to expand his own understandings, hence the co-creation of insights – insights for both the practitioner and the guide.

The reality wall

It is one thing to holding creative tension, resolving it is quite another. In a rational world it is easy to see how performance could be improved. However, the world is not rational. It is governed by norms and assumptions grounded in issues of authority, tradition and embodiment – *the reality wall*. These norms that govern everyday practice are not easy to appreciate simply because they are normal. The guide helps the practitioner understand these norms and ways in which they might be shifted towards a more desirable state of affairs. However, such is the constraining power of these forces, the practitioner may choose to rationalise the contradiction or tension and decide to let matters lie, particularly if the practitioner is fearful of consequences. She may fear disapproval and sanction. Smyth (1987, p. 40) notes, 'Most of us, unless we feel uncomfortable, shaken, or forced to look at ourselves, are unlikely to change. It is far easier to accept our current conditions and adopt the least line of resistance.' Lieberman (1989, p. 88 – cited by Day 1993) writes, 'Working in bureaucratic settings has taught everyone to be compliant, to be rule governed, not to ask questions, seek alternatives or deal with competing values.' Day (1993) asserts that reflection will bring the practitioner into tension with prevailing dominant organisational values, suggesting that reflection will struggle to make an impact unless the organisation is sympathetic to more collaborative ways of working.

In Kieffer's (1984) study of empowerment of grass root community leaders in the USA, participants referred with great emotional intensity to the importance of the external enabler to support their struggle against more powerful others who were motivated to maintain the status quo. The practitioner connects with her guide as a representative of the wider community, the gatekeeper and guide to this new world. In order to do this, the guide must connect with the practitioner in terms of her existing reality and, simultaneously in terms of a potential new reality. As Fay (1987, pp. 265–6) writes,

Coming to a radically new self-conception is hardly ever a process that occurs simply by reading some theoretical work; rather it requires an environment of trust and support in which one's own preconceptions and feeling can be properly made conscious to oneself, in which one can think through one's experiences in terms of a radically new vocabulary which expresses a fundamentally different conceptualisation of the world in which one can see the particular and concrete ways that one unwittingly collaborates in producing one's own misery and in which one can gain emotional strength to accept and act on one's new insights.

Misery sounds an exaggeration but I meet few practitioners who are happy with 'their lot', especially under current working conditions of 'more for less' that characterises healthcare organisations that leaves practitioners tired and demoralised. The guide may struggle with the trauma stories the practitioner reveals, and it becomes an ethical issue to urge the practitioner to take action and then watch them stumble and fall against the hard edge of reality. The key is not to fix the problem for the practitioners but to guide them to see ways they can fix it for themselves.

The guide's role is to help plant seeds of doubt in tune with desirable practice and to water them so the seeds grow and blossom, weeding away old ideas that are no longer tenable. Through continuity of guidance, new ideas can quickly be put into practice and subsequently reflected on. If the seeds don't take because the soil is stony, then the stone is chipped away slowly, until the moment when the new seed takes hold. Then the practitioner can emerge transformed into a new horizon.

Margolis (1993) considers that new ideas compete with existing ideas. The success of adopting new ideas depends on the robustness of existing ones and the force of argument available to support the new idea. Practitioners are likely to feel anxious when their 'old ways' are challenged. They are caught between defending self from this anxiety and opening self to new possibilities. However, in exploring new, more congruent ways, the practitioner may experience a crisis of isolation or separateness (Isaacs 1993) whereby group norms and ways of relating must shift. This may overflow into personal lives as practitioners find their voices and speak out. Isaacs (1993, p. 38) writes, 'Such loosening of rigid thought patterns frees energy that now permits new levels of intelligence and creativity.'

Contracting

Guided reflection is collaborative – a way of working together towards a mutual set of expectations where the roles of both parties are clearly understood and agreed. Contracts need to be written as if a charter for learning and reviewed constantly. It should always form a dynamic background to guided reflection, enabling objective confrontation when expectations are strained or broken.

What issues need to be contracted?

The practitioner accepts responsibility for using the learning space in the most appropriate and effective way. Reflective practice is student centred, and the implications of what that means in terms of authority and control are vast. As such, the agenda for what should be brought into this space is negotiated, although it should always concern practice. Guided reflection is not counselling or therapy, although inevitably deep aspects of self will be legitimately revealed that requires the guide to be skilled in therapeutic work. The guide must know his own boundaries and limitations and know how to draw the line of involvement and refer elsewhere if necessary. It is an important consideration, because what the practitioner reveals is not known beforehand. It is imperative that the guide does not wear a 'Mr fix-it' hat or adopt parental-type behaviours that, in my experience, are typical of teacher–student relationships within nursing. The learning agenda will vary between learning situations, for example, clinical supervision and the pre-registration classroom. Either way, trust is vital but it is more likely to be taken seriously in clinical supervision than the pre-registration classroom due to teachers' assumed control of the learning agenda, considering previous learnt patterns of teacher–student relationships. Trust takes time, as does the learner and guide appreciating their respective roles. A potent ingredient of trust is confidentiality. What is shared within guided reflection should stay within the community of inquiry. Loose tongues will almost certainly reverberate with potentially serious consequences for group performance.

Finding the path

Essential reading for all reflective practitioners and guides is Pirsig's *Zen and the Art of Motorcycle Maintenance: An Enquiry into Values*. He writes about climbing mountains that resonates strongly with the practitioner finding her own way to write a narrative and indeed learn through reflection:

> Some practitioners travel into the mountains accompanied by experienced guides who know the best and least dangerous routes by which they arrive at their destination. Still others, inexperienced and untrusting attempt to make their own routes. Few of these are successful, but occasionally some, by sheer will and luck and grace, do make it. Once there, they become more aware than any of the others that there's no single or fixed number of routes. There are as many routes as there are individuals. (Pirsig 1974, p. 191)

Being an experienced guide, I am sometimes caught out by assuming that it is easy for others to write a narrative. My natural posture is not to prescribe the path but encourage others to explore the best route for themselves. Naturally I offer my rope as a safety harness. Recently I kept saying to one student, 'just practice it and it will come'. And of course it doesn't just come. I recognised my frustration that she could not get it, a blind spot that emerged when another student recognised her own difficulty in getting it. Sometimes people do need to be shown the path and stick to it and that's OK! It is a creative tension between prescription and finding your own way.

The nature of guidance

I suspect the qualities of the effective guide have become obvious through a linear reading of the text so far. The guide is mindful of self within the learning space, mindful of his own assumptions and suspending these assumptions in order to listen and respond dialogically to the learner's reflections in the most appropriate way. Guidance is the enthusiastic and intense balance of challenge and support. Inevitably, revealing and exploring self creates anxiety, as deeper parts of self become exposed. The guide holds the practitioner to face up to anxiety rather than to defend against it. In this respect the guide becomes part of the practitioner's defence system, a surrogate defence system: a supportive hand across Schön's (1987) metaphoric swamplands until harder former ground is felt. The guide is comfortable being with the practitioner in this way. In my experience, this is not a big deal, a big psychotherapeutic drama. It is a mindful, caring way of being in dialogue whereby the guide is non-attached to the other, connected to them yet separate from them. The guide is skilled at not absorbing the practitioner's suffering.

Lisa, a Macmillan support nurse in guided reflection with me, noted:

> I felt that being challenged is an essential element of guidance, providing you feel comfortable in your environment and at ease with your guide. The challenge element encouraged me to think further than I had been and to deal with issues in a way I would not have considered before. (unpublished journal notes)

The balance of high challenge, high support can be visualised using the challenge/support grid (Figure 6.1). Ideally, the practitioners would score their guide 10/10 for both challenge and support. Perfect balance. The optimum learning environment. If you guide reflection – what score would your practitioners judge you? If you are a practitioner – what score would you judge him?

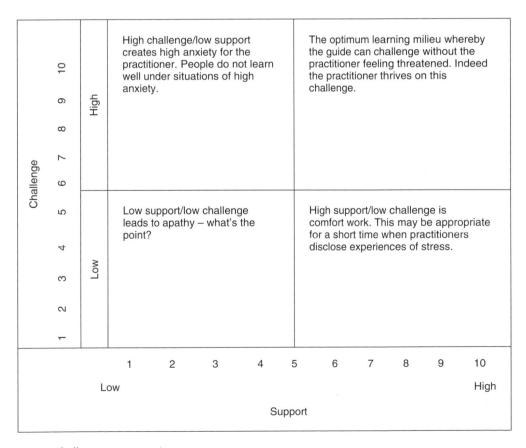

Figure 6.1   Challenge–support axis.

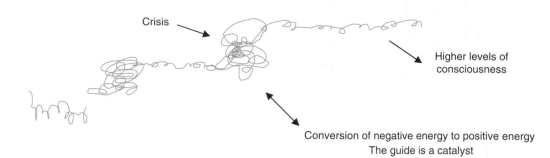

Crisis

Higher levels of
consciousness

Conversion of negative energy to positive energy
The guide is a catalyst

Figure 6.2   Converting negative energy to positive energy.

Remoralisation

I have alluded to the fact that many practitioners are demoralised working within unsympathetic organisations. Being able to tell a trauma story to someone you trust who truly listens is healing simply in the telling. The guide's cathartic response – 'tell me your story' opening a space to understand and transformation as possible. Being heard the practitioners are remoralised (Frank 2002a), a self that has often become demoralised through loss of care, both the care they give and the care they receive.

The guide intends to create a safe place for the practitioner to explore her feelings, encouraging going to deeper places where the root of unhelpful feelings lie, understanding and letting them go. In doing so, the guide works as a catalyst, helping the practitioner convert negative feelings into positive energy for taking action (Hall 1964). The conversion of negative energy into positive energy for taking action can be understood within Prigogine and Stengers' (1984) theory of dissipative structures cited by Margaret Newman (1994). In my sketch (Figure 6.2, inspired by Newman 1994, p. 38), the single curly line represents effective self-organisation continuing until it hits a crisis, represented by a mass of curly lines. In crisis, normal patterns of self-organisation fail, resulting in anxiety (negative energy). Being open systems, practitioners can convert this energy with the environment and create positive energy for taking action based on a reorganisation of self as necessary to resolve the crisis and emerge at a higher level of consciousness; that is, until the next crisis.

As a guide I listen intently for the turning points. In paying attention I hear more than words, as if the feelings associated with the words flow out as energy waves. The energy is a tension, often locked into the person's body. Listening is a form of massage, easing tension and releasing energy. In one recent group supervision session, an experienced district nurse shared a story that concerned her distress at being caught between two people at work who both leaned on her for support. After she had shared her story and contemplated a way to resolve her conflict she had a headache, as if the stress was working its way out of the body.

Pulling free

Often in guided reflection sessions, I ask the practitioners to imagine I am pulling out the negative feeling from within their body. I ask them to imagine a rope extending into their body connected to their feelings. Hand over hand I pull the imaginary rope until I pull it free and stamp on it. It is an extraordinary effective cathartic technique.

People are often ambivalent to learn because any significant learning involves a certain amount of pain, either pain connected with learning itself or giving up previous learning (Rogers 1969). Rogers notes that the first type of ambivalence is illustrated by the small child who is learning to walk. He stumbles, he falls, he hurts himself. It is a painful process. Yet the satisfaction of developing his potential far outweighs the bumps and bruises.

Conclusion

Guidance enhances the learning potential of reflection. Indeed without guidance, novice reflective practitioners would struggle to learn from this approach. It is likely that exposure to reflection will take place within formal settings facilitated by supervisors or teachers. The quality of this guidance is vital. Guidance is not unproblematic. It is contextual and strongly influenced by the relationship between the guide and practitioner notably in situations where embodied patterns of relationship have led to traditional subordinate-type relationships. For example, the guides may view themselves as an authority and demand compliance, impose the practitioner's agenda and even determine what insights the practitioner has gained.

Chapter 7

Weaving and performing narrative: the fifth and sixth dialogical movements

We now move into the narrative and performance turns. The fifth and sixth dialogical movements are reviewed in the same chapter because the narrative is always written with a view to performance. In this sense the movements become one. However, I explore them as successive movements.

Fifth dialogical movement

The fifth dialogical movement weaves together the first four movements into a coherent reflexive narrative that adequately plots the unfolding journey towards self-realisation, however that might be expressed. Reflexive narratives aim to inform the reader of the author's reflexive journey and open a dialogical space for its audience towards social action. Factors that have constrained this journey are clearly explicated. What started as 'doodles in my journal' or *story text* is woven into *narrative text* to capture a moment in time. The narrative continues to evolve through dialogue with its audience, into a *substantive narrative* (see Table 7.1).

Methodology

Reflexive narrative is 'a journey of self-inquiry and transformation towards self-realisation'. My development of this methodology stems many years and is the focus of the *Guided Reflection: A Narrative Approach to Advancing Practice* (Johns 2010a). Now in its second edition, this book explores the creative edge of this methodology. Narrative has a significant theoretical basis through diverse intellectual traditions such as anthropology, psychoanalysis, literary criticism and performance (Mattingly 1998). To this list I would add hermeneutics, critical social science, feminism, chaos theory and ancient traditions. Mattingly's work, in particular, offers a useful overview of narrative.

Becoming a Reflective Practitioner, Fourth Edition. Christopher Johns.
© 2013 John Wiley & Sons, Ltd. Published 2013 by John Wiley & Sons, Ltd.

Table 7.1   The shaping of text through the six dialogical movements

Story text	Reflective text	Narrative text	Substantive narrative
Dialogical movement 1	Dialogical movements 2, 3 and 4	Dialogical movement 5	Dialogical movement 6

Narrative form

As I sit in front of the computer screen, so many ideas and insights bombard me. Punching in certain words evoke meaning. It is being open to the words, letting the words flow through me, as if they pattern themselves below the threshold of conscious thought. It is intuitive, a kind of poetic prose. It is tuning down the left brain and letting the creative juices run free. It is chaos theory, letting go of control as if the writing is self-organising, 'penetrating beyond what is superficial or obvious' (Carson 2008, p. 205).

Reflexive narrative is constructed through layers of (reflected-on) experience. This may be multiple experiences extending over years, or simply be one experience linked to the past and the future by paying attention to the model for structured reflection (MSR) cues: 'how does this experience link with past experiences' and 'given the situation again, how might I respond differently?' Reflexivity is always in the author's mind towards constructing a chain of experiences linked together to reveal the plot of being and becoming. Each experience or link leaves a trace that is picked up in subsequent experiences creating the reflexive movement (Dewey 1933).

The narrative is best patterned around transitional moments or *turning points*. These points communicate insights that are pivotal in the journey of becoming or moments of significant resistance to becoming. They give the narrative its sense of drama unfolding.

Wheatley (1999, p. 126) writes,

> to see patterns, we have to step back from the problem [text] and gain perspective. Shapes are not discerned from close range. They require distance and time to show themselves. Pattern recognition requires that we sit together reflectively and patiently. I say patiently not just because patterns take time to form, but because we are trying to see the world differently and there are many years of blindness to overcome.

In other words, the mind is not trained to seeing reflexive patterns.

The reflexive narrative is written as experienced around key insights and themes in becoming. This sets the background for subsequent experiences to be woven into the emerging pattern of becoming. Guiding practitioners in narrative construction I find that the practitioner has often reflected on many experiences without finding any discerning pattern. To help make sense of the journey so far, I suggest drawing a line under the experiences to date and retrospectively analysing these experiences as a whole to find linkage and pattern as the basis for reflexive development. It may be that life is experienced randomly with unrelated threads and the narrative has little linkage between experiences. This would suggest a weak narrative plot – so if my plot is to 'ease suffering in people with terminal illness' then you would expect some linkage between experiences.

Gradually the disciplined and committed practitioner becomes increasingly mindful of self in practice to the point where practice *is* narrative unfolding. Then the threads are lived and patterned continuously.

Given the complexity of the whole, it is not possible to capture the wholeness of everything. Narrative is always fragmentary, focusing on significant issues pulled out from the whole and yet in relation to the whole. As Fay (1987, p. 168) writes, 'No narrative of actual human lives can ever be characterised as the "genuine one"; the results of human activities are forever occurring, so that any narrative about them must be inherently fragmentary and tentative.'

Writing self always intends to capture reality as far as possible and yet within the realisation that this is only representational of reality rather than reality itself. In other words, such capture is not naïve. This is the mimetic position in contrast with an anti-mimetic position that acknowledges any effort to capture reality as futile (Mattingly 1998). I describe this as *mimetic tension*. Whilst a story tends to be as mimetic as possible, a narrative restructures a story to plot the becoming. This lends itself more to artistic license and creativity.

Creativity

Narrative is creative art. Okri (1997, p. 22) writes, 'the artist should never lose the spirit of play.' Let us dwell with such words and sense their significance as we begin to craft our narratives. Play reminds me of children in the sand, being imaginative, finding the flow of creative life without censor. Play should be fun! Yet there are rules to play the game.

Okri puts play and discipline into balance – 'an ideal creative genius would be one who knew how to consciously initiate great play, as well as how to harness great discipline, towards the most sublime endeavours . . . with smile in the soul' (pp. 22–3).

Symbols, images and metaphors are significant forms for holding meaning. Tuffnell and Crickmay (2004, p. 41) write, 'An image evokes a world, a solar system of connections and meanings, of associations, qualities, textures and memories . . . an image forms a bridge between what's inside us and what is outside . . . it brings us more fully into a felt relationship with the world.'

Images are imaginative and creative. A variety of media can be utilised: metaphor, poetry, art, dramatic prose, storyboard, photographs, nature, music, installation, movement, film and dance to represent meaning, often with a commentary that reflexively links the whole together. This is pertinent for narrative subject to academic scrutiny that often demands explanation of events in contrast with the writer's legitimate claim to *show not tell*, where the narrative pattern reveals meaning to the discerning reader.

These different media forms give texture to the narrative. They engage the reader's imagination more than the dry words of prosaic intellectual language. Parker (2002, p. 104) writes, 'Art and aesthetic expression unite us and contribute to our wholeness. They are essential means of communication and move us all toward increased wellbeing.' The potential of narrative for well-being reflects the cathartic impact of writing and reflection. It is a way of working through emotion and trauma. Fordham (2010) used the idea of 'the net' as a metaphor and image to represent organisational services through which homeless people fell through. She envisaged her role as a specialist nurse working with the homeless as a 'net weaver'. In an earlier paper (Fordham 2008) she used the metaphor of a 'bridge' to span the homelessness void. In a similar vein, Jarrett (2008) used the idea of 'opening space' in her work with disabled people, literally opening space for their physical disability and opening space metaphorically for living more satisfying lives.

Fiction

At times I expand reality or write fiction if I consider it will help to dramatise the point I want to make. However, fiction is always based on real experience. For example, in Anthea,[1] I wrote a fictional piece about a woman with terminal breast cancer experience of returning home after an inappropriate hospital admission. The fiction enabled me to explore controversial issues in home care. The fiction part originated from real issues that women with breast cancer had disclosed to me in my work as a community complementary therapist. Fiction for the sake of it would threaten the narrative's authenticity.

Coherence

Fundamentally there is no prescription for constructing a narrative. Narrative writing is learnt through reflection on the process of constructing it and yet a narrative must be coherent. Reflection is self-inquiry, an inherent sense making of self towards a coherent world. Wheatley and Keller-Rogers (1996, p. 890) write, 'every self makes sense. It creates a world and an identity that feels coherent to itself. From infinite possibilities, it chooses what to notice and how to respond. As we look at any living being, we are observing its particular coherence, the logic it has used to create itself.' The idea of *coherent to itself* challenges any idea of imposing criteria on narrative coherence – that to be coherent it must conform to this or that idea. Such an approach is merely an attempt to control and prescribe a narrative – a technical rational trap. Narrative is chaotic simply because life is. From a chaotic perspective, life is self-organising. As such, so is narrative, being a reflection of lived experience. Wheatley and Keller-Rogers (1996, p. 38) write,

> in self-organisation, structures emerge. They are not imposed. They spring from the process of doing the work. These structures will be useful but only temporary. We can expect them to emerge and recede as needed. It is not the design of a specific structure that requires our attention but rather the conditions that will support the emergence of necessary structures.

Hence, whilst on one hand, it is natural to seek criteria for coherence (what makes a valid narrative) from a technical rational perspective in which the practitioner has been socialised, on the other hand, imposed criteria may force the narrative to fit the criteria rather than the other way round. Once the narrative becomes normalised through an established set of criteria, does it lose its creative impetus (Clough 2000)? The risk is that it becomes a discipline of fitting the narrative to criteria.

Having said that there is no prescription for reflexive narrative, the six dialogical movements does set out a path to follow, yet without imposing how the path is best followed. I previously described the dialogical movements as dialogical layers, as if one layer built on the previous one. This is certainly applicable, but movement suggests a more fluid dynamic state of the six movements in dynamic interplay.

My inquiry into potential criteria has been extensive, identifying criteria for each dialogical movement (see Johns 2010a). Whilst this inquiry helped me grasp the idea of coherence, it also enabled me to loosen the reins to view criteria as merely markers rather than prescriptors. Narrative is a liberating structure for reflexive self-inquiry and expression, and as a liberating structure its form must be determined by the author. This is not to advocate 'anything goes'. Reflexive narrative must be compellingly crafted. A number of writers have influenced my approach to coherence, for example, Richardson's (2000) work as set out in Johns (2010a). Okri has most inspired my approach to narrative. Interpreting his work, I can set out some compelling guidelines for narrative:

- that narrative should plant seeds in the reader's mind;
- that narrative should be both enchanting and challenging, where beauty and horror lie side by side;
- that narrative should be transgressive, always challenging the taken for granted, the complacent, the oppressive state of affairs;
- that narrative should always be reflexive and transformational;
- that the reader does half the work.

Whilst Okri sets out some criteria against which the adequacy of narrative might be judged, developing guided reflection or narrative with Master's and doctoral students demands a more thorough appreciation of what constitutes adequate narrative. Auto-ethnography seemed a natural fit with its emphasis on self-inquiry, if less so with reflexivity. This is not the space to develop these ideas – they are developed in the second edition of *Guided Reflection: A Narrative Approach to Advancing Practice*, dedicated as it is to guided reflection as a research process.

I dialogue with Ellis (2004) (in italics):

E: *Does the narrative have the possibility for changing the world?*

CJ: I view narrative as reflexive in enabling practitioners to become who they desire to be. In realising self, they change themselves. In changing themselves they change the world.

E: *Good auto-ethnographic writing should motivate cultural criticism.*

CJ: I view narrative as 'critical' – that in order to change self, then the nature of reality and the assumptions that govern this reality are exposed, understood and worked towards shifting to support a more desirable state of affairs.

E: *Narratives must be hopeful, well-written and well-plotted stories that show memorable characters and unforgettable scenes.*

CJ: Narrative must be compelling and engaging to draw the reader into the text, as if they were present within the scenario, feeling it as well as thinking it; leaving indelible marks and planted seeds to explode at later moments in terms of their own experiences and social action.

Sixth dialogical movement

Meaning is not something the author creates within the text for the reader to simply pull out. Such a view is naïve. Clearly the reader draws meaning out for themselves. As Okri (1997, p. 41) asserts,

> The writer does one half of the work, but the reader does the other. The reader's mind becomes the screen, the place, the era. To a large extent, readers create the world from words, they invent the reality they read. Reading, therefore, is a co-production between writer and reader.

I wonder to the extent that such claims hold fast for narrative written as self-inquiry and transformation. Okri asks that writers should 'serve truth, be humble, and finely craft their words arrowed to the deepest points of the reader's hearts and minds – they should be silent, leave the stage and let the imagination of the world give sanctuary' (p. 42).

To serve truth is an utter requirement even if the narrative is fiction, a finely crafted fiction based on insights. Perhaps this is necessary when the words are too sharp, arrowed at oppressive systems who may take strident offence if they can detect the author. The ethics of narrative are a swampy field.

Truth is a contested idea depending on your perspective of knowledge (Wilber 1998). Wilber identified four quadrants or paradigms of knowing. He divides these quadrants into the subjective and objective paths. The subjective path is characterised by I and We, whereas the objective path is characterised by It. From a knowledge perspective in health care, the objective path is dominant in its efforts to know and control the world where bias is managed so knowledge is not contaminated by subjectivity. Reflective knowing belongs in the subjective path. It's claim for truth is *authenticity*. However, this begs the question how might authenticity be known? Of course such a question stems from those buried deep in the It world. Authenticity is sensed rather than measured. It is absolutely pointless to write a narrative if not based on genuine intent. If this happened, then someone has missed the point.

As a narrative reader I generally take for granted the authenticity of the narrative unless it doesn't ring true, a different perspective to being sceptical of the narrative's authenticity until it rings true. Gadamer (1975) asks that the reader not take offence, not project meanings into the text but read it with an open mind in order to enter into the text and learn from it. Okri (1997) asks that readers bring the best of themselves to meet the best in the writer's work. Noble sentiments. If only we were all so open-minded and concerned for the truth (Wilber 1998, p. 97).

When the status quo of the dominant is threatened then such pleas fall on closed ears. So I disguise names and places even within the narratives. I speak my own truth through my stories but am careful not to hurt. Where I criticise I intend it to be moral and constructive. People dying should always be at the centre of best care. There is no compromise. No contradictions can be tolerated.

Yet, how our censors pull us back and impose their own rules. I return as I so often do to the words of Virginia Woolf (1945, p. 105):

> So long as you write what you wish to write that is all that matters; and whether it matters for ages or only for a few hours, nobody can say. But to sacrifice a hair of the head of your vision, a shade of its colour, in deference to some professor with a measuring rod up his sleeve is the most abject treachery.

Change value of narrative

The value of narratives to inform and influence work practices is reflected by Ted Maddex. Maddex (2002, p. 21) writes, 'I found that the more I journalled, the more I started to use narratives in my teaching, in meetings – telling stories of experiences with patients to make my points more real.' Fordham (2012) writes of the influence of taking her experiences of working with homeless people into the executive meetings and disturbing the gathered professionals with the reality of homelessness, in contrast with a view of homelessness as statistics. As the Virgin banking poster declared 'people are not numbers to crunch'. Narratives wake up people to reality and confront blindness and complacency. As Mattingly (1998, p. 8) writes, 'It [narrative] casts events in a particular light that allow the audience to infer something about what it is really like to be in that story.' Narratives engage people on a sensory level, drawing them into the text to the extent that they imagine experiencing the situation for themselves. Again, Mattingly (1998, p. 8) writes, 'Narrative offers meaning through evocation, image, mystery of the unsaid. It persuades by seducing the listener or reader into the world it portrays, unfolding events in a suspense-laden time in which one wonders what will happen next.'

Conclusion

Constructing a narrative is like following a stream and seeing where it flows. It seeks to capture the drama of the unfolding journey of becoming, of realisation. Like experience itself it can never be formulaic even as we seek to impose order in the world. However, the demand for coherence does impose some structure to the steam banks.

Note

1   Anthea is currently unpublished.

Chapter 8
The reflective curriculum

The text, up to this point, has been concerned with establishing a reflective learning environment. The idea of curriculum takes the text into a formal curriculum for developing professional practitioners at both pre-registration and post-registration levels. I intend playing with both the macro and micro curriculum environment, playing with ideas largely untested.

The prescriptive nature of a professional curriculum tends to determine the route and pace of the journey of becoming. A reflective curriculum offers the opportunity for more flexibility, to wander off the beaten paths and explore the surrounding areas knowing that guides are available to optimise the learning routes. More significantly, learning through reflection is deeply meaningful simply because it is the individual's journey of becoming a nurse. As such, each step along the journey becomes significant rather than simply looking at the outcomes. Each step is an event in itself not merely a means towards the end. This paying attention to experience creates the reflexive momentum. As Pirsig (1974, p. 208) writes, 'to live only for some future goal is shallow. It's the sides of the mountain which sustains life, not the top. Here's where things grow.'

All professional curricula have to respond to the demand of governing bodies, for example, the Nursing and Midwifery Council (NMC) for approval of the nursing programme where specific regulations and outcomes must be met. In addition approval of programmes is determined by university validation events and the demand of the National Health Service (NHS) trusts within the vagaries of tendering. NHS nurse education contracts are big money! As such, the reflective curriculum is not a blank canvass. It is a contested political canvass.

There will also be strong diverse views within the faculty. Without doubt, a truly reflective curriculum is a radical idea that evokes strong feelings for and against it. In my experience, the voices against outweigh the voices for reflective curriculum fuelled by lack of knowledge as to how a reflective curriculum will work in practice. Reflective practice tends to be bolted onto the existing curriculum as if another teaching technology. Teachers set and control the agenda, prescribing the reflective approach and setting reflective assignments focused on using a model of reflection rather than the insights gained. Besides issues of control, teachers are likely to resist a reflective curriculum because they lack knowledge of reflection and are themselves not reflective. Of course, the teacher, the curriculum, has to ask itself, why do we want reflective practice in the curriculum? Is it simply to teach reflective skills as if these are significant to being an effective practitioner?

Becoming a Reflective Practitioner, Fourth Edition. Christopher Johns.
© 2013 John Wiley & Sons, Ltd. Published 2013 by John Wiley & Sons, Ltd.

Is reflective practice a hegemonic discourse of reflection in nursing (Cotton 2001)? What are the consequences of a reflective curriculum?

Is reflective curriculum simply bolted onto the dominant hegemonic structures and therefore the discourse of reflection is no more than a subculture, because its consequence is democratising the classroom and even learning outcomes?

The odds are stacked against.

The community of inquiry

The reflective curriculum is a community of inquiry based on the principles of collaboration and dialogue. It is a community where people come together to explore a mutual interest. As Wheatley and Kellner-Rogers (1996, p. 70) identify, 'It springs to life from agreements among individuals on how best to live together.' The community shifts in response as people seek to find better ways of living together. In doing so any rules appear to give the community solidity shift giving the community its dynamic, co-creative and reflexive nature.

Collaboration

Within the broad idea of the community of inquiry, student practitioners and teachers collaborate to ensure the optimum learning environment towards enabling students to qualify as registered practitioners and be effective in their newly registered roles. Each individual takes responsibility for her own performance and for the group as a whole. This is the bottom line. Without responsibility the group will fail. Hooks (1994, p. 152) writes,

> That's the difference education as the practice of freedom makes. The bottom-line assumption has to be that everyone in the classroom has to act responsibly. That has to be the starting point – that we are able to act responsibly together to create a learning environment. All too often we have been trained as professors to assume students are not capable of acting responsibly, that is we don't exert control over them, then there's just going to be mayhem.

Peers

Collaboration extends to peers. Peers are an invaluable resource to each other, relating to each other's experiences in such a way that they offer solutions to each other's problems. The group gives voice to student experiences. If one student shared an experience within her group, other students will immediately be able to relate to it in terms of their own experiences. Wheatley and Kellner-Rogers (1996, p. 53) write,

> When we link up with others, we open ourselves to yet another paradox. While surrendering some of our freedom, we open ourselves to even more creative forms of expression. This stage of being has been described as communion, because we are preserved as our selves but are shorn of our separateness or aloneness. What we bring to others remains our self-expression. Yet the meaning of who we are changes through our communion with them. We are identifiable as our selves. But we have discovered new meaning and different contributions, and we are no longer the same.

Learning becomes co-creative.

Isaacs (1993, p. 24), in a more political vein, writes,

> Given the nature of global and institutional problems, thinking alone at whatever level of leadership is no longer adequate. The problems are too complex, the interdependencies too intricate, and the consequences of isolation and fragmentation too devastating. Human beings everywhere are being forced to develop collaborative thought and coordinated action.

Put another way, learning is a political collective endeavour. Nursing is inter-professional and societal. And yet, I sense that communion between nurses is shallow. Nurses are generally apolitical, as if their training has not prepared them to stomp the organisational stage. Practitioner identity needs to be developed to embrace an image of nurses and nursing as powerful within organisational life.

However, the teacher/guide is mindful that collaboration can intimidate the student no matter how much the guide might emphasise collaboration. Students bring their learnt learning experiences that have been strongly imbued by non-reflective modes of learning. The shift from passivity to agency can seem threatening if not frankly over-whelming. As Hooks (1994, p. 143) writes, 'The difficulty getting students to take responsibility is that they have already learnt that they are not the ones with legitimate authority. Students have learnt the left brain approach and expect to be taught in the manner they are accustomed to.' However, the guide is mindful of this transitional period and sensitive to power relations between self and other(s). He acknowledges the ideological basis of his teaching, mindful not to impose collaboration in any hegemonic or contradictory way.

Potential benefits of a reflective curriculum

Teaching and learning through reflective practice can claim a number of benefits that are generally lacking in the non-reflective curriculum:

- It is 'whole-brain' teaching enabling the development of right brain attributes: intuition, perception, imagination and creativity, notably through art.
- It juxtaposes theory in relation to emerging issues from practice – hence the student will find theory more relevant and meaningful and hence assimilate it within personal knowing.
- It develops learning on an intuitive level and thus may seem more suited to experienced practitioners. However, it also enables the development of intuition.
- It accesses the swampy lowlands where real issues lie rather than focus on hard high ground of abstract concepts. Many students may struggle in the real world because of the complexity of practice; reflection gives direct focus to their experience and enables them to make sense of contradictions and develop problem-solving and survival skills. It also acknowledges and accepts their difficulties.
- It values and honours everyday practice as the ground for learning as befits a practice discipline.
- It is values based – constantly challenging and clarifying vision and purpose – balancing 'being a nurse' with 'doing nursing', addressing such issues as ethics, relationships, compassion, knowing self that are not traditionally taught within a theory-led curriculum.

- It enables the teaching of skills such as ethics, relationship, caring, compassion, thera-peutic use of self and poise that are essential to effective nursing practice.
- It naturally moves towards radical learning through performance.
- It is based in the real world, seeking understanding and meaning of why things are as they are.
- It is problem solving – focusing on areas of contradiction, ethics, politics, tradition, power and change – enabling practitioners to become political, empowered and assertive.
- It makes a difference to practice through its reflexive focus of gaining and applying insights to new experiences. In this way we get 'joined-up learning'.
- It prepares practitioners for lifelong learning and ongoing supervision roles.
- It enables practitioners to develop an assertive, political and collective voice (don't mess with me; I am a nurse!).
- It is supportive, dynamic and engaging. And fun!

Potential constraints to the reflective curriculum

- Students may feel threatened by the intense gaze particularly if they lack commitment to practice or study. It is less prescriptive and therefore more 'adult' and requires more responsibility and self-direction.
- It is harder work than conventional learning – because it requires the critique and juxtaposition of theory with practice.
- The teacher or guide may not be good enough – stuck in traditional modes of teaching leading to issues of control and viewing reflection as an educational technology rather than an organic evolving process.
- Teachers may feel threatened due to destructuring and democratising the classroom.

Theory–practice gap

In a practice discipline such as nursing it is self-evident that we learn through doing. We may have theories of how to do it but that doesn't mean we know what it is to nurse. As such, nursing curriculum traditionally has blocks of theory and blocks of practice but that doesn't mean the twain shall meet. It is legend that nurses learn one thing in the classroom and another thing in clinical practice – what has been historically described as the theory–practice gap. Every story or reflection on experience on clinical practice is a microcosm of the whole of nursing. Within each experience significant aspects of nurs-ing can be pulled out as a focus for attention yet always set against a background of the whole culture of nursing. What is significant lies on the surface of the experience. Different aspects of the story can be pulled out from the story canvass and explored against the story's contextual and wider theoretical, philosophical and background – the constant dialogue of the particular with the universal – the third and fourth dialogical movements.

The problem with theory prior to practice is that the student has nothing to hang the theory upon or as Ausubel (1967) notes, 'a hook to hang your hat on.' As such, it is difficult to assimilate theory into personal knowing. It remains 'out there' as an abstract idea. The problem with theory after practice is to let students loose with little idea about what they might be trying to achieve with patients.

Beck (1997, p. 123) writes,

> Suppose we want to know how a marathon runner feels; if we run two blocks, or two miles or five miles, we will know something about running these distances, but we won't yet know anything about running a marathon. We can recite theories about marathons; we can describe tables about the physiology of marathon runners; we can pile up endless information about marathon running; but it doesn't mean we know what it is. We can only know when we are the one doing it. We only know our lives when we experience them directly. This we can call running in place, being present as we are, right here and now.

Running in place might be considered a euphemism for reflective practice. Guided reflection leads to praxis – the constant interplay between ideas about practice and practiced as lived. The illusion of the theory–practice gap is obliterated.

Imagining the shape of a reflective curriculum

What would the basic structure of a reflective curriculum look like? In Figure 8.1, I have identified four elements that constitute the reflective curriculum:

- clinical practice
- reflection (holding creative tension between desirable practitioner identity and lived reality of becoming a registered practitioner)

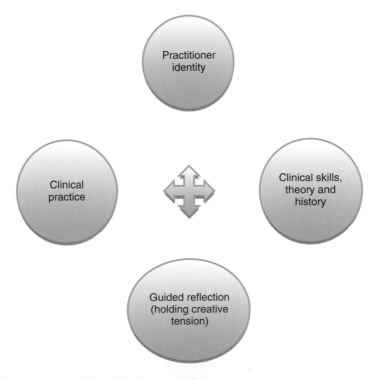

Figure 8.1   The basic structure of the reflective curriculum.

- clinical skills teaching, theory and history of nursing
- practitioner identity (vision of being a registered nurse).

The model is simple and spans the whole training period. Ideally, students entering nursing would have completed a credited diploma in human anatomy and physiology at college, rather than cramp the curriculum with basic theory. Space within the curriculum for guided reflection is created with a reduction in traditional classroom teaching on topics that are better learnt within guided reflection, although short lectures on topics can be picked up and applied to practice within guided reflection.

It would seem reasonable that a practice discipline has practice at the core of its curriculum. Practice is the apprenticeship, the learning of the craft of nursing mentored by nurses in practice. To use my own experience as a clinical teacher, I found that mentoring was a hit and miss affair. Perhaps this has become more problematic with the pressure on clinical staff in a stressed clinical environment due to less staff and a greater workload due to increased turnover and more acutely dependent patients. In response to financial restraint, qualified staff have been replaced by healthcare assistants. As a consequence, qualified staff become tied into the more technical aspects of care, limiting their ability to role-model what is usually described as basic nursing care. Fewer qualified staff means less mentors, who under pressure, may view the supernumerary student more as a pair of hands.

However, as if recognising the problem, NHS trusts associated with the University of Bedfordshire are demanding a greater presence of the nurse tutors in clinical areas. However, the neglect of their clinical role may leave reluctant and resistant nurse teachers scratching their heads as to how best they fulfil this role. And of course it will have a budgetary impact. When I became the director of a BSc palliative care programme in 1998, the first thing I arranged was my clinical placement in a hospice and dedicated 1 day a week to ensure I was credible, as a practitioner, to teach palliative care besides supporting both staff and students as appropriate. I also had another motive in that I needed to collect real stories as the basis for my teaching.

If students are to learn most effectively through their everyday clinical practice, then the value of reflective practice is self-evident. As such, mentors in clinical practice would be reflective practitioners, role modelling reflection as a way of being in practice. It would be like offering a running commentary of their narrative practice with patient care. It is noticeable when I teach clinical supervision to experienced healthcare professionals that professions that have seriously incorporated reflection into curriculum are better equipped for supervisory roles than those professions, such as nursing, that have not. Of course, this is a generalisation. This would require mentoring preparation and support programmes to have a significant reflective core by reflection on the practice of mentoring students in practice. As I will return to later, guided reflection could shape the final year of professional training. Given the general precarious state of mentoring in clinical practice, it becomes more incumbent of the faculty to design a reflective curriculum to ensure that students can learn through their clinical experience.

I would advocate a return to clinical teaching for clinical skills followed by reflection. This would get teachers back into clinical practice at least 1 day per week to facilitate students and support the practice team. There is nothing like the real stuff to develop person-centred learning. One risk with simulation teaching is that if you talk to a doll object long enough, that's the way you will be with patients and families.

Guided reflection groups

As a rule of thumb, student practitioners would spend 4–6 hours per week (2 or 3 × 2 hours) in guided reflection throughout the programme in contracted small groups of 10 (the number is flexible) facilitated by a personal mentor.

A number of pointers:

- Each student practitioner takes responsibility for his or her own performance and the performance of the whole group.
- The student practitioners would bring at least two reflected-on experiences to share each week. One experience would focus on something that went well (self-affirming) and one that went less well (problematic).
- The group would continue either throughout the whole 3-year programme with one mentor or for 1 year with subsequent change of mentor.
- The groups would review its performance each week in terms of learning outcomes and group process to ensure its effectiveness (see Box 8.1).
- The agenda is set by the student experiences with set curriculum objectives. The whole curriculum can be covered within any single experience; it is just a question of what is pulled out from the whole for the focus of learning set against the background of the whole.
- Relevant theory (including lecture notes) is accessed, critiqued and assimilated as appropriate. People will bring theory into texts and dialogue, opening a critical group-think on the significance of that theory to the particular practice being explored, and then opening the theory up into a more general consideration.
- The student practitioners will keep an ongoing learning journal (this would almost certainly be linked to the formal acknowledgement of meeting learning outcomes as stipulated in the case of nursing by the NMC).

Rather paradoxically, guides don't set out to teach people. They intend to open a learning space so student practitioners can learn for themselves. This teaching posture reflects a fundamental shift of responsibility and control in the learning relationship between the

Box 8.1

In his book *Becoming a Critically Reflective Teacher*, Brookfield (1996) offers many examples of being a critical reflective teacher in terms of the curriculum and classroom politics and democratising the learning space. For example (p. 115), he offers 'the classroom critical incident questionnaire' whereby he poses a number of questions to the student:

- At what moment in the class this week did you feel most engaged with what was happening?
- At what moment in the class this week did you feel most distanced from what was happening?
- What action that anyone (teacher or student) took in class did you find most affirming or helpful?
- What action that anyone (teacher or student) took in class this week did you find the most puzzling?
- What about the class surprised you the most? (This could be something about your own reactions to what went on, or something that someone did, or anything else that occurs to you.)

The guide invites the student to submit these anonymously. He then analyses the responses and gives feedback next session and invites dialogue. In time, the students rise responsibly to the democratic ideal. Brookfield recognises the benefits of this approach to build trust, to alert the group to problems before a disaster occurs and to give the guide feedback about ways he might develop his facilitation.

student and the teacher. Indeed, the guide will encourage people *not to know* and in doing so to cultivate a curious and challenging attitude to both personal and extant knowing. When people think they know, they stop learning and close to possibilities (Lao Tzu 1999). Based on their own experiences, the student practitioners are more likely to find their own way with challenge and support. Reflexive learning enables, in a direct way, learning from one situation to inform the next.

The teacher/guide checks himself at every turn not to fall back into a dominant teacher mode of being. When hegemony has been the norm, diversity must be actively worked towards. It can never be assumed simply because we might say 'this group is collaborative based on mutual respect'. Fine words 'out there' but they have to be lived and at first we may not know how to live them. Saying a classroom is safe doesn't make it safe.

Dialogue

To reiterate,[1] guidance talk is dialogue. Dialogue is a particular type of talk between people, possibly of differing opinions, constructively oriented towards consensus. The emphasis is on the process of working towards rather than achieving consensus. In other words, dialogue is about process not outcomes. Get the process right and the right outcomes will tumble out.

In my experience dialogue is a rare thing. I sit in meetings and observe patterns of talk, and it is nothing like what Isaacs describes. Sometimes talk resembles debate or discussion characterised by people trying to make and win the point. I do not think people are good at listening when concerned with making their own point.

Student practitioners and guides must learn to dialogue. The key to dialogue is to listen carefully with respect (see Chapter 1 for 'rules' of dialogue). This can be demonstrated by feeding back to the speaker what you have heard and how your own words are linked and to explore the underlying assumptions that govern peoples' views.

The talking stick

One way to facilitate dialogue is to use the *talking stick* as a way of orchestrating talk within the council. It is a microphone; so when one holds the talking stick, everyone listens. The person holding the stick talks into the circle with no thought of influencing others but to speak the truth. Because they sit at one point of the circle, they only represent one viewpoint. Those who listen look into the open fire with an open heart and mind – and what is meant for their spirits will come to them and what is not will pass away. It gives empowerment by first noting your name – 'I am Chris and I will speak. . . .' And finishing 'I am Chris and I have spoken.' The stick teaches about options and choices and that each person has a unique disposition. The stick can be decorated with specific meaningful emblems (Lee 1994, p. 122).

At the Inaugural Reflective Practice Gathering in Zakynthos in 2011, the group of 17 international participants experienced 4 days of dialogue. Initially the talking stick was used for 2 days until participants learnt the etiquette of dialogue. The stick was then put aside. It was interesting to see how individuals within the group confronted those who reverted to old ways. Using the stick facilitated more considered speech farther than 'off-the-cuff' remarks or commentary. As such, a greater sense of focus and continuity was achieved.

As a guide, I usually wait for peers within the group to respond to another student practitioner's sharing of experience before myself, not because I am unduly humble or courteous, but because I know that my voice is acknowledged as the expert voice. The student practitioners know that, so let's not play at collaborative games. The student practitioners want to hear my voice and learn from it. As a guide, knowing how to assert one's own voice is like tuning into the community's wavelength – not easy with large groups, and yet groups settle and create norms. The astute guide is always checking out the control of the community through practitioner feedback, and yet the practitioner needs to feel able to voice true feedback if the community is to achieve optimum performance.

Through working in intense guided reflection over 3 years, I envisage the student practitioner will exit the programme deeply reflective and mindful of self within clinical practice. She will be assertive, politically aware, adept at conflict management and able to frame and respond to problems. She will be clinically poised, compassionate and skilled in person-centred practice. She will be responsible for ensuring her ongoing clinical effectiveness.

Skilled guides

Clearly, guided reflection requires skilled guides. I have previously explored reasons why reflection needs to be guided (Chapter 6). The guide points the way forward, sometimes leading on the front foot and at other times on the back foot, mindful of the group's performance and learning outcomes. As suggested, guidance demands a wide range of knowledge yet without setting self up as the expert. Guides or teachers will require an intense development to function effectively within the community of inquiry. This can be achieved by establishing teacher-guided reflection groups initially expertly facilitated and subsequently peer led, where each teacher takes responsibility for his or her own perform-ance and the performance of the group as a whole, in other words, mirroring the student groups.

Storytelling

Before inviting student practitioners to share their stories, I always share one of my own to role-model taking the risk and to offer my expertise. Remind yourself of my story concerning Tom and Joan (Chapter 3). I have often shared this story in guided reflection to both pre- and post-registration nurses. It evokes passion, guilt and outrage. Yet the same nurses who express such strong emotion seem to be chained by their inappropriate models, seemingly unable to break free although they know there are more congruent ways of responding to clinical practice. Perhaps that is the guilt, knowing that they too slip unwittingly into routines that diminish person-hood and inadvertently cause suffer-ing. The story helps practitioners to expose their own creative tension. In time, people who live contradictory lives become alienated from self in the struggle to maintain the illusion. Jourard (1971) informs that people who are alienated from self are unable to use themselves in any therapeutic way and hence are no longer able to care beyond a perfunctory response to the other as an object.

Because stories are personal, there is a risk that its audience will avoid being critical for *at least* two reasons. Firstly, it is difficult to be critical of storytellers when their stories are emotional and oppressive. The natural response of listeners is emotional, to sympathise rather than be critical. Secondly, there is a collusive strategy to make the audience space safe by avoiding difficult issues so they do not have to face difficult issues in telling their own stories. As such, I problematise myself – critiquing myself in terms of not just what I do but my background behind it. In doing so I model story sharing and open the space for a critical listening.

Art workshops

Art workshops are vital within the reflective curriculum to open and stir the imaginative, creative and intuitive mind. I have explored the value of storyboard and poetry as forms of narrative representation. In Chapter 2 – I used the photograph of a building in Boulder Colorado quoting Georgia O'Keefe that is worth repeating: 'I could say things with colors and shapes that I had no words for.' I find that people are often either verbal or visual. I am verbal, although living with an artist, I have been inspired and encouraged to engage art more overtly in my more recent narratives through photography and installation.

The construction of a narrative as art is an exciting reflective development, pioneered by artist teachers such as Cameron *et al* (2008) and Gaydos (2008). Cameron *et al* worked with Canadian pre-registration students. They write,

> the purpose of the aesthetic assignment is to invite students to participate in a journey that stretches and challenges self in the paradoxes of life experiences. The students begin to engage in a form of 'academic play' which gives them permission to 'think outside the box' and leads them to ponder, analyze and develop their own perspectives. They apply the theoretical underpinnings of a critical social theory, which includes the values of justice and equity, inclusion, empowerment and respect as related to 'lived experience' of their clients. Expression through art brings to life suppressed and repressed feelings, attitudes and beliefs and increases insights and self-awareness. (p. 115)

In their chapter, the results of this project are beautifully illustrated in colour plates. Gaydos used collage with midwives on a maternity unit in the USA to help them reconnect with their values after a severe period of disruption. The results are deeply symbolic. Gaydos (p. 168) cites Eliade (1991, p. 12): 'the symbol reveals certain aspects of reality – the deepest aspects – which defy other means of knowledge.'

Performance

The performance turn opens a creative space within the curriculum. I know that reading a narrative engages students in meaningful learning. This is proven time and time again as I share my stories in the classroom, in workshops, in conferences. In developing performance I consider ways to engage the audience more actively in the performance.

Jane's rap

In two performances of Jane's rap, I engaged drama and psychiatric students to read the empathic poems that represented the voice of eight self-harm patients referred to within the text. I read the voice of Jane, a staff nurse working within the accident and emergency

(A&E) department. Jane used reflexive methodology for her BSc post-registration degree. Her topic was her attitude towards self-harm patients. She recognised her attitude was negative and wanted to develop a more positive attitude. As her research supervisor, we met eight times using guided reflection. At each session she reflected on her experiences of nursing self-harm patients. The result was a reflexive narrative (Groom and Johns 2002/2010). Such was the potential educational value of this work for A&E staff and psychiatric nurses; I developed the text into performance and commissioned a writer to write empathic poems to represent the voice of each self-harm patient (Johns and Marlin 2010).

The feedback from both drama and psychiatric students was very positive. Some of the drama students had a history of self-harm, and reading their poems was cathartic. It led to a deeper understanding of themselves. Participating in the performance was a powerful drama lesson through tuning into the poems. What was the persons' experience? It was a more powerful experience for the psychiatric students, offering real insight into self-harm. The students dialogued with the audience and between themselves following each performance. In another performance with drama students in the USA, the audience included student nurses. The feedback was 'I have learnt more about self-harm and A&E in one hour than in any previous theory class.'

Imagine

The logical move is to engage students in drama workshops, perhaps sharing curriculum with other practice disciplines and with drama faculty. Take a topic like stroke. The traditional approach would be to set learning objectives and then sequentially move through anatomy and physiology, aetiology, signs and symptoms, medical treatment and patient care. No different than with a host of other medical conditions.

Now imagine, taking a class of 50 students, dividing the class into 5 groups of 10. Imagine a 1-day workshop working with drama and dance teachers, perhaps a shared class with drama students that introduces the group to drama technique. Imagine setting out five projects around medical disorders such as stroke, depression, myocardial infarction, receiving chemotherapy and dementia. Imagine prepping the group to talk to stroke patients, nurses, doctors and other healthcare workers, and families to gain peoples' perspectives of living with and treating stroke. Imagine the student practitioners reading about stroke and then putting together a performance around caring for a stroke patient to their colleagues. A second drama workshop is done to put the performance together. No lecture. The students take responsibility. The performance is stunning. They say 'we have learnt so much.' The other four projects are equally brilliant. The buzz about the place is great. Learning is profound and fun. What odds the students learn more through performance than lecture?

The rub

Traditional teachers are likely to resist the truly reflective curriculum for at least three reasons:

- They have been socialised into a set of assumptions that support a traditional teacher-led technical rational curriculum. This approach has not privileged students' voices. As such, the truly reflective curriculum is beyond their scope.

- They are not reflective on their own practice and lack both reflective and facilitative skills. As Hooks (1994) writes, 'Focusing on experience allows students to claim a knowledge base from which they can speak' (p. 148). '[However] many professors are critical of the inclusion of confessional narrative in the classroom, where students are doing a lot of the talking because they lack the skill needed to facilitate dialogue' (p. 151).
- They are fearful of losing control of the curriculum and being exposed as lacking expertise across a wide range of topics.
- They have become comfortable and complacent in their teaching roles within a non-reflective culture that has made virtually no demand for teachers to demonstrate teaching excellence.

Given the expected resistance at both an institutional and personal level, how might pressure to shift to a reflective curriculum be applied? Perhaps by NHS trusts who contract nurse education. However, this is unlikely within a transactional culture that seeks conformity to competencies. Perhaps it requires a return to an apprenticeship-type, hospital-based education. Perhaps the NMC would be willing to pilot such a scheme? I am aware of recent innovations in Canadian nurse education around 44 stories that encapsulates the scope of nurse education.[2]

If the education system resists widespread adoption of the reflective curriculum, then individual teachers or collective groups can tinker around the edges and begin to create bubbles of reflective teaching. They can make their voices heard within curriculum and course planning. However, those who buck the system run the risk of marginalisation (Brookfield 1996).

Reading through my text I sense I paint first an optimistic picture for a reflective curriculum and then a pessimistic picture of organisational resistance grounded in tradition, authority and embodiment (Fay 1987). Yet things are possible from an individual teacher's perspective as I try to illuminate through a series of vignettes.

Journal entry 1

I have eight students on the rehabilitation module on placement at Burford. My role as a lecturer–practitioner is to provide both the theoretical input and supervise their clinical practice. They have a learning contract whereby they must demonstrate through reflection how they have met them during the placement. Looking at past examples, these are very descriptive. I decide to teach this module as guided reflection. For the previous cohort, I had constructed stories from my own practice at Burford to stimulate their reflection and feed in relevant theory as appropriate, ensuring that the learning outcomes for the module were covered. This time I share one story as a trigger for reflection and then suggest for the remaining sessions that they bring in their own reflections. I know the patient they reflect on, giving me inside information. Although I know the theoretical literature (I did write the extensive reading list), I ask the students to note any particular relevant literature as part of their reflection (ever mindful of the practice–theory gap). Our library is well stocked, and we had 10 sessions. Learning can be so productive and so much fun for students and myself. I had no sense of students being disadvantaged within the group due to learning style even though I insisted that each student formally prepared to share at least one experience. It was evident how one story sparked so many others, helping me realise that students learnt from listening to and reflecting on other students' stories as much as they did presenting their own stories.

Journal entry 2

A first-year student nurse suggests that students always focus on negative experiences for two reasons: firstly, that's what teachers expect, and secondly, how can you reflect on a positive experience? He gave an example of a male patient thanking him for giving him a bath. 'What is there to reflect upon?'
I ask 'how do you mean?'
I mean 'it was not a problem.'
In my response a number of questions tumbled out:

- How did that make you feel?
- Why is it important to feel like that?
- How do you feel if patients don't thank you?
- Does it make you feel differently towards them (than those who do thank you)?
- If you feel negative towards the patient, are you less available?
- Do male patients like being bathed/touched by male nurses?
- How do you feel about bathing women patients?
- What was significant in bathing him?
- What assumptions govern your practice?

These questions (and perhaps many more) seem obvious yet it was not the student's natural way to think. What is normal on the surface becomes potentially problematic when the surface of the experience is scratched to expose deeper significance. The student's experience suggests the need for guidance perceptive enough to pose these types of questions, especially for practitioners who lack reflective or clinical experience. Such a rich teaching opportunity stems from one line: 'A male patient thanked me for helping him bath.'

Honour thy mother

The value of sharing a story as a trigger for reflection is illustrated by Margaret Graham.[3] She writes, 'A liberty Chris, thank you and apologies if I have got some of this so very wrong.'

Shame: disgrace, humiliation, embarrassment, indignity, ignominy, make uncomfortable, discredit. I felt moved, frustrated and humbled when listening to your performance of 'My Mother's Death'[4] at the 15th International Reflective Practice Conference 2009. When listening, I asked myself: what is my role as an educator in answering this call for social action?

The performance changed my way of knowing as I have struggled with the social action element within my own reflections and I now write as if a small unfurling of the sail.

I wonder at the purpose behind Chris's story.

I wonder about my teaching – do I collude in a notion that we teach students and then they know and do? Feelings of disempowerment.

On November day we read the story, with a group of 12–13 students in a lab session. The clinical room was grey, somewhat cold with the artificial fluorescent light, the light barely penetrating through the soulless vertical blinds across the windows, yet giving a glimpse of a wintery sun. The sound of the wind swirled through the barely open window. The only colour was the multitude of student bodies. I know that many of the students work part-time in nursing homes at the weekend. I began with a short introduction and explained the author's position and tentatively invited volunteers to help with reading. I offered to read the first page. Volunteers offered to read page by page. I was somewhat nervous reading; I felt the narrative could be devoid of the occasion in the theatre where I originally heard Chris perform. There were no props to aid the performance – no evocative background music, no charismatic voice of Chris, no stage presence, no poignant black and white images of Kay, Chris's mum.

As we circled, read and listened, I hoped what I sensed was happening was a positive response. Earlier, when preparing to read and copying the published narrative, I wondered about the impact of engaging students through narrative. The thought 'was I sending lambs to the slaughter' confronted me with my maternal inclination to protect the students – protect them from what? I read, she read, he read, we all listened and at the end silence. I resisted the urge to speak out. I suggested we dwelt with what we have heard. Several minutes later I saw eyes sparkle with tears and some distress.

We held the space and I purposefully followed Virginia Woolf's thoughtful idea that 'one can only show how one came to hold whatever opinion one holds. One can only give one's audience the chance to draw their own conclusions.'

As I looked through the window in silence on the dull winter day, a leaf slowly wafted down, suspended in mid-air and then collided with all the other leaves, and it seemed to me a significant representation of my thoughts as I question my role as an educator.

I asked the students: what would you say to Chris Johns in response to his story?

They wrote comments in their reflective lab reports, quickly written words like ripples in a rock pool that vibrate outwards to change the world.

Student reflections on listening and dialoguing with the text:

- I was completely embarrassed to be a member of the nursing profession.
- It is good to read articles like this every so often as it brings me back down to earth to recognise the most basic needs of the patient.
- It makes me think how do I treat patients and what can I do for people. How long does it take to be gentle and help with mouth care/how long does it take to call a person by the right name?
- The smallest gesture matters; we can change things and we can make a big difference.
- It was a huge eye opener; it is sad to see the easiest of tasks, cleaning a person's mouth and brushing their hair, is seen as less important as doing the stores.
- It really opened my eyes how upset he was and for his mother.
- It is a daunting task, a daunting issue of the workplace that we are preparing to enter.
- Johns's article opened my eyes to the neglected, little things; a smile or the three phrases that you suggested in the text, I am going to start using them now.
- I felt shocked, disgusted at the lack of empathy. I felt sadness for the family.
- The article gave me a chance to evaluate my own performance as a care assistant and student nurse while I always try to be kind and empathise with family members; it is easy to become very task and routine focused; it allowed me to be aware that this can happen, and to be aware of recognising the possibilities is beneficial.
- It is really easy to fall into the ways of services.

- My experience of people dying has been so different, so positive.
- I work in a nursing home and I try to work hard and wonder can I change anything but now I can – a little look can change everything.
- The thoughts and feelings raised here help me be aware of how I can be a better role model for junior students.
- This article is so much more than the quantitative and qualitative research and evidence that we have to read.
- Only one comment: I would like to hear the comments from the staff in the care home.
- Such a good article – I am really glad the reality to which I am aware is now being challenged.
- It highlights what is going on but we are afraid to talk about.
- It helped me realise the changes that I need to make in my practice while caring for the patient; I need to also be aware of the family's needs.
- I don't think I will ever forget this article and feel that every nurse should read it. It supports the need for dramatic change in nursing homes – thank you Mr Johns.
- The article is one that I will keep throughout my career and read frequently; I know that the day it fails to shock me or move me, it may be time to assess my own level of care – a really moving piece.
- I found this article very effective as a student; I vow not to let myself fall into that routine of task-centred care as I know that I am one nut in the machine that can change.
- After reading the article everyone became moved, the story moved me, the silence in the room was so powerful. We are the nursing generation of change.
- Can we change? A drastic situation like this should be described, and the story should be sent to all nursing homes to help re-motivate us.
- This story should be sent to every hospital and nursing home; nurses should have a chance to hear it and stop and think.
- I felt that nursing is a powerful profession that can influence the actual lives of others and a great deal of thought is required in the littlest of tasks.
- A learning experience that I will never ever, ever forget – the use of language was fantastic.

The reading seems to have had an influence on their perceptions of nursing older persons. It also acted as a trigger for change. Chris describes this as embodied knowing – knowing that changes them. The story was so ordinary, yet extraordinary on this November day, part of the rhythm of life. The heart of the story – the question of the quality of care for nursing older people – what are our responsibilities and what actions are we taking? WHO research (2002) with older people concludes that freedom from all forms of abuse and violence must be a common goal for all societies of the 21st century.

In Ireland we have experienced a public investigation into the treatment of older people in nursing homes. The harrowing account has led to the publication of the Health Service Executive HIQA (2009) standards guiding care and a robust process for the inspection of homes. The Irish Nursing Board has responded with standards for professional guidance of those working with older people (An Bord Altranais 2009).

These policy documents are expected to inform my teaching. Indeed, Taoiseach's office has asked whether such material is covered in our curriculum.

Using stories in teaching reveals the tension between facilitating learning and managing content. Managing this tension is a veritable juggling act between 'ticking the boxes, covering the content and creating a space for meaningful learning.'

Yet such stories reflect the whole: from the whole we can pull out aspects of care yet always against a background of the whole. Relevant theory can be fed in as appropriate enabling students to link ideas with practice. I am impressed how the story gripped the students. I sense my role as an educator to open spaces for reflection through such stories, triggering their own stories – stories of shame. We need to search and find this humanity.

Virginia Woolf (1945, p. 127) writes,

> for the reading of these books seem to perform a curious couching operation on the senses; one sees more intensely afterward, the world seems bared of its covering and given an intenser life. Learning should be memorable. As for the students, it was a learning experience I will never ever forget. I will keep trying to explore story telling within the limiting confines of the system and perhaps ripples will become waves. Stories are empowering – we all leave the room richer for the experience.

Journal entry 3

November 2011. First-year MSc leadership in healthcare programme. Twelve student leaders gather in the community of inquiry. It is the fifth session of this unit that explores the creative tension between one's vision of leadership and one's reality of living leadership. Holding creative tension is core to all reflective practice learning. The reflective effort is towards resolving the tension so leadership can be realised as something lived rather than as an ideal. In this process, factors that constrain leadership are revealed.

Rick [yet again] raises concern with what is expected of the second assignment. Patiently, I explain it requires a reflection on a specific experience that explores the creative tension between realising your vision of leadership and an understanding of your current reality. I sense his anxiety – his need to know exactly what is required. I ask (perhaps slightly less patiently) 'what is your problem?' It stems from his uncertainty with reflective writing – his ability to 'get it'.

When we explore this difficulty, certain points emerge. Firstly, he, like some of the other student leaders, is not keeping his reflective journals between sessions (every 2 weeks). After leaving each session, they get caught up in their everyday work-worlds. This is not uncommon for students commencing this programme; their normal everyday world is unreflective. Lucy, defensively, asserts she does reflect, but does this in her head. I make the point that she needs to write it down – that something deeper happens when we write it down and move into disciplined reflection. She agrees that in writing she is more attentive to the experience. The student practitioners agree that they must become disciplined to set aside time to write and reflect. The connection between this activity, at this early stage of the programme, and becoming a mindful leader is vital. I state my frustration that they are not writing their journals. I know it is early days and this is a familiar pattern but, slipping into an unhelpful parental mode, I nag them to take responsibility for their learning. Not good dialogue! Yet I know from experience, that the more they invest in systematic (and serious) reflection at this stage, the more they will benefit from the programme and succeed at assignments. We agree to spend the next 30 minutes of the session writing and reflecting to get into a reflective groove. We agree that every leader will bring two experiences; one self-affirming and one problematic to the next session.

Lucy shares an experience. I confront her with the cues in the model for structured reflection (MSR) (role modelling the exploration of cues with the whole group, reinforcing the value of each cue). How did people feel within the situation? How did she feel within the situation? How does she feel now? She laughs nervously. Her feelings are not easily expressed. I use a word for her to consider – anger? Reluctantly, she admits she did feel angry at her colleague. I ask, 'So why is it difficult to admit?' She is uncertain. I persist. 'Well anger isn't easy to admit. I know I need to be more poised.' I throw it open to the group. One of her peers says, 'Could you be less angry given the situation again?' Anger is an embodied response. I suggest she works through the 'influences grid' (Figure 3.4). A culture of conflict avoidance and emotional detachment emerges: better not to get involved, turn a blind eye to injustice, rationalise that it is not her sphere of responsibility – behaviours that are governed by socialised patterns of authority, tradition and embodiment. Lucy reveals how issues of anxiety, control and authority weave a toxic mix to demoralise staff. She is confronted with the moral need to act as a leader. Does she have the argument and courage to achieve this? We will pick it up next session. The group buzzes in response.

Gregg reveals his discomfort that a staff member known to be 'difficult' has been turned down for training. The group helps him explore his options for action drawing on his leadership vision. He struggles to articulate his vision groping with different theoretical ideas. His vision is out there, not inside him as yet. The group acknowledges that it is the same for them. Vision takes time to form and longer to be lived in any meaningful way – the shift from words on paper and words lived in everyday practice. In relation to Lucy and Gregg's experiences, the group explores the organisational backgrounds of their workplaces, deepening its mutual understanding of the tension between the transactional and transformational (Table 14.1).

MSc leadership in healthcare programme spans 28 months consisting of a number of taught units around specific leadership attributes. These units are largely project based requiring a deep reflection of leadership of the projects. The whole programme is constructed as a community of inquiry taught entirely through guided reflection holding creative tension between the student leaders' evolving vision of leadership and their reality of becoming a leader in practice. The taught programme is a woven spiral around the dissertation of constructing a narrative of being and becoming a leader using a reflexive narrative methodology (Figure 8.2). The novel format of the dissertation did not fit within normal academic regulations. Yet I was able to defend its inclusion at validation from the perspective of reflective learning. The regulations were not changed but simply bent to accommodate this deviation – a question of making the case and standing your ground.

Journal entry 4

I am invited by a group of second-year nursing students to talk to them about reflection. They say how frustrated they are with reflection. It has no value. They cannot see the point and resent wasting curriculum time on it. Reflection is a chore with little value except to answer reflective-type assignments. Carrot and stick education. We have 2 hours.

I said 'let me tell you a story.' It concerns my practice with a patient called Violet.[5] I read from my text for about 20 minutes. I always commence with a story especially if I expect the student practitioners to write and tell their own stories. This role-models what

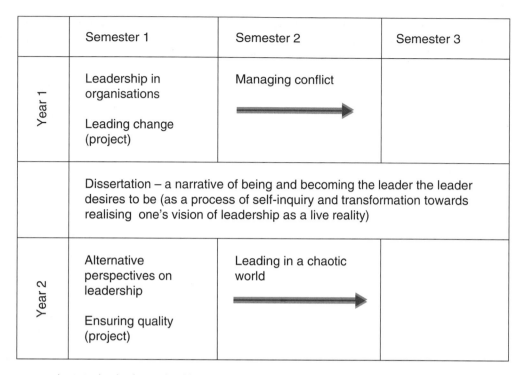

	Semester 1	Semester 2	Semester 3
Year 1	Leadership in organisations Leading change (project)	Managing conflict ───────►	
	Dissertation – a narrative of being and becoming the leader the leader desires to be (as a process of self-inquiry and transformation towards realising one's vision of leadership as a live reality)		
Year 2	Alternative perspectives on leadership Ensuring quality (project)	Leading in a chaotic world ───────►	

Figure 8.2   The MSc leadership in healthcare programme outline.

a story might look like and my risk of sharing it. Within the story, I problematise myself, and focus the problem as *the turning point*, the moment of most significant insight and potential transformation. In addition, I always pose the MSR reflective cue: 'how might I respond differently given the situation again?' I might not answer the cue, simply to pose it, stimulates the audience to consider this cue for themselves: 'if that was me, how might have responded?'

Afterwards I invite comments, both about the content in terms of their own nascent stories of practice and about the structure of the text. The students say that the text was engaging to the extent that some felt they actually experienced the situation. Two students, bold enough to reveal, share similar stories. It is as if we sit around a campfire telling our stories – what I term *campfire* teaching (Johns 2010a).

A further 20 minutes pass. I invite them to write a story. I give them 15 minutes. After an initial flurry of comments between them, the room is very quiet as pens race across pages.

I then talk through the MSR (Box 3.1) and the way the cues have influenced my story. I say 'there is the story on the surface – what are the assumptions that govern my practice?' I make a point of emphasising my experience as a contextual moment situated in history – a personal, social, cultural, professional, political, environmental, professional, gendered history. In other words everything that constitutes this moment in time. It is also recognising our roots, that nursing, or any profession, evolves from its history, its tradition. I say 'it's like peeling back an onion skin to reveal deeper contextual layers.' A bit deep for them, but I wanted them to think about that, that reflection is deeper than the stories we tell.

I share how I've not used some of the cues and explore how these might have extended or even changed the story. At the same time I prompt the student practitioners to apply the cues to their own stories and, as possible, to draw out any insight.

I then invite them to share their stories. The 2 hours have passed. The students stay on, wanting to talk generally about reflective practice. Many of them (although not all) said they had no idea that reflection could be so creative and exciting. Their creative impulse has been unleashed. They exclaim 'why haven't we been taught reflection like this?' I reply, 'The problem of accommodating reflection within a nursing programme grounded in technical rational approach to knowing. What happens is that reflection is distorted to fit in within the dominant attitude of instrumental learning. It becomes bolted on rather than radically influences the curriculum. Perhaps not surprising because it requires a radically different approach from teachers.' They are frustrated. I am being politically subversive to disturb the system. For the reflective practitioner all action is ultimately political towards creating a better world, although what constitutes a better world is contestable.

I explain that their reflective assignments are designed to measure their application of a reflective model supported by references (a pseudo-intellectual game) with no credit for aesthetic expression. I feel that assignments should be written around insights gained or what I have learnt (see Figure 8.3 as an example of a potential reflective practice grading profile). The students say that they play the game. 'What game is that?' I inquire. 'Guess what is in teacher's head – that way at least you pass.' What kind of education is that? 'If I had submitted my story as an assignment would I pass?' 'No' is the general consensus; 'it doesn't tick the boxes.' Education is no more than ticking the boxes.

Some days later, their course teacher and head of curriculum development for pre-registration nursing approaches me and feeds back the students' enthusiastic response. The power of students' voices could not be easily discounted. She is convinced of a need for a new approach to reflection within the curriculum. She asks if I would lead a specialist subgroup for the curriculum revalidation for degree nurse training.

I agree but that's another story. To my colleagues, I explain that the existing approach to teaching reflective practice is not good enough. That it led to student dissatisfaction with reflective practice. It simply cannot be bolted on. I outline the model (Figure 8.1) and it is rejected as impractical. I try to explain that there is ample space within the curriculum because what is normally taught can now be taught through guided reflection. Below the surface I feel the resistance – that teachers are threatened by reflective practice at this deeper level of significance. I hit the reality wall. A few teachers who support this approach soften the blow. I simply said 'so be it.'

What they got was more of the same.

I recognised that two fundamental things needed addressing to implement a truly reflective curriculum:

- How can teachers become reflective given that teachers must themselves be reflective to guide reflection in others?
- How can teachers best facilitate reflection?

Teachers resist reflection because they are not reflective. They see it as a threat to their own competence as a teacher. They view it as radical to give students a voice that threatens their classroom control. They are wrapped up in conventional theory-driven curriculum grounded in the delivery of extensive ideas, caught up in practice of aims of objectives and so on.

	Weighting	Fail	Pass
			Increasing criticality and creativity →
Clear expression of insights evidenced through reflections on specific experiences	30	Understanding and analysis of knowledge base is limited and superficial to support claimed insights.	The experiences chosen for inclusion are central to the insights. They are analysed competently and creatively to support the emergence of insights.
Consideration of ethical factors around the notion of the right thing to do and congruence with my values	10	Little evidence of an ethical understanding for practice. Inadequate reflection on the impact of one's values and intentions to guide practice.	A robust insight into the value of ethics and values to guide practice showing a clear appreciation of the nature of ethical dilemmas.
Consideration of personal factors, including past experiences, that were influencing my responses	10	Little evidence of appreciating the impact of personal factors and previous experiences in shaping responses.	The significance of personal factors and past experiences in influencing clinical judgment and action is critically analysed, revealing a deep sense of self.
Critical juxtaposition between an informing literature and insights	20	Limited range of literature explored with over-reliance on secondary sources. Weak dialogue between the literature and insights resulting in unconvincing juxtaposition.	A broad range of primary sources is evident with good critical analysis and juxtaposition leading to compelling and creative insight development.
Consideration of how insights will inform my future practice	10	Unconvincing claims as to how insights might shift practice with insubstantial consideration of the ability of self to act on insights.	A clear exposition of the way insights might or has shifted practice alongside an appreciation of those factors that might constrain responding in new ways.
The paper is presented in a suitable, aesthetic and scholarly manner	20	The structure is fragmented. Written expression makes some of the arguments difficult to access. Lack of appropriate signposting and planning. Does not engage the reader. Careless referencing.	Written expression and presentation is clear and concise. Paper is well structured and flows creatively and coherently throughout around insights and engages the reader in its creative form.
	100		

Module: Reflective Practice   [Code:]

Name of student

1st marker   2nd marker

Figure 8.3   Professional doctorate (PD) osteopathy – assignment criteria for reflective essays (second draft).

They have few classroom skills in dialogue. They lack courage, imagination and risk. They treat students as generally irresponsible adopting a maternal pedagogical stance – critical and comforting parents to potentially naughty and hurt children. Teachers are judgemental and derisive of poor students. Listening to teacher banter. One teacher says to another, 'that student can't have more than one functioning brain neurone'; the other replies, 'you're being generous'. General laughter. I want to say (but don't), 'perhaps it is your poor teaching that is the problem.' The transactional world always blames the individual, not the system that has failed this student and no doubt many others.

Teachers lack practice credibility and are often far removed from everyday clinical issues. Teachers have poor leadership. I sense teachers' hackles rising as they read this. The natural defence to the threatened ego – and yet if we do not know ourselves as teachers, there is no hope for any radical curriculum. We get more of the same insipid stuff.

Judging reflective writing

I recently explored with a group of third-year adult branch nursing students about their experience with reflection. I had read the group one of my stories. One student exclaimed 'that's just how I see reflection but when I wrote like that I was told it was too descriptive.' They complained that teachers constantly say 'the work is too descriptive.'

They were expected to use a model for reflection and yet the cues had not been explored with them in any depth. It is superficial and possibly harmful to say their effort was inadequate.

Academic reflective writing should focus on what insights/learning have I gained juxtaposed with a relevant literature? (The literature could be wide ranging from philosophical texts, newspapers, novels, etc.)

In other words, academic reflective writing should not focus on the reflective process, although description of the event and specific reflective cues will naturally be used within an exploration of insights/learning gained. Academic work that utilises art medium always requires a commentary whereby insights are clearly set out. In Figure 8.3 I set out a potential assessment grid whereby I have identified key criteria and weighting. Of course, such judgement is a speculative and moveable feast. The key is the balance between criticality and creativity. The second draft reflects greater weighting to the creative and scholarly presentation of the paper.

Programmes

In 1992 I set up the 'becoming a reflective and effective practitioner' programme at the University of Luton (now Bedfordshire) (60 credits and level 3, equivalent of four units). The programme was constructed as 20×3-hour sessions – a mixture of workshops around specific topics and guided reflection sessions delivered over 30 weeks. It was a truly innovative programme that accepted nurses and midwives across diverse backgrounds.

The students had three assignments:

1 Reflect on a single experience, using the MSR, and critically explore the insights gained.
2 Develop a personal theory of reflection based on theories of reflection and your own experience during this programme.

3 Reflect on the reflexive development of your expertise during the programme drawing on (at least) three experiences.

An analysis of assignment 3 consistently demonstrated the extent of learning achieved through this programme, as evidenced in the narratives written by Clare, Jim and Simon (Chapters 10–12). Other published narratives from this programme are Johns and Hardy (2005), Morgan and Johns (2005), and Johns and Joiner (2010) (Johns 2010a). Jill (Chapter 9) wrote her narrative as the final assignment of the BSc palliative care degree.

Conclusion

The reflective curriculum is a vast subject. Essentially it turns on its head the traditional relationship between teachers and students and between theory and practice. Reflective learning cannot simply be bolted on to existing curriculum from a technical rational perspective. Yet, it can be implemented by reflective minded teachers, if they are brave and savvy enough.

Notes

1 I outlined dialogue in Chapter 1.
2 MJ McGraw, personal communication.
3 Margaret is a PhD student within the school of reflective practice, performance and narrative inquiry at the University of Bedfordshire.
4 Johns C (2009b) Reflections on my mother dying: a story of caring shame. *Journal of Holistic Nursing* 27(2): 136–40.
5 Unpublished narrative.

Chapter 9

Reflection on touch and the environment

Jill undertook the BSc palliative care programme at the University of Bedfordshire. The assignment for the holistic practice module asked her to reflect on the development of three aspects of her practice. She works as a night staff nurse in a hospice and chose to write three exemplars around one patient, Sally, concerning touch, the environment and spirituality – all concerned with a broader question – how can we create places of healing? Touch and environment are the focus of these two brief narratives, although both are infused with a sense of the spiritual. You might assume that the use of touch is fundamental to nursing practice and yet how mindful and skilled are nurses at using touch? You might also assume that every practitioner should be skilled in using touch as an expression of caring, mindful of its benefit and wary of its intrusion, whether bathing, comforting, massaging or whatever.

Jill's text raises significant issues for anybody who claims to care. It points to assumptions grounded in tradition, authority and embodiment that rise like demons to blight nursing's therapeutic quest. Jill does not state her vision. It is implied in her words, enabling the reader to grasp the creative tension that flows through the text.

Touch

This narrative concerns my experience with Sally who struggled to accept her horrific circumstances as life slipped away. Sally was diagnosed with acute lymphoblastic leukeamia 2 years ago. She underwent a bone marrow transplant, which completely cured her illness. Eighteen months later she developed cutaneous T-cell lymphoma caused by graft versus host disease. There has only been one other case like this reported in the world! Filled with astounded disbelief Sally was left to suffer the consequences of this devastating condition with the knowledge that no curative treatment is available.

On admission to the hospice Sally is in the terminal phase of her illness. Using selective literature, I enhance and substantiate my intuitive awareness that many skills used in palliative care are not formally taught in nursing school but acquired during life experience and personal study. I aim to explore the depths and meaning of touch to gain insight

Becoming a Reflective Practitioner, Fourth Edition. Christopher Johns.
© 2013 John Wiley & Sons, Ltd. Published 2013 by John Wiley & Sons, Ltd.

into its therapeutic value. By reflecting on my thoughts, feelings and reactions of the care I administer, I aim to gain insight to improve my nursing.

The evening reports continues: 'Her skin is burnt all over, each movement causes pain creating many difficulties with her care. She is having trouble coming to terms with her condition.'

The words reverberate; perhaps it is us who is having the trouble. I say nothing.

My mind troubled, I leave the office and wander along the corridor greeting patients and informing them that I am here tonight. A penetrating nauseous vapour fills the air leading towards an open door. Standing at the doorway my eyes transfix onto the small wispy figure covered only by a thin linen sheet. Her face, peaceful in sleep, disfigured by ferocious, sore red patches that connect and weave their way into every crease and feature of beauty. The main attack centres on her eyes producing a monstrous appearance of two cracked shivering starfish oozing from tentacles. Small mounds of decaying skin cling desperately all around her head reluctant to completely give up and let go. Goose pimples emerge on my arms; my body shudders coldly ending the momentary glance.

On autopilot, I continue to the next room. Disgust and horror overwhelm my mind as I smile at the clean-shaven unblemished tanned face of the gentleman sitting comfortably reading. Conversation readily flows, we discuss the beautiful view from the window but my brain struggles to dismiss the suffering in the previous room.

Sally calls for assistance. She requests I cream a very sensitive sore area on her back. As my hand approaches an invisible layer of heat 3 inches from her body penetrates my skin. Like entering a hot oven I carefully make contact with her slippery flesh. The cream dissolves into oil and trickles onto the sheets. With gentle circular movements my fingers attempt to coat the raw burning tissues of Sally's back, lubricating the rippled surfaces. Feelings of sadness and hesitance are replaced by pleasurable sensations. The moist warmth infuses through the dryness of my hands creating suppleness and ease. In silence, I continue covering any area of need, enjoying the experience of Sally's relaxation radiating through my fingertips.

'That's wonderful,' she whispers. 'You're not wearing gloves.'

Startled I question, 'Should I be?'

'Well I'm not contagious but everyone wears them because it's so revolting.'

Sally's reply is nonchalant.

Checking for approval, I ask, 'Would you prefer that I wear gloves?'

With eyes closed Sally relaxes, smiles and mouths, 'No, no it's lovely.'

Continuing our intimate interaction until the peacefulness of sleep encompasses Sally, I leave feeling enriched by this encounter.

Returning to the office, thoughts of gratitude swell my mind. How privileged I am to work in an environment that values and prioritises time with patients. Gone are the days when I was considered a time-waster! De Hennezel (1998, p. 61) speaks to me: 'how often are nurses rebuked for wasting time when they follow their heart's natural instinct and give a little of their simple presence to the sick.' Even in a hospice I sense the underlying culture that we do things to people rather than essentially be with people.

As morning slowly emerges, I draw back the curtains enabling Sally to witness the beauty of the sunrise over the lake. She smiles whilst beckoning me to her, taking my arm she thanks me for last night. Our eyes meet as I reassure her that I also benefited by creaming my neglected hands.

Sally rushes into conversation about her history and prognosis. As if frightened that I might leave her, she holds my hand tight. With resentfulness she recounts her story, bewildered how or why she has to suffer such torment. Restrained by her grasp I can only listen, no words are available to explain or bring comfort. Normal responses of stroking the hair or hugging are inappropriate due to causing excruciating pain. Motionless, I stand as the painful darts of information enter my heart, and compassion is portrayed through facial expression and contact. Consumed into the depths of reality and truth, I feel Sally's pain opening, disturbing craters in my soul. My mind wanders to things I should put right and others that I want to do before I die (Autton 1996). Slowly an awareness of death is expressed, as De Hennezel (1998) observed many times. Like panning for gold I sieve through each word. Trickling down the mountains of despair is a tiny but clear meandering stream of hope and desire. The simplicity of Sally's needs brings tears to my eyes. Lowering my head, a spontaneous kiss reaches her erupting cheek; fragments of her scabby skin cohere to my lips but I only feel love. Sally mouths a return gesture, smiling we squeeze hands and disengage.

'See you later,' I whisper, leaving her space. Sally nods closing her eyes.

Sally's history in report left me dumbstruck. What could I say to her that would make a difference, alleviate anguish and help her find peace? As Autton (1996, p. 121) agrees, 'In some circumstances words can be more of a hindrance than a help.'

By using touch, I relayed my feelings to Sally (Talton 1995). I had the intention of achieving connection with Sally through physical contact. Sympathy and empathy can be exchanged by touch as Edwards (1998) explains citing Wyshcogrod (p. 801): 'fellow feelings that you and I are one.' I wanted Sally to know I cared, to break down the barriers of being strangers and facilitate her journey of acceptance. Estabrooks and Morse (1992) use the beautiful phrase 'bumping souls', which sums up what I wanted to achieve. Sally and I 'tuned in' to each other through the caring touch (Fredriksson 1999). I find amazing peace inside me that so much can be gained without the use of words!

Touch has been categorised as task oriented, caring and protective (Fredriksson 1999, Talton 1995). Task touch is the most commonly used by nurses and does not always have the intent to communicate in a positive manner. It can be defined by 'hurried, rough, jarred movements' relaying 'frustration, anger, or impatience' (Fredriksson 1999, p. 2). I find this comment disturbing and not true in the hospice. Because of the horrific condition of Sally's skin I was very wary of how I apply the cream. Taking time to register Sally's reaction to my contact and constantly reassessing our intention, I was able to ensure that we understood each other. To make the mistake of hurting Sally would create fear of me administering treatment and in turn cause anxiety instead of ease (Davidhizar and Giger 1997).

The disgust I felt on first seeing Sally produced intense guilt. The T-cell lymphoma had totally consumed her skin into a revolting, stinking mess. I suppose it would have been normal to reach for gloves. However, I felt they would create a barrier within the touching process, preventing skin-to-skin contact. I wanted to communicate my acceptance of Sally despite her disfigured body. Autton (1996) describes how reassuring physical contact can be transferred by healing massage. Transmissions of pain and touch have joint nerve pathways (Talton 1995). The gentle movements of my fingers on Sally's back initiated relaxation and eventually sleep. What better way, during the night, can there be of dealing with personal mental trauma? So often, as hospice nurses, we turn to sedatives to induce sleep but I am learning that giving time to patients is more effective and rewarding. This can be demonstrated clearly in the way that Sally acted in the morning.

If I had created a barrier by wearing gloves, would Sally have received my message? No, I think it would have intensified her feelings of self-repulsion and ugliness. I didn't even consider using gloves. Sadly, when I tried to discuss this with my colleagues, they dismissed the idea and requested that we should all wear aprons as well to protect our clothes! My words fell on stony ground, as if I have touched something deeply threatening they inherently recoiled from. When they look at Sally do they only see disgust rather than this suffering woman? If we choose to work in hospice then such attitude must be confronted, yet with compassion, understanding that this is not easy work. We need to reorient our values to being with rather than doing to.

Writing this reflective narrative has heightened my awareness of the physical and therapeutic areas of touch. Chang (2001) observes, 'touching is an integral part of human life' (p. 2). Within the nursing environment using touch is a normal, frequent method of administering care both physically and psychologically. Nurses are also allowed to enter the private zones of the individual through intimate touch due to societal agreement (Hickman and Holmes 1994). However, consideration must always be given to ethnic background, personal history and social connotations to ensure that touch is appropriate and authentic (Talton 1995). Turton (1989) reminds practitioners to be mindful of their use of touch and its therapeutic impact. Ochs (2001) suggests that we should always ask permission before touching patients or family. I find it more agreeable to continually assess the person's reactions (Talton 1995). The meaning of touch is personal and can only be translated by the recipient (Chang 2001).

Surprisingly, Estabrooks and Morse (1992) note, 'One of the most neglected areas of touch in nursing research is the investigation of the touching behaviours of nurses.' These authors suggest that nurses develop their own touching style through individual life experience and training. It is a comfort to know that touching can be a learned behaviour, especially when observing those who appear to have a comfortable natural ability of its proper use (Estabrooks and Morse 1992).

Commentary

Reading the text, what emerges as significant for you the reader? On the surface it is a narrative about the significance of being with Sally. Underneath, and yet barely mentioned, the text is about an environment that constrains being with patients, which I feel is particularly significant.

Jill alludes to the idea that massaging Sally might be considered 'time wasting', drawing on words by De Hennezel for support. She points to the underlying culture of nursing where being with patients is not considered proper work. Perhaps one reason is that nurses feel ill-equipped for such emotional work. De Hennezel (1998, p. 61) writes, 'many of the people I've met at the bedside of the dying feel themselves to be useless and ill at ease in this situation of just being there and not doing anything.' You might wonder where such attitudes stem from. My glib answer is 'deep in nursing lore' whereby nurses were instructed to maintain a professional detachment from patients (Menzies-Lyth 1988), reflecting a subordination to the medical model that separated mind from body and focuses on disease processes. The contradiction with any claim to holistic nursing is obvious.

The disgust expressed by Jill's colleagues is disturbing. It resonates with the idea of body work as dirty work – the body work behind the screens (Lawler 1991), with the need to protect self from both its physical and emotional impact. The apron protects not just the body but forms an emotional barrier, as if it is death itself touching me. Jill does not reflect on her response to her colleagues' disgust. We could speculate endlessly about that.

Jill's own initial disgust at Sally's blistered and festering skin is a powerful confession. Sally had learnt that her skin was disgusting for the nurses to treat. She had embodied that knowing. Hence she expected Jill to wear gloves whilst applying cream. Jill hadn't even considered wearing gloves (or so she says) because she knew, tacitly, that wearing gloves would be rejecting Sally.

As practitioners go about their practice they touch people in different ways. Sally emphasises that touch is a vital part of healing, not just physical touch but also the sense of touching someone in an emotional way. Turton (1989) reminds us that 'To put our hand on someone's shoulder or take someone's arm are such apparently simple and commonplace acts that we can easily forget that touch is the most important sense in human growth and development' (p. 42).

Sally's text prompts me to question my own practice, notably, 'Do I convey disgust in my posture?'

Jill's attention to Sally was an act of remoralisation, inspired by the work of Frank (2002a). Frank, who was being treated for cancer, describes his experience with a blood technician: 'As this technician went about her work I remarked how skilful she was compared to some other technicians. She then said something to me that had a direct reference to my complaint but also elevated the occasion to a wholly different plane – "Remember," she said slowly, "everyone who touches you affects your healing." That technician [amongst many] is the one who drew me into a relation of care, in the full sense of *remoralisation*. She recognised, and she found a way to express that recognition, that she was not just extracting blood as a part of a diagnostic procedure, but was also affecting a change in who I was as a result of touching me' (p. 18).

Frank makes the point that caring 'is not a substance or thing . . . not merely the taking of blood but is possible only within "relations of caring . . . not as a puzzle to be solved but as a mystery"' (p. 13). Frank asks what did the technician mean by using the words 'touch' and 'healing'? The words capture the sense of caring: the mutual exchange as something in Frank touched the technician, that she was open to and could listen to his suffering. From this perspective, touch to be recognised as caring is more than a technical thing. Indeed, being touched without a sense of being cared for, without a sense of intimacy is demoralising, the sense of being treated as an object. It is the antithesis of caring. For Frank, this experience was remoralising – that the technician placed him firmly on his healing journey. In other words, the role of any caregiver is to remoralise the patient, to help him or her grow through the illness experience, to emerge as more whole having been cut to pieces by the cancer experience, even for patients who are dying, who feel torn apart. Touch is then healing.

Jones and Jones (1996, pp. 184–5) write, 'Touch is the harmonic healing the grieving spirit craves. A gentle touch on the back, the shoulder, the head, the hand tells the receiver more than what can be expressed. Hands held can quickly heal and bind together more than months of psychotherapy. Touch is the great gift of self that offers immediate renewal and certain connection for both the receiver and giver.'

Environment (Jill)

Slowly washing my hands in the cream enamel basin my eyes wander around Sally's room through the mirror above the sink. Wilting, shrivelled stems interspersed by youthful blooms hang from vases. Stagnating in discoloured water they silently scream for attention. Twisted chocolate wrappers hide between magazines haphazardly balanced on the bedside table. Walkman cables, compact discs and tubes of cream create a 'modern' work of art. 'Get well' cards lie abandoned, children's drawings huddle in a corner and photos of loved-ones faces face the window.

An unintentional arena of chaos faces me as I turn around, feelings of claustrophobia creep inside my body. I need some space. Each item of furniture is overburdened with unnecessary clutter. The floor extends storage pads and dressings; red 'infected' linen bags openly display their contents.

Reaching for a paper towel I dry my hands carefully ensuring that nothing is knocked from the nearby shelf. Gadgets of hygiene engulf the small wash area whilst the sad magnolia walls absorb the atmosphere of dull isolation and neglect. Sally is asleep so I tiptoe away.

Standing outside the hospice a refreshing night breeze hits my skin. A stabbing tightness tightens my chest; Sally finds even ripples of air painful on her burning flesh. She is cocooned in the moist 'foul smelling' warmth of her room. Aromas of freshly mown grass fill my nostrils but Sally's sense of smell has become numbed by continuous stench. Confined to her bed through weakness but craving independence, she is rendered helpless in personally changing her surroundings. I wonder how she would arrange things if able?

Entering the main entrance a beautiful arrangement of fresh flowers adorn the foyer. 'Welcome' signs invite my arrival and homely décor instils comfort. Windows proudly display wonderful views of nature, a lake, gardens, wildlife and an abundance of glorious, towering protective trees. The corridor turns revealing a quiet area of cosiness to relax, chat with family or befriend other patients. Visually nothing to fear is apparent except the word 'hospice' all around the building!

An intoxicating fetid odour invisibly digests the air, as I get closer to Sally's room. 'Can't sleep,' she whispers as I move blankets and clothes by her bedside. 'Can I tidy your room?' slips from my mouth. Smiling Sally giggles, 'Where will you start?'

Mesmerised by activity, Sally remains quiet. Within half an hour her environment evokes order, cleanliness and thoughtful comfort. Nursing supplies are secretly hidden in cupboards. Smeared surfaces now shine with approval. Photos smile at Sally from wardrobe doors and cards hang appreciably over head displaying their messages of comfort. Wiping tears of joy from Sally's eyes I ask if the room is to her liking, nodding contentedly Sally pours into conversation centred on memorabilia. Time rushes by, twilight creeps across the sky bringing a new day. Exhausted Sally drifts leisurely into the land of dreams.

How many times do I ignore the irritating untidiness of patient's rooms? Actually the answer is never. Mess constantly annoys me but I don't always clean it up! Neither do I consistently take time to consider how patients feel about their surroundings.

Sally craved her independence, but it had been snatched from her. She would have loved to keep her room tidy, bright and cheerful. Her pleasure when seeing her room tidy and family photos smiling at her confirmed it. Yet why had we allowed her room to get in such a mess? It suggests we do not pay much attention to the impact of the environment on her well-being. Florence Nightingale turns in her grave.

Sally is vulnerable and silent. The intra-subjective world of the patient is discussed by Sumner (2001), who claims the patient becomes vulnerable, in need of help due to illness. Summer states, 'the patient comes to the illness-induced interaction hopeful that this exquisite vulnerability will be acknowledged' (p. 4). Hope that this will happen comes from 'a yearning for a recognition or consideration by others of unmet needs' (p. 4). Morse and Dobernect (1995) mention the determination of the patient to endure the unpleasant 'side effects' of illness (cited by Sumner 2001, p. 4), in this case the mess in her room.

I felt she had lost something of her identity in the mess and that she had become part of the mess.

Loss is described by Robinson and McKenna (1998) as having three attributes:

- Loss signifies that someone or something one has had or ought to have had in the future, has been taken away;
- that which is taken away must have been valued by the person experiencing the loss;
- the meaning of loss is determined individually, subjectively and contextually by the person experiencing it (p. 7).

Each point is salient regards Sally. A sense of guilt burdens me that we had let her room get into such a mess. Chris challenges me in the group: 'how do I ensure that all staff respect the patient's environment?' 'Can I be influential in changing attitudes?' I like to think so, but I already have a reputation for complaining about care issues. People tend to agree with me but nothing gets changed as if the place is infected with inertia. A focus for future experiences, that is, if I persist with reflection after the course is completed. The value of reflection is to lift these things into consciousness, things we take for granted or get complacent about, but then we also get complacent about reflection. We need to establish a regular reflection group at the hospice where such issues can be aired openly and acted upon.

The daily nursing rituals of ward rounds, checking that everything is 'ship-shape' has long gone (Biley and Wright 1997). In an investigation by Rogers *et al* (2000) on the sources of dissatisfaction with hospital care, the environment comes right at the bottom of the list! This research included 229 people but only 6 complained about untidiness, or dirty bathrooms. Am I to believe that hospitals and hospices are very tidy, clean places? Unfortunately we nearly all have personal stories to tell, or have heard disturbing reports to the contrary. Is it good that people are so grateful of our care that they feel unable to express their concerns? Sometimes I feel that in nursing we have gone from one extreme to another. For example, identifying the task of cleaning to a particular person usually, in my opinion, gets the job done, whereas relying on individual commitment unfortunately often doesn't! This is a good example of why the stench from Sally's room had not been dealt with. Everyone had to be aware of its existence, with the exception of Sally, but nobody took responsibility to act.

The sense of smell is the most immediate of our senses due to the olfactory nerve being directly connected to the brain (Davis 2000). Smell is also the most fleeting of the senses, fading occurs when one is exposed to a smell for a long time (Davis 2000, p. 279). Sally sadly had become a victim of this. I know that Bergamot is one of the most effective deodorising oils (Davis 2000), so why didn't I take the time to discover this oil and use it? Davis also informs that Bergamot is an 'uplifting' oil producing a relaxing atmosphere for the anxious, depressed person (p. 57). Although Sally had lost her sense of smell she still could have absorbed the oil into her bloodstream through inhalation via the lungs (Davis 2000, p. 281). Music can be used to improve the nursing environment and has been demonstrated to decrease pain, reduce anxiety and promote relaxation (McCaffrey 2002). Sally obviously appreciated music, a walkman and compact discs were in her room. Given the potential effectiveness of this non-invasive pleasure, 'it should be offered to all hospital patients in all situations that are known to be stressful' (Evans 2002,

p. 9). Music improves the mood of patients and may reduce the need for sedatives (Evans 2002, p. 9).

My mind fills with a picture of Sally's room. The light is dimmed, Bergamot penetrates the air and soft sounds ripple in the background. Serenity. How easy it is to produce a peaceful haven. So why didn't I achieve this for Sally?

The environment has an enormous impact on both patients and their families. Wuest (1997) argues that a broader conceptualisation of environment needs to become a focus for nursing action. I second that!

Conclusion

Jill's narratives of touch and environment are transgressive in confronting individual and collective practice. Through her rich evocative description she draws the reader's attention to significant aspects of person-centred practice that may be hidden in the technological glare of practise. Her dialogue with theory is limited but adequate to frame the issues in a wider compelling literature.

Chapter 10

The emotional cost of caring

Reflection brings us face to face with ourselves.
There is nowhere to hide as we gaze into the mirror,
that is, unless, we turn our head away,
bury it in the sand,
failing ourselves and those we serve.

Simon writes[1]

I work as a charge nurse on a medical ward. Nursing is a demanding profession. The commitment we invest in our roles provides us with our greatest source of reward – the ability to use our position to aid others. This interpersonal aspect of nursing when encountering people at their most vulnerable is the foundation of our practice and its fulfilment is the foundation of our satisfaction even though the price of constant exposure to emotionally challenging situations can be high. Can we avoid this expense? Or can we grow through it? Can we become overexposed to death and dying, resulting in emotional detachment that undermines holistic care and prevents us from using ourselves in therapeutic way or learning from the experience?

By reflecting on my involvement with Bill, a 40-year-old man who died of cancer, I am attempting to discover the factors that influenced my feelings and actions.

Standing at a shade over 6 ft tall, weighing a muscular 14 stone, the smiling face on the photograph provided a shocking contrast to the image of its owner sleeping in the bed. I use the word shocking in response to how cancer specialises in the distortion of features and expressions more rapidly than a cosmetic surgeon's knife and in a fashion that only first-hand witnesses could believe. When the bones, normally concealed beneath a physique developed through good living and exercise, become not only visible but the dominating feature in Bill's experience, it becomes a cruel irony of nature that many years of development can be so undone at a rate that growth can never equal.

We described Bill as cachexic, a single word to describe so much. As professionals we are very comfortable and familiar with our terminology. It becomes very easy to use and the words can soften their meaning. This is a user-friendly language that cannot portray what it describes. Cachexia is defined as abnormally low weight, weakness and general bodily decline associated with chronic disease, most notably cancer.

In reality, however, it is the image that Jane (Bill's wife) tries to spare her sons – Joe and Tim – from seeing, fearing nightmares and difficult 'why?' questions. It is the sight

Becoming a Reflective Practitioner, Fourth Edition. Christopher Johns.
© 2013 John Wiley & Sons, Ltd. Published 2013 by John Wiley & Sons, Ltd.

of a loving son, a devoted husband and doting father reduced to a living skeleton barely able to acknowledge everything in a life that is dear to him and those who love him struggling with their pain.

Bill was admitted to our ward when symptoms of his lung cancer began to overwhelm him and his family. It had been a short disease process typical in its presentation and diagnosis. The dry cough that had failed to respond to linctus annoyed Jane so much that she wore down Bill's reluctance and persuaded him to go to the general practitioner (GP) who sent Bill for a chest X-ray. The film showed a shadow that in turn resulted in bronchoscopic biopsy and diagnosis. Simple, systematic and effective intervention. It is the impact that has the medical profession floundering like a bully having its bluff called; 'so what are you going to do now?' You can almost sense the taunt.

Radiotherapy was marginally successful in reducing the size of the shadow. Isn't *shadow* an easy word to use, avoiding the dreaded 'C' word but managing to remain mysterious, sinister, and often, for the patient, ambiguous? But tragically, its postponement of the inevitable was its only consequence. Subsequent community management with the input of Macmillan nurses had kept Bill at home until uncontrollable pain and nausea necessitated admission to the hospital. The original plan was to achieve symptom control to facilitate discharge as soon as possible. However, the best laid plans of mice and men. . . .

Bill could feel the pain through his chest wall. A subcutaneous syringe driver containing diamorphine and cyclizine was used to manage his pain and nausea. These drugs were initially effective, but the diamorphine needed to be increased within hours to achieve adequate pain control.

Bill had lost his appetite and was unable to keep fluids down long enough for them to be of any value. He looked dry and blood tests confirmed this impression. An intravenous infusion was commenced to correct his dehydration. Secondary to his reduced fluid intake Bill experienced oral candida and some painful oral ulcers. Anti-fungal and ulcer medications were prescribed and regular mouth care was provided. Bill was nursed on a pressure-reducing mattress.

Over the next couple of days Bill's condition stabilised and improved enough for him to have visit from his sons. They were aged 8 and 12 years old. Jane had protected them as much as possible by shielding them from seeing their father when he had looked so unwell. During this period, over three to four shifts, I got to know Bill quite well. He was intelligent and articulate, and we shared mutual interests in sport and music. We shared a similar sense of humour and managed to make each other laugh frequently. I wished I had the opportunity to know Bill for longer. Bill and I were disagreeing about England's World Cup chances as I left the ward for 2 days off. Bill invited me to call round and see him when he was at home as we were aiming for discharge in the next 2 days. I replied that I would try but I knew deep down that I wouldn't. Not because I doubted that Bill would get home, but once a patient goes home we prepare for the next one. Our busy schedules are exactly that and how much time and involvement should one invest? I sense Carmack's (1997) challenge of balancing engagement and detachment – and yet how can I be detached when clearly I seek engagement? I see no way of drawing a line that marks a limit to engagement. It is absurd to suggest otherwise. The skill is to develop a greater sense of poise if I am to be available to patients like Bill and his family (Johns 2009a).

On one occasion, whilst completing some paperwork, I found myself watching Bill as his family visited. The indelible image was that of seeing the boys at the foot of his bed and simultaneously touch their dad's feet as their mum hugged him. The boys so needed the physical contact but seemed reserved and hesitant until Bill held out his arms and the boys rushed to him and held him tightly. They seemed scared to let go, and Bill, eyes closed, tried to absorb and retain every precious moment, knowing how valuable time was.

Later that evening, I checked on my sleeping son and cried as I recalled what I had seen earlier. My emotions were a combination of anger at how peoples' lives are so sense-lessly destroyed and fear generated where the fine line between life and death is made so visible and where our own mortality is questioned.

Returning from my days off, I noted that Bill had been transferred into the side room. I immediately asked the nurse looking after Bill what had happened? She informed me that Bill was close to death. He had become increasingly dyspnoeic due to the develop-ment of an extensive pleural infusion. A pleural aspiration had been performed, which had alleviated some of his breathlessness. However, the effusion was a sign of general deterioration that warranted increased analgesia and a sedative to control his developing agitation. Bill's deterioration was rapid, the disease's only concession to Jane's feelings – 'he's not in pain, is he?' Jane urgently inquired. Before I could respond, Jane continued, 'I wish we could have him home.' I responded by saying that Bill was asleep and peaceful, indicating that the medication was effective and that we were continually assessing his condition. Jane was obviously distressed that Bill had not got home as she repeated her statement to herself shaking her head and crying. 'I think Bill's main concern was to have you all here.' I responded, looking towards the sons, trying to highlight to them how important their presence was to their dad. I continued: 'Holding his hand and talking to him is the most you can do regardless of where you are.' Jane forced a smile in my direc-tion and nodded in agreement. She turned her attention to Bill and her sons. Feeling somewhat uncomfortable with the ensuing silence, I asked a typically English question 'Can I get you a cup of tea or anything?'

Bill's family visited at regular intervals as he slipped into unconsciousness. I continued to let the family know that I was there for them should they need anything. Within an hour Bill died. I stood silently, deprived of the sanctuary of offering tea. I withdrew to allow the family privacy. Jane was very protective of her sons and through her grief she remained strong for them. They were distraught and through their tears betrayed a vacant, disbelieving look; in this instant they were experiencing emotions with demands beyond their tender years. Their sobbing provided a heart-breaking image and I was revisited by the twin impostors of anger and fear and a feeling of frustration at my helplessness.

I offered my condolence simply by expressing how sorry I was and instinctively touched Tim's arm as he stood next to me. Jane took my hand and thanked me for all I had done. I repeated how sorry I was and said how I liked Bill a lot. She seemed to appreciate this and smiled. I was glad that I told Jane this. I felt for some reason that this was important to me as I knew that I would not get another chance to hint at the impact looking after Bill was having on me. The practical aspects were discussed with Bill's brother-in-law and provided a sense of relief that comes with taking refuge in practices over which we have some control.

Reflecting back on this story, Bill required a subtle balance of physical and psychologi-cal care typical in palliative nursing. But its influence on me as a person, and subsequently as a nurse, was atypical. I found myself experiencing fear, helplessness, inadequacy, anger and levels of distress that I had not felt since my earliest nursing exposure to death and dying. Farrar (1992) recognised these emotions in novices. However, my experience is far beyond novice so why do I seem to be regressing? I initially perceived these feelings to be barriers to effective care as they can elevate stress levels and compromise my ability to carry out clinical care objectively. In providing psychological support I have always felt it prudent to keep some distance between my empathy and my personal feelings, a kind of conditional empathy whose extent is determined by my feelings of discomfort and my emotional self-defence. In short, the experience has exposed barriers in my attitudes that, unless resolved, will impact negatively on my practice.

My reflection illuminates the darkest areas of my practice and reveals the source of my fear, anger and frustration, and guides me in my attempts to learn from them and apply my understandings in practice. Bill and I had much in common that stimulated me to empathise to the extent that I was forced to confront my own personal experience of loss and my own mortality. I felt helpless at not being able to alter the course of Bill's prognosis or lessen the impact on his wife and sons. These are perfectly normal human responses but need to be fully understood to turn them into positive emotions, rather than areas for personal conflict and distress. The majority of my nursing practice has been in care of the elderly environment, and my dealings with palliative care in my own age group have been limited. In managing the needs of the older patient, I can see that I could have more easily employed coping mechanisms that dilute the personal impact and subsequently lessen the felt distress. This is not to say that terminal disease is any less tragic for the people involved or that it requires any less skill or commitment on the nurse's behalf. But I am able to rationalise the event and see it more objectively. In examining my thoughts related to my own mortality, it is clear to me that it is a subject that I have actively avoided. McSherry (1996) details the importance of discovering our attitudes to mortality in order to resolve our barriers to death and dying. The experience of observing the trauma of Bill's sons brings back memories of my own father's death that I have not allowed to impact on my nursing due to the upset that they still evoke. Reisetter and Thomas (1986) consider that these are the very emotions that we need to expose and incorporate into our practice. In avoiding applying my own experience into my practice, I am denying a major source of personal knowing. Utilising this knowing would enhance my care as I could use my subsequent increased capacity for empathy to understand my patients' needs more acutely and view this closeness as a bridge rather than as a barrier.

Applying my own anxiety and fear of death and dying to provide a door to another's actions and thoughts rather than a subject to be dispelled immediately on appearance gives me the opportunity to provide true holistic care. The question 'how would I feel if that were me?' should not only be accepted but encouraged if holism is our objective. In revisiting my father's illness, I am reminded of the doctors, nurses and therapist that we came into contact with and the way they made me feel. Whispering at the foot of the bed, head shaking when reading the notes and being stared at by curious student nurses are memories that I seldom, if ever, relate to my own ideas of nursing. Do I whisper over my patients, leave patients perplexed and terrified with the shake of my head or the raising of an eyebrow, or forget the individual's right not to be a source of medical curiosity? I wish that I could cast the first stone at these sins but in reality I fear that I cannot. I worry that a lack of true empathy that can prevail when we lessen our humanness leads to a provision of care guided by a form of nursing 'autopilot' that demands little from us. I am equally reminded of the staff who respected my father and our family with their time, skills and most of all their understanding that meant so much to us so much of the time.

I want to leave a positive impression of my caring on those with whom I come into contact and recognise the factors that reduce this possibility. I hope that Jane's memories of Bill's hospital care are reassuring. I will then have achieved something. At times I feel like a voyeur, impotent, unable to achieve practical goals that would make myself or Bill's family feel better. The danger of containing these feelings is that I carry them around with me into the next similar scenario, immediately creating a barrier.

I have never been 'taught' to use myself in a therapeutic way or to deal with feelings that such work evoked. Such realisation seems shocking given the nature of suffering. Yet suffering has never been the focus of nursing work. Indeed, it might be argued that the patient's suffering has been avoided within the partial lens of the medical model and task approaches to practice. My realisation resonates with James's (1989) compelling observation that *emotional labour* is generally unrecognised, viewed as unskilled, and as such, not taught.

Through reflection I am now in better shape to use my frustration and anger to enhance my care. Being able to value the care I give reduces my frustration and allows me to accept my limitations, whilst my anger can be channelled into striving to improve in all areas of practice. Anger experienced by patients is often part of the grieving process (Kübler-Ross 1969), but its impact can be damaging if there is no justifiable recipient to direct it at. In harnessing memories of my own anger when experiencing my father's illness, I can detect this in difficult and aggressive people and avoid dismissing them as irritating or their behaviour as meaningless.

The anger I felt at seeing a man deprived of the opportunity to love his sons, enjoy and nurture their growth has to be managed and resolved to avoid extreme levels of stress and potential burnout. In response to this I am committed to working with our palliative care team to establish a support network for ward nurses to explore, share and hopefully resolve emotional fallout from our work. I am now a more complete nurse through knowing Bill. Reflection has been enlightening, supportive and rewarding.

Challenged by my guide, I wonder to what extent I would like to have responded differently given the situation again? Certainly to be more poised. I am certainly more conscious of creating a ward environment to facilitate holistic care. As a leader, I now see a bigger picture and have become more sensitive to staff who struggle with the emotional demand of our practice. This is most noticeable in shift reports when I always ask the nurse how is the person and family feeling and how do you feel about them?

Commentary

Simon's narrative blends emotions and reasoning. I image that few practitioners will not feel the emotion and transformation within and between the words. For many nurses working on busy medical wards Simon's story will be well known. Simon's narrative is a search for meaning in the suffering and joy he experienced. It reflects the complex nature of holistic practice. Perhaps he might have stood back and asked what is holistic nursing? Is it realistic given his experience? Without doubt, 'the self of the practitioner' is his primary therapeutic tool within any claim to person-centred practice. It follows that 'the self' needs to be kept sharp enough to cut the cloth in skilful action. No mean feat unless we offer watered down holistic practice.

The idea we can separate the personal self from the professional self is challenged by Simon's story. Morse (1991) identifies the risk of 'over-involvement' whereby the therapeutic gaze becomes blurred through entanglement with the other. This is always a risk when the practitioner does not know himself or herself well enough. Becoming over-involved may be a necessary learning journey, for how else can I come to know myself? The fear is 'getting in too deep'. The metaphor suggests drowning, of becoming submerged in another's suffering. Yet Simon was willing to 'go there' and dwell with Bill and his family. In dwelling with the family and letting go of the urge to 'fix it' for them, he could explore the depths of their suffering with them. That he absorbed their suffering and suffered himself is human nature. None of us are immune from that but through guided reflection he was able to make sense of his emotions and grow through the experience. He was able to use the energy from suffering positively. As Rinpoche (1992) writes, 'when we try and defend ourselves from suffering, we only suffer more and don't learn what we can from the experience' (p. 316). Reisetter and Thomas (1986) showed a significant relationship between high-quality palliative care, reduced stress levels and the individual nurse's ability to draw on personal experience of death and dying. This would seem to suggest that practitioners who have the motivation and ability to reflect on their experience as a method of development are better equipped to respond effectively to the needs of their patients. In contrast, Atkinson *et al* (1990) detail the way people deal with personal loss by viewing it in abstract terms that 'prevent us from internalising and personalising questions surrounding our mortality and death.' Practitioners who are able to utilise their own experience to enhance their personal knowing are in a better position to respond to the needs of their patients and the impact upon themselves, and understand the feelings, attitudes and prejudices that influence behaviour.

Most relationships fall within a person's 'normal' intimacy boundaries and are not problematic. But as Simon experiences, experience sometimes falls outside normal boundaries, resulting in anxiety. Menzies-Lyth (1988) writes,

> The core of the anxiety situation for the nurse lies in her relationship with the patient. The closer and more concentrated this relationship, the more the nurse is likely to experience this anxiety . . . a necessary psychological task for the entrant into any profession that works with people is the development of adequate professional detachment. (pp. 51–4)

An alternative and more coherent view is for the practitioner to develop an adequate professional involvement whereby the practitioner can acknowledge the limitations of her ability to ease suffering rather than adopt a detached posture. The risk of detachment is a loss of intimacy and a denial of self as caring (Benner and Wrubel 1989).

Jones and Jones (1996, pp. 183–4) write,

> Uncomfortable with the griever's uncertainty about life, deep sadness, encounter with death, and changed self, we turn away when we are needed most. Look at times when, perhaps, you have turned away – what were you avoiding? Most likely it was your own uncertainty, your own sadness, your own changes, your own mortality.

As a consequence of reading this narrative, practitioners will inevitably reflect on their own feelings and practice with dying patients and their families when next at work. Teachers may use the narrative to spark dialogue with students concerning the nature and difficulties of palliative care. The narrative is a powerful 'call for action' when caring on medical wards is threatened by diminishing resources. Initiatives such as the Liverpool Care Pathway are helpful to draw attention to dying patients but I suspect that such tools become little more than a prescriptive checklist. They may even discourage the practitioner from seeing the person.

Note

1   This narrative was constructed as an assignment whilst undertaking the 'becoming a reflective and effective practitioner' post-registration undergraduate programme at the University of Bedfordshire. The programme was designed with 60 credits spanning two semesters.

Chapter 11
Life begins at 40

Clare writes

It was Pitkin (1932) who coined the phrase 'life begins at 40' and how right he was. The first day I attended the 'Becoming a reflective and effective practitioner course' also happened to be my 40th birthday and when my life as a reflective practitioner was to begin, although at that point in time, I could not have envisaged the significant impact and influence the course would have on me.

What follows is the story of how my practice has developed as a result and an analysis of factors that constrained my development. This will be illustrated through a series of experiences I wrote in my reflective journal which, when viewed alone, are perhaps not of great significance. However, like a child's dot-to-dot picture, it is only when the dots are joined together that a tangible picture becomes clear.

At the beginning of the course I recorded my feelings and thoughts at the end of the day on a separate piece of paper in my journal. I felt I was reflecting. This made me question why I needed to be on an 8-month course to do this. It was only when I began to share my experiences within the group did I realise that all I was doing was stating what had happened and how I had felt. It was when I was challenged and *forced* to examine my feelings and view the situation from different perspectives that I started to learn from my experiences. However, it still took some weeks and a comment from Chris, the course tutor, who informed me that 'an effective practitioner is an informed practitioner', for me to ashamedly acknowledge to myself that knowledge acquisition does not happen magically but does in fact require a degree of effort on my part.

Electrocardiographs (ECGs)

Within my current practice, one of my clinical responsibilities is to perform electrocardiographs (ECGs) for all the inpatient units of the hospital. Initially I found this interesting. However, once the novelty had worn off, I viewed it as a task that had to be done. My lack of enthusiasm was quite evident in my journal entries until one day following an attempt to perform an ECG, my journal entry was very different:

> When I arrived on the ward I was shown in to the ladies bedroom. I introduced myself and started to explain the procedure. The nurse interrupted me, stating that I was wasting my time:

Becoming a Reflective Practitioner, Fourth Edition. Christopher Johns.
© 2013 John Wiley & Sons, Ltd. Published 2013 by John Wiley & Sons, Ltd.

'she doesn't understand a word you are saying, she has dementia'. My anger levels rose but I carried on trying not to let my feelings show. The lady looked at me with watery pale blue eyes and, speaking in a language of her own, was trying to tell me something but I was unable to understand her; she kept tugging at my arm, getting more frustrated with tears falling down her cheeks. I reassured her that I would not be performing the ECG and left the ward. The image of her eyes stayed with me, had they once been sparkling deep blue, full of life and what had those eyes seen in their 82 years of existence? I felt disgust with the nurse for treating her with disparagement and disrespect, but I also had to acknowledge the uncomfortable feelings within myself about my view of performing an ECG as a tedious task and had appreciated the privilege of entering into this intimate relationship. . . .

The impact this experience had on me was immense; it enforced me to examine my attitudes, beliefs and focus my thoughts upon the nurse–patient relationship, especially the challenges faced when the patients' ability to communicate is compromised.

What sense do I make of this? Morse (1991) states that the nurse–patient relationship is established as 'the result of interplay or covert negotiations until a mutually satisfying relationship is reached'. She discusses the types of relationships that exist and divides them into two categories: mutual or unilateral. The latter she describes as being asynchronous, with one person unwilling or unable to develop the relationship to the desired level of the other. Morse (1991) provides an example of why mutual involvement is not possible; that is, when a patient is unconscious or in a psychotic state. Due to the fact that the lady with blue eyes was suffering from dementia automatically forced her into a unilateral relationship.

Rao (1993) believes the act of communication comprises all of the ways that people send and receive messages. However, Miller (2002) draws to our attention that most people do not think about the way they communicate on a day-to-day basis and are often unaware of how they relate to others; yet communication is essential to our development as social beings, and it is the ability to communicate that enables the development of short- and long-term relationships. What happens then if the ability to communicate becomes impaired? Bush (2003) suggests that people who cannot communicate or who communicate inappropriately are often marginalised by society and run the risk of social alienation and diminished function and that as a result of the frustration of being unable to make needs and feelings understood by others, challenging behaviour and behavioural disturbances can occur. It has been proposed by Lliffe and Drennan (2001) that communication with the patient suffering from dementia may be the key to understanding and resolving behaviour disturbances. One method of communicating with people with dementia is validation therapy. This was developed by Feil (1993) and attempts to help persons deal with their feelings by validating them, subsequently helping them to move from their inner world to the shared reality of the present. It is claimed that validation therapy promotes communication with the severely confused older persons on their own terms, on subjects and issues that are chosen and are important to them, assuming that all the words and actions of a person with dementia have a real sense of purpose and value.

Picking up the story, as a consequence of confronting and examining my feelings, my attitude towards performing ECGs altered. I no longer viewed it just a task that had to be done as quickly as possible but recognised that although only brief, I was engaging in a relationship with another person who should be given time and respect. Having shifted my viewpoint, I found that I once again I found performing ECGs a positive experience. I was mindful of this when I received an ECG request from one of the wards that specialises in treating elderly people who are more severely confused, suffering from dementia or other organic brain disorders. The name on the ECG request seemed vaguely familiar; however, I was not prepared for the shock when I was introduced to the lady. Sitting slumped to one side with saliva dribbling out of the corner of her mouth was a lady with whom I had contact with about a year ago when she received a course of elecrtoconvulsive therapy (ECT) to which she responded well. My last memory of her was of a bright, smiling, physically fit lady in her 50s who was able to return back to her work, which incidentally was as a healthcare assistant on one of the other elderly wards. This is an extract from my journal entry for that day.

> When I first saw her the shock was immense, like a jolt of electricity had surged through my body, causing my skin to prickle and take a sharp intake of breath. It took me a moment to recover. What message had my face portrayed and had she seen it? How lonely must it be to be trapped inside a body, unable to communicate verbally, and how must it feel to be reliant upon nurses, with whom you had once worked along side with, to feed, wash and dress you . . . what is it about this situation that I find so uncomfortable? I perform ECGs on other patients who are unable to communicate verbally and do not feel the same. Perhaps the sadness I feel is that she is too young to be treated on an elderly mental health ward and that her own profession has in some way let her down. . . .

I remembered Chris had recommended an article about silent advocacy (Gadow 1980) and I set about finding it. However, it was then that I started to question my motives for doing this. Was it that being more informed about a situation helps me to become a more effective practitioner or was it to help me resolve my uncomfortable feelings and feel better in myself?

It was this conflict that I shared with the group at the next session. I began by sharing the experience and discussing the conflicts I faced, which was helpful. The focus of the discussion wandered slightly with issues around communicating with patients with communication difficulties examined. One of the group members made a comment about how some nurses, without realising it, treated people as objects and lost sight of the person and challenged me on one aspect of my practice: ECT. I was defensive and categorically stated that within the ECT department, people were treated with respect, dignity and as individuals.

This comment niggled away at me. During the next two ECT sessions I metaphorically took a step back and observed with more critical eyes how we regarded and treated the patients receiving ECT. I was reassured that the mental health nursing team did show respect for the patient, taking time to explain procedures and provide reassurance, although once the patient was asleep the focus of them as a person was lost. One thing that struck me was the amount of people that are present during treatment; on that day seven people, including the patient, were present in the treatment room (Figure 11.1). Conversations took place that excluded the patient.

At the next team meeting I shared this experience and my observations. In order to generate discussion I posed some questions. How would you like to be treated if you were to receive ECT? What aspects of our practice are positive and what areas could we improve upon?

In order to gain a better understanding, I suggested we recreate the scenario as fully as possible to experience first hand being on the trolley with people attaching various monitoring equipment to you. Benner (2003) highlights that good nursing practice requires ongoing clinical knowledge development through experiential learning. However, it is not automatic and requires openness, attentiveness and responsible engaged learning on the part of the practitioner. One of the team members was not a willing participant

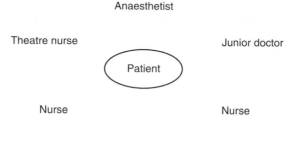

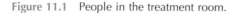

Figure 11.1   People in the treatment room.

at first but did join in and at the end of the session commented that she had never thought about it from the patient's point of view.

We discussed this exercise within the next team meeting. We all felt it was worthwhile and that it gave us a better understanding of how the patients feel before they are anaesthetised. What struck us all was how vulnerable and intimidating it felt lying on the trolley with so many people surrounding you. From this we considered ways we could improve our practice, limiting the amount of people surrounding the patient until they are asleep, encouraging the doctors to have discussions about treatment regimes out of earshot of the patients, and instead of having the radio on, play more soothing and relaxing music. This exercise was only carried out with the mental health nursing staff who felt it would be beneficial for the whole treatment team to undergo this, particularly with the theatre nurse and the anaesthetist who, by the nature of their work, spend the majority of the time with unconscious patients. As Morse (1991) highlights, nurses working in operating rooms use a strategy of depersonalisation which includes transforming not only the person into a patient but also the patient into a case.

According to Sisson (1990), hearing is the last sense to go when a person becomes unconscious. Studies of patients' memories of their unconscious state indicate that they heard and understood various conversations that took place while they were unconscious (Lawrence 1995, Podurgiel 1990, Tosch 1988). It is imperative, as Leigh (2001) points out, that health professionals evaluate the way in which they communicate with unconscious patients. Russell's (1999) study concludes that hospitals are often noisy, which can make the patient anxious, whereas reassurance and explanations by nurses help them to feel safe, secure and feel less vulnerable. This study also found that where nurses became overinvolved with technical equipment and the physical aspects of care, this reduced the level of communication with the patient. While Podurgiel (1990) and Green (1996) both recommend that personalised care should be given, through the use of effective communication strategies such as speaking directly to the patient and using touch to enhance communication and express emotional support, Dyer (1995) cautions that touch is a two-way process, and permission should be sought before a nurse invades a patient's personal space.

At the end of an ECT session I shared our experiential experience with the theatre nurse, hoping that she would be receptive to the idea of participating in a similar exercise with the anaesthetist. 'Whatever did you want to do a thing like that for?' was her cynical reply. I attempted to explain that I felt it was important to view the care we gave from the patients' perspective. She ridiculed such an idea: 'What a load of poppycock, how do they know what they need, we are the anaesthesiology specialists not them, so how can they possibly know what they need and I certainly do not need to lay on a theatre trolley to know how to do my job.'

She left the department with very ruffled feathers and I felt irritated and disappointed as this extract from my journal entry shows.

> My emotions are all in a muddle like a big ball of spaghetti lying heavily and uncomfortably in the pit of my stomach. I have experienced these feelings before. When I was a child in primary school there was one particular teacher who, no matter how hard I tried to please and gain her approval, she always knocked me back, leaving me feeling angry and frustrated and confused. Only now I am not a schoolgirl. I am a professional practitioner and believe in what I am trying to achieve. Why do I always let her get to me? Why do I feel intimidated by her and unable to assert myself with her when I can with other people . . .?'

When I read this extract in the guided reflection group, Chris, in his ubiquitous coaxing manner, simply asked, 'so why do you let her get to you?' A silence descended over the group as I contemplated this question. Was it a simple identification with a teacher from primary school? How could I know that? I connected this experience to another experience that concerned a junior doctor who was constantly late and on one occasion did not show up at all. I had no hesitation in letting the doctor know my feelings.

Chris asked, 'how can you change things?'

I couldn't imagine how I could.

Using transactional analysis (TA) (Berne 1961) to examine the pattern of communication between myself and the theatre nurse, I discovered where the breakdown of communication lay. The theatre nurse's response was not the adult response I had invited. Instead, it was a cynical dismissive response I linked with the primary school teacher. It conjured up similar feelings that left me seething. I became the 'hurt child'. I had spoken to her as an adult, she responded as a critical parent. Stewart and Joines (1987) describe this as a crossed transaction. *Cross* is an apt description of how I felt! Looking again at how I communicate with the theatre nurse, it became evident that I often revert into 'child mode' in response to her 'critical parent mode'.

Chris asks, 'So how can you stop reverting to a hurt child mode?'

I confessed 'I don't know.'

Chris asks, 'Imagine the situation again – how might you respond differently?'

I mused 'he's using the MSR cues'. It reminded me of star wars and using the force. Uncanny. I smiled 'smack her in the teeth!' The group laughed. The spell was broken.

Applying the TA framework was most helpful using the labels of critical parent and hurt child – it enabled me to visualise the relationship between myself and the theatre nurse and, perhaps most significantly, engendered the feelings associated with those labels. It was illuminating and challenging, and prompted me to examine my patterns of communication with other members of the team towards promoting more effective collaborative working.

Insight

The point of reflection is gaining insight. Am I more available to my patients? I have been starkly reminded of my vision to realise person-centred nursing. I had become complacent! Practice had become routinised as if I was on auto-pilot most of the time. What a wake-up call! My concern for patients was relit. I learnt something about myself and my communication skills improved. Perhaps, most significantly, I acted to create a more therapeutic environment. Checking out insights is significant because it helps to solidify learning.

One of the biggest factors that hindered my development was myself. At the beginning my attitude was arrogant, and the reasons for attending the course were influenced by the educational credits that could be obtained. Although I consistently kept a reflective journal, my entries were descriptive, inexpressive and once written, were not returned to. I am not sure when exactly my transformation happened as it was a gradual process. However, I remember feeling uncomfortable when other members of the group shared their journal entries. The words of a teacher who taught spelling came back to me. He said, 'If you cheat you are only deceiving yourself and it will be you who has to face the consequences.' I felt like an impostor and my atheism would be exposed at any minute.

This journey has been lonely at times, but having under gone a complete transformation of my attitude and realised the power that reflection has to change and improve practice, I wanted to share this enlightenment and sought after converting my colleagues to my newfound faith. However, in my passionate and overzealous approach, what I in fact achieved was to alienate my colleagues, not bring them on board. I realised that in order for me to have any influence, a drastic modification of my approach was needed.

There were times on this journey that I became exhausted, and on occasions I wished I could remove my reflective lenses and view things through my old eyes. Reflecting daily on my practice constantly highlighted areas that need modification or change.

Has attending this course helped me to become an effective practitioner? The answer is unequivocally yes. Although I am a novice in the world of reflection, I realise the potential reflective practice has on shaping the future of our profession whereby we can begin to value our practical expertise as a profession (Bulman 2004). In a relatively short period of time I have under gone a revolution of myself as a practitioner. For me, one of the immense values of this course was that the process of reflection was guided. Being in the reflective group helped me to remain focused and motivated me to continue on my journey. If my reflective journey had not been guided, then I feel it may well have been more of a magical mystery tour.

Reflection

Many practitioners, like Clare, are initially resistant to the idea of reflective practice. She had the idea that reflection was just writing things on a bit of paper. I expect many practitioners feel like Clare, especially if they are just asked to write and not have the opportunity to share their writings in expertly guided sessions. When Clare broke through her resistance to experience the transformational potential of reflection, it was a revelation.

Clare took her insights into the group guided reflection for dialogue, especially in relation to her difficult feelings about the theatre nurse. She felt helpless. In the group, the 'spell was broken' as if by magic. And that is often the way it works. Clare reframed her relationship with this person without further difficulty. That is as far as we know. Tomorrow is another today.

Inserting excerpts from her journal gives the narrative richness and authenticity. Reflect on the evocative richness of Clare's language: 'the lady looked at me with watery pale blue eyes and, speaking in a language of her own, was trying to tell me something. . . .'

And later in the same passage, 'the image of those eyes stayed with me: had they once been sparkling and deep blue, full of life, and what had those eyes seen in their 82 years of existence?'

It is not easy to see people as objects when you look into their eyes. Perhaps one reason nurses avoid eye contact. A disturbing thought.

Again in the same passage, 'I felt disgust with the nurse for treating her with disparagement and disrespect, but I also had to acknowledge the uncomfortable feelings within myself. . . .'

In this passage I sense the cathartic impact of writing. The experience transformed her.

Chapter 12

Balancing the wind or a lot of hot air

Writing a narrative is a creative act. Yet finding the right style can perplex writers. I find it helpful to read widely, absorbing the writer's narrative style. Fiction and autobiographies are most inspiring. One writer who inspires my narrative writing is Jeannette Winterson. In *Lighthousekeeping* (Winterson 2005) she writes, 'A beginning, a middle and an end is the proper way to tell a story. But I have difficulty with that method' (p. 23). As I have learnt for myself, the flow of the creative mind doesn't work that way. I wonder who told Jeannette that was the proper way? A thought as you read Jim's narrative.

Jim writes

If you take the Christian bible and put it in the wind and rain, soon the paper on which the words are printed will disintegrate and the words are gone. Our bible is the wind.

(Anon, Native American)

My journey towards becoming a reflective practitioner has been exciting, challenging and cathartic. I have travelled nomadically through theory and practice in my effort to regain the vision I once had as a fresh-faced nursing student, a vision that has become clouded by the bureaucracy and politics of mental health nursing.

Reflection (following Johns 2009a) is learning through my everyday experiences towards gaining insight. The learning potential is the contradiction or creative tension between my vision of practice and the way I actually practice.

Reflection is not without its critics. Mackintosh (1998) argues it is a flawed and a passing fad which will be replaced by another. However, I come to praise Caesar not to kill him. I will attempt to show the reader how reflection has enabled me to develop my practice. My patient, Mary, has given me permission to talk about her in this narrative. There is no happy or sad conclusion for her. This narrative is merely my quest to find some answers to life's complicated questions for the sake of Mary and all the Marys I

Becoming a Reflective Practitioner, Fourth Edition. Christopher Johns.
© 2013 John Wiley & Sons, Ltd. Published 2013 by John Wiley & Sons, Ltd.

have yet to meet. As Mary says, 'life is not like the movies . . . maybe there will be a sequel'.

Names have been changed to protect the innocent or guilty.

Mary

The sun filters through the patio windows. Wogan in the background prattling on about this and that (have I really become a tog?). Strange! Radio 2: who would ever have that on at 7:30 in the morning. Wogan plays 'White Man in Hammersmith Palais' by the Clash (Strummer and Jones 1978). As Joe Strummer sings, my mind wanders back to the late 1970s when, as a pimply faced youth with freshly bleached spiky hair, I wandered down the Kings Road in London, deaf, hoarse and exhilarated having just seen The Clash perform at the Hammersmith Palais.

Inspired, Terry Wogan turned off, I place my 'Best of the Clash' record on the turntable, pump up the volume as much as acceptable. A 'fluffy moment', the iron in front of me, I set it on 'linen' and prepare to press my suit – Matalan, £40, navy blue, wash 'n' wear. I bought it when I commenced as acting ward manager on an older person's ward for mental health. I am due to take the lead in a multidisciplinary team (MDT) meeting later this morning. I feel I need to make a good impression. My insecurity bites.

Twenty-five years from the release of the Clash; from safety pins in ears, bondage trousers and leather jacket to a £40 Matalan suit. Have I really become the establishment? A different uniform for a different time, but what of the uniform of the mind? Have I changed that much inside and if so, how did it sneak up on me without me even knowing? Can I find me again within a job I love yet still be accepted by my peers and fight for the right of patients?

Mary has been known to the mental health services for about 5 years. She saw her nephew who she raised murdered by another member of the family. Her own mother had died when Mary was with relatives in New York. During her time there she had been trapped on a burning train whilst riding the subway. The clinical diagnosis: post-traumatic stress and psychotic depression. Physically this manifests as chronic facial pain. Many treatments had been tried – dental treatment, analgesia, X-rays, referrals to pain clinic, electroconvulsive therapy (ECT) – none of which has had a satisfactory outcome for Mary. On two of her many admissions, whilst on leave, Mary had succumbed in desperation to overdosing her prescribed medication. As a consequence she was placed under Section 3 of the Mental Health Act that allows the authorities to detain her in hospital for six months.

This resulted in Mary being nursed on a high level of observation, granting me the opportunity as her key worker to engage with her in plenty of conversation. I knew her and she trusted me. Therefore, negative comments such as 'She's putting it on', 'It's all in her mind', 'She's not helping herself' and 'She's attention seeking', which are flippantly bandied around by my fellow professionals, give offence (the right hump!). As Mary's key worker, I could argue that I knew more about what makes her tick than other members of the MDT. At the meeting today I need to get 'our' point of view across and advocate her needs.

My trusty suit may just assist in this process. I m going to be one of them in a room full of 'suits'. Playing the game – the game identified by (Stein 1978). The object of the game is for the nurse to be bold, intuitive and be responsible for making significant recommendations whilst at the same time appearing passive so that it appears that the doctor made the decision. The game is designed to preserve the doctor's authority. The reward for the nurse is the doctor's patronage. Failure to play is 'hell to pay'. Through earlier reflections, I have become more mindful of this game and my part within it, becoming better able to express my opinions without being passive or subordinate. The game sucks. It insults my self-respect to play it. Yet I play it. I play it because I fear the consequences of not playing it, not so much for myself, but for the Marys.

The pain clinic referral

The referral to the pain clinic by the senior house officer (SHO) has been overlooked. Everyone had assumed this had been done. Frustration went from simmer to boiling, anger vented at the nursing team. Hackles on the back of my neck start to rise. It was the doctor's responsibility, why should we have to chase after them? The doctors close ranks – the finger of blame pointed towards myself. They are trying to put me in my place.

I feel the tension as I struggle to stay in the right place to advocate for Mary and for myself. My collar is too tight. My integrity hung out to dry! Dear reader, you may think that as an old punk rocker I would relish 'hell to pay', but there is something very sinister about the way nurses are oppressed. Maybe if I was wearing bondage trousers I could have overthrown the establishment. Perhaps it is 'the suit' that keeps me in place.

Benner (1984) argues that in the initial stages of learning we are acutely aware of what we are doing and our failings. Put another way, being consciously incompetent, knowing that you are struggling with something, and the frustrations that ensue. In not knowing how to deal with something, it is always best having one's arsenal, somebody or something to aid me. My arsenal was a battery of reflective tools and guidance within the guided reflection sessions. But most of all it was being open and honest with myself, as I have always endeavoured to be with patients like Mary. No longer hiding behind my 'funny man' posture and cropped shock of bleached hair. No longer trivialising academic effort. I had to grow up and take responsibility for myself supported by a cup of jasmine tea at the ceremonious tea party that infused each guided reflection session and a glass or two of beloved 'Stella Artois' to shift the blockages when reflection become stuck.

Mary's family

Mary's family mysteriously appears for 15 minutes on pension day. They had agreed at an early family meeting to pay Mary's bills whilst she was undergoing her healing process. Several months later Mary was £750 in arrears with her rent and utility bills – yet more stressors adding to her distress and depressive state. She was unwilling or unable to challenge her family. Should I intervene on her behalf? If so how?

Weighing up the situation considering everybody's perspective (ethical mapping), I conclude I should act but not directly. I contacted Age Concern who offer an advocacy service. This action was paternalistic, acting on behalf of Mary when she was being harmed and was unable to act for herself. Benjamin and Curtis (1986) set out three factors that must be justified to warrant acting for the other person:

- Harm – Mary was being harmed.
- Autonomy – Mary was unable to make decisions or act on her own behalf.
- Ratification – Mary would thank me for my actions when she was able to.

My decision to contact Age Concern avoided me coming into direct conflict with Mary's family. Was I too close to the situation, emotionally entangled and losing my objectivity? It's tough to sit by and watch helpless people be abused.

Writing in my journal as this situation played itself out enabled me to freeze the moment and view it more objectively from different angles, digesting and dissecting it, bringing the experience back into focus, surfacing and working through my mixed emotions of anger towards the family, sadness and pity towards Mary, and residual feelings of anger at my colleagues. All stuff bubbling away inside my body cauldron. It's hot in there – what was that about getting out of the kitchen if you can't stand the heat?

This is not the language I would use when at work. It (the journal) does not judge, criticise or threaten to use my words against me at a later date. Holly (1989) believes keeping a journal enables development of an educational archive, to aid insight and enrichment in future practice. Ferruci (1982) argues that journal writing stimulates the 'interchange between the conscious and the unconscious' – how true I have found that to be. Burrows (1995) thinks journals are too time-consuming. Burnard (1995) thinks that they are too superficial. I wonder if they keep journals. My journal allows me to express my anger, thereby diffusing it, allowing me space to deal with events in a more reasonable and professional way. Do I mean professional? Let it go. Johnny Rotten once sang about anger being an energy. I channel my energy using it as momentum to press forward to finding a positive outcome for Mary. I don't like feeling angry – for others would then perceive me as unprofessional (buying into an idea that professionals are impassive or are good at wearing masks to deceive). Buddha states that anger will never disappear so long as there are thoughts of resentment. I sense my residual resentment at the consultant for not hearing me and at the relatives for abusing Mary . . . and the list goes on. Anger and resentment are self-harming. As one American chat show host said, 'Remember, when you point the finger at another in anger, you have three fingers pointing back at you'. Wish I could remember his name.

I write in my journal, 'They (the family) don't give a damn about Mary, they are fleecing her blind. I need to be more assertive and shed my fear of conflict'.

Reading this out in the guided reflection session, I feel embarrassed as if I am some kind of failure. The punk rocker brought to his knees. Exposed as a fraud. Yet the group are amazingly supportive. They all recognise the conflict avoider in themselves, giving credence to research (Cavanagh 1991) that conflict avoidance is the primary mode of being for nurses and nurse managers. What are we frightened of? Why are we so willing to ditch the patient to ensure peace with the relatives and patronage of doctors? Surely dialogue is a better way – being open and honest, or as Chris says, being tough on the issues and soft on the people.

Chris talks me through the assertive action ladder to see at what level my blocks are (see Figure 18.4). Blocked at rungs 3 and 4 – lacking confidence in my authority vís-a-vís others, and with making a good argument, at least in a language that is heard. For certain, it is not easy being assertive in a power-driven hierarchy with the pendulum of punishment swinging, ready to take your head off.

I digress. Getting back to the meeting. During a break for coffee and a smoke, as these meetings last several hours, my mobile phone rings. Elvis Costello (1983) ring tone . . . 'every day I write the book' seems a fitting tone . . . it's my Mum. 'Dad has been to the urologist. It's his prostate . . . they want him to have more tests'.

Sensing her concerns, 'Sorry mum I'm at a meeting, ring you later'.

CANCER – the very thought burns into my being. I need time to take stock. Ethical dilemma – my father's medical records are confidential yet I can gain access. He will have to wait a fortnight for his results but, at the push of a few buttons on the computer, I can get them tomorrow. I contact Dawn, the specialist urology nurse. She has assisted me in the past with clients on my ward. She listens, explains possible treatments, gives me statistics – 60% plus of all men in my father's age range – 70 plus – have prostate cancer and are blissfully unaware of the situation. It's slow growing. Reassuring she says, 'He will probably die of something else before the cancer gets him.' Dawn never pulls her punches – again honesty. We arrange to meet later in the week.

The urology team are now aware that the man under their care is my dad, not just another patient. At least I feel I have done something for now. I also share this dilemma at the guided reflection session. Waterworth (1995) argues that such workshops allow nothing more than a forum for expressing negativity. In my experience this is not so. The session supports and guides and nurtures creativity. So Waterworth, stick that in your pipe! Of course Chris would argue, 'Where is Waterworth coming from, what is the basis for her claim?' And it's true, I partially read stuff and draw hasty conclusions. Stick that in my pipe!

Back at the meeting. The consultant advocates further use of ECT to raise Mary's mood. He argues that the Mary's (psychosomatic) facial pain will be addressed.

I chirp up, 'What about stronger pain killers?' 'I'm not prescribing anything else until the consultant pain specialist has seen her.'

I tap my fingers in frustration. More delay. My eyes burn into the SHO. He avoids my gaze – I smell his guilt.

Cut to several weeks later.

Mary has been having two ECT sessions per week. No change in her facial pain. Little positive change in affect. No word from the pain consultant. The wheels of the NHS turn slowly. My frustration increases. The ends of my fingers will soon be worn thin.

Friday I set up the ECT on my ward. The anaesthetists are on rotation. I check the list. Dr Zaphon. Something jolts my attention. A 5-minute check on the computer. Yes! Yes! Dr Zaphon is the consultant in pain specialist, the one and only scarlet pimpernel (they seek him here, etc.) and he is walking right into my sticky web! By pure chance, destiny, good luck, say what you will, I have the opportunity to affect change and move Mary up his waiting list. Imagine the scenario: 'Good morning Dr Zaphon, would you like a cup of tea?' Learnt behaviour. Hitler is raining bombs around my patient's head yet still the English make a cup of tea.

Dr Zaphon comes with a formidable reputation: 'I am the Boss and what I say goes.' I sense the challenge that awaits me. Be careful Jim, he is a right one for putting people down and making complaint if you cross him, so say my pals from theatres. Little room for manoeuvre. I imagine the scenario: 'Dr Zaphon, while you are here can I please draw your attention to a referral we made some months ago (suitable fawning posture). His face like thunder, assuming the stance of the critical parent. I do not wish to be perceived as pushy, must remember the game. I can't simply change the rules and expect him to be different. It would only lead to conflict as we cross vectors of communication.

Through the thick veil of self-concern I see Mary and remind myself: 'What do we do our jobs for? So sorry if my patient gets in the way of a smooth day at the office.'

I mentioned Mary and got short change. A curt response: 'I'm not wearing my pain hat, here to do ECT. Focus on the task ahead.'

He is giving me the right hump, again trying to put the little nurse in his place. But the old Jim is still there – a voice in my head says 'focus the anger', reflecting in the moment, drawing upon the assertive action ladder, playing the game, acknowledge the doctor's position, back to the job in hand.

Part of the ECT procedure is to give the doctor a brief history of the patient prior to treatment. Adjust the tie, make good eye contact, positive stance (show your professionalism Jim, blind him with your personality). Back and forward from controlled self, pushy and yielding, finding the balance, being adult, not being put into child mode. Anticipating the situation gave me the chance for my 'scheming self' (rung 5 on the assertiveness action ladder for the uninitiated) to come to fore. What better optimum conditions to maximise my effectiveness would I ever get? My vision is focused. I understand intuitively the boundaries and my authority within the game. I have the right to assert myself on behalf of Mary. I am empowered and by being coercive maybe I can just make him listen. So much for my ruminations, what about the real event?

The procedure went smoothly. I like to create a positive atmosphere for clients and staff alike, but this morning I use more manipulative tactics. Dr Zaphon likes jazz. I had found this out earlier from Geoff from the anaesthetic team when jazz pianist legend Oscar Peterson was on the stereo.

Whilst Mary is being recovered and I'm thanking the team, I turn the conversation to the choice of music. I mention that my father had once met Oscar Peterson at a showcase in the mid 1970s. Dr Zaphon's eyes lit up. I recount this experience and mention my dad has recently been seen by the urologist, casually mentioning the urologist by his first name, and saying how delighted my father was with his care. Using the first name term of reference I aligned myself on first name terms with Dr Zaphon's peers. Levelling the playing field. Light banter and a second apology for confusing Dr Zaphon's remit this morning. The previous tense atmosphere is diffused.

Dr Zaphon had been on call the previous night; three emergency caesareans and a road traffic accident had contributed to his tetchiness. He said he would look into Mary's referral but made no promises, stating that he is a busy man and my client is just one of many. He would ask his secretary to arrange something. Buddha's teachings come to mind 'to utter pretty words without acting on them is like a fine flower without a fragrance'.

I feel better. I have used a newly acquired skill, an art form, and understood it. I played the game skilfully and yet I had still played the game. Patterns of relating are deeply embodied and not easily shifted. But I feel stronger, the balance has shifted.

'Ring, ring' . . . 'Hello, older adults mental health, Jim here, how can I help you?'

'I am Dr Zaphon's secretary. I have an appointment for next Tuesday for Mary. Do you think you can make it as well? You must have left an impression, he never changes his mind.'

Will wonders never cease? Excuse me if I feel slightly smug.

Jones and Jones (1996) say that before we can help another we must first address our own bruises, and in doing so, we become real, we become who we must be. The truth of these words flood through me. I cannot help Mary until I had helped myself. That is why we fail patients because we fail ourselves. Reflection is enlightening, empowering and ultimately transforming. If we remain stuck in oppressive patterns of relationship we simply cannot grow. Instead we fester and rot, stewing in our oppression and misery. I climb out of the box I was put in.

The suit has now been resigned to the charity shop. The bondage trousers, although not suitable for work, still make the odd weekend appearance much to the annoyance of my partner. But without her support this journey would not have been possible. Better than safety pins to hold my trousers together. I have forgotten now who said that we are the sum of many parts, possibly something I read many moons ago whilst training to be a nurse. Bit like this narrative really, more than the sum of its parts when taking as a whole. At least I think so. I'm still learning, not just to play the game, but to shape the game towards a better state of affairs for myself and my patients. A game that has its basis in values and integrity. I'm not always agreeing with points of views and climbing the ladder to work on that assertiveness thing. Demanding in dulcet tones my right to have a voice and be heard. As Voltaire said, 'I may not like what you say but will defend to the death your right to say it.' Again I can't finger the source. Sorry Chris.

I still listen to the Clash but have to sit in the conservatory, but at least my partner now appreciates the lyrical delights of Elvis Costello. Her son is upstairs with a friend.

'Aaron, will you turn that bloody rubbish down!' Hip hop, what's that ball about then? Time to reflect. Intolerance to other views and arrogance that I am right are such destructive negative events. As I read back through this work I acknowledge all the assumptions I have made. I first wrote pseudo-assumptions but that is daft. Assumptions are assumptions although their basis may be questionable. But that's the point of reflection, to reveal assumptions and ask that question: What is their basis? And is that basis right?

Schön and his ilk came from disciplines outside my field of practice. Just because punk music and Native American ideology is not nursing, is it less relevant to inform our values and practice? I would argue that it adds flavour and new perspectives. So when Chris enthusiastically says, 'look what I've found in Native American dancing philosophies', why should I doubt? Get out of the box for it is a coffin.

As I sit in my self-built Japanese tea house (roof structure ongoing . . . you can't rush these things), sipping jasmine tea (thanks Chris), I see baby blackbirds follow their mother, eager for the worms and insects – learning, growing, waiting for the chance to break free and fly from the nest. I too (when my belly is full of worms and juicy bugs) will find the right time and strength to make my own way in the nursing world, not held back by politics or traditions. I am getting there. Reflection has expanded my view of the world. My horizons are infinitely broader. I can breathe more fully. I am enriched through this process. Less bondage.

So back to Mary and my journey to ease her suffering. 'What about acupuncture? Is there a policy? How much would it cost? Would she (the object, not patient), who is taking up valuable time in the MDT meeting, accept it?'

'She has said to me on many occasions, she would try anything. She even stated to me that she regrets the offer from her parents to have all her teeth out for her 21st birthday – apparently that was commonplace for Scottish working class of her generation.'

'They will bring back foot binding next,' says some unhelpful wag.

I could not help but see the humour. To find humour in a negative situation has for me always been beneficial. It relieves tension, creates bonding and does not show up on the monthly fiscal deficit.

Reflection

When I first read Jim's narrative, I was absorbed by his 'punkish' narrative style. It cocks a hoop at academic tradition. It snaps the professor's measuring rod. His humour is engaging, suggesting the value of humour in narrative. The more engaging the narrative the more influence it has to change people and the world. It is a significant aesthetic for the reflective writer to consider. You sense the artist at play with a smile on his face. If nothing else, then the writing has worked in transforming the seriousness, the mundane, the frustrating, the boredom of work into play and fun (Okri 1997).

Jim highlights the balance of the epistemological and ontological when he writes: 'My arsenal was a battery of reflective tools and guidance but most of all it was being open and honest with myself.'

The deeply personal aspect of reflection is captured in his words: 'No longer hiding behind my 'funny man' posture and cropped shock of bleached hair. No longer trivialising academic effort. I had to grow up and take responsibility for myself.'

And then, as if to balance this seriousness, 'supported by a cup of jasmine tea . . . and a glass or two of the beloved Stella Artois to shift the blockages when reflection becomes stuck.'

Pulling out just phrases of Jim's narrative highlights its profound nature that may be missed as you skip across its surface. Reflective reading is engaging with – a meeting of minds and souls – a co-creation.

Chapter 13

A reflective framework for clinical practice

In 1989 I became general manager of Burford Community Hospital. It is a significant moment because it marks the gestation of ideas within this book. My role also encompassed Head of the Burford Nursing Development Unit (Burford NDU) and Lecturer/ practitioner with Oxford Polytechnic (now Oxford Brookes University). Prior to this appointment I had been senior nurse at Brackley Cottage Hospital where many of the ideas that grew at Burford spawned. The NDU had been established by Alan Pearson (1983) as a testing bed to prove the therapeutic value of nursing.

Of great concern was my resolve to implement reflective practice as something lived within clinical practice. This work became framed as *The Burford NDU Model: Caring in Practice*, initially published as that title in 1994 (Johns 1994).

The Burford NDU model: caring in practice

The Burford NDU model is both a reflective and person-centred approach to clinical practice. It was a time when nursing models were fashionable, fuelled by a plethora of nursing models from the USA. This reflected an era where nursing sought a theoretical identity and credibility as a profession emerging from the shadows of medical domination. I might add, an era that has since faded away.

The overall pattern of the model is illustrated in Figure 13.1. At the core of the model is a valid vision for practice operationalised through four systems set within an organisational culture, all constructed to support the realisation of the vision as a lived reality. The two most significant elements of organisational culture are leadership and the learning organisation – both topics covered elsewhere in the text.

Vision

The heart of the Burford NDU model is a vision or philosophy for practice. A vision gives purpose and direction to clinical practice. A vision is not static, merely words pinned on

Becoming a Reflective Practitioner, Fourth Edition. Christopher Johns.
© 2013 John Wiley & Sons, Ltd. Published 2013 by John Wiley & Sons, Ltd.

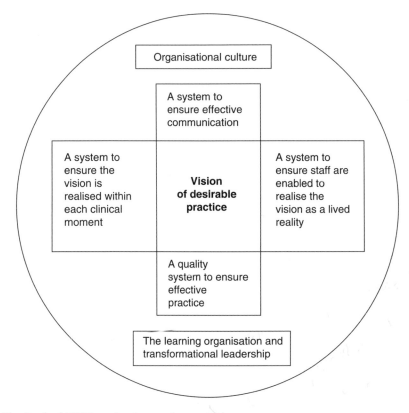

Figure 13.1 The Burford NDU: caring in practice mandala.

some notice board or buried in some dark file. It is an organic living thing that continually evolves. It sets up the learning organisation (Senge 1990), intent upon realising the vision as a lived reality. By *living* I mean it is something embodied, shifting to accommodate new meanings and ideas. A vision is the bedrock of practice, a springboard to guide all aspects of clinical practice and practice development. Where groups of practitioners work together it is self-evident that they need to share a common belief system that gives purpose and direction to practice and learning to ensure a consistent and congruent approach towards patients and families.

Senge (1990, pp. 206, 208) writes, 'When people truly share a vision they are connected, bound together by a common aspiration. Visions are exhilarating . . . they create the "spark", the excitement that *lifts* an organisation out of the mundane.' The words *lifts* – lifting people into a higher consciousness.

In writing a vision, practitioners connect to their caring beliefs and values. In doing so they become empowered. Building a shared vision involves unearthing shared beliefs and values about the nature of practice that fosters genuine commitment rather than compliance (Senge 1990). Leaders learn the counterproductiveness of trying to dictate a vision, no matter how heartfelt. As such, constructing a vision must always be a bottom-up approach to change that enables practitioners to grasp their own destiny rather than have it imposed on them. Then practitioners become active creators of their own practice and take responsibility for realising their beliefs in practice. Vision sets up both resistance and possibility.

Shortly after arriving at Burford, I challenged staff to reflect on the meaning of care within the hospital. I asked them to tell me about the hospital's philosophy. They struggled to articulate this. At that time, the hospital philosophy was 'imported', based on the philosophy of the Loeb Center in New York (Alfano 1971, Hall 1964). Hall's work was a vision of nursing as the primary therapy in its own right, alongside a complementary role to medicine. In 1982, when Pearson (1983) had introduced this philosophy, it made sense in terms of his vision to establish nursing beds. Pearson had departed Burford 3 years previously to my appointment. Now, from the nurses' responses, it was apparent that the Loeb Center vision had faded. It was no longer *alive*. I realised that an 'imported' philosophy imposes a reality on practitioners which denies the expression of their own. Dare I say, the complexity of the model seemed to evoke an anti-intellectual recoil.

In response, I facilitated the construction of a vision that reflected individual practitioners' beliefs as a statement of collaborative intent that gave meaning and direction to our collective practice (Johns 2009a). I invited all practitioners (not just nurses) to post their values of caring at the hospital on a public notice board (I eventually needed two notice boards). One month later, I typed the extensive set of values and circulated them to each member of staff. I then facilitated a series of community meetings to discuss these value statements, leading to a composite statement that everyone could agree. It was written in a relatively jargon-free language to give it access to our patients and families. The process took 4 months to complete.

The value of this exercise was to open a learning space where everyone had the opportunity to express their views and counters any ideological imposition on my behalf as leader of the group. Of course, there was resistance from people who, it emerged, had even resisted Pearson. However, the majority held sway.

The 4th edition (Box 13.1) has been amended from the original to reflect the development of my own understanding of person-centred practice, evolving in light of reflection of its value to adequately represent the nature of clinical practice. I added 'a culture of transformational leadership' to the 3rd edition (Johns 2009a). I now write 'a culture of reflective leadership' (see Chapter 14). The focus on suffering was a profound statement to make at this time, lifting the focus from disease to suffering.

Box 13.1   Burford vision for clinical practice (4th edition)

We believe that caring is grounded in the core therapeutic of easing suffering and enabling the growth of the other through his/her health–illness experience whether towards recovery or death. The practitioner is mindful of intent and is available to work with the person and the person's family in relationship, on the basis of empathic connection, compassion and mutual understanding, where the person's life pattern and health needs are appreciated and effectively responded to.

Caring is seamless across healthcare settings and responds to and promotes both the local community's and society's expectations of effective service. In this respect, we accept a responsibility to develop a culture of reflective leadership and the learning organisation that continually strives to anticipate and develop practice to ensure its efficacy and quality. By appropriate monitoring and sharing, we contribute to the development of the societal value of nursing and health care generally.

Our caring is enhanced when I work in relationship with our (multi) professional colleagues on the basis of mutual respect and care for each other within our respective roles. This means being free to share our feelings openly but appropriately, acknowledging that as persons, we are stressed and have differences of opinion at times. This is the basis of the therapeutic team that is essential to reciprocate and support our caring to patients.

(March 2003, amended 2012)

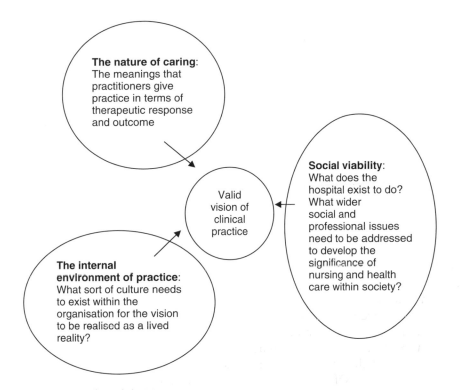

Figure 13.2 Cornerstone of a valid vision.

Valid vision

To be *valid*, a vision for practice needs to address the three cornerstones (Johns 2009a)[1] (Figure 13.2).

The nature of caring

So, what is person-centred practice? Holism is built upon the premise that the whole is greater than the sum of its parts (Smuts 1927). As such the person must be seen as a whole person rather than the sum of his parts. Put another way, the parts must always be seen against a background of the whole person. Now, I would challenge this perspective, suggesting that any reference to parts, still reflects a body-split that detracts from the whole irreducible person. Hence I prefer the idea of person-centred nursing, where the meanings the person gives to their health–illness experience become the focus of care.

Recent experiences of being a partner attending an angiogram have strongly reinforced the way nursing reduces the person receiving care into an object and completely disregard the relative.

The nurse we first met, wearing blues, did not introduce herself. She ignored me. She carried a clipboard and fired a series of perfunctory questions at my partner. Not once did she ask how my partner felt, a quiet astonishing fact given the risk of mortality with stent insertion. The risk of such mindless behaviour is to increase rather than reduce suffering.

Suffering

Suffering is a disruption of the spirit. It manifests on the physical, emotional, psychological and spiritual planes. People suffer because they are afraid and feel alone. Hence, at the heart of easing suffering is connection – connection with self by listening to our own stories and connection with others who listen to our stories and say through skilful, wise and compassionate words and actions, 'You are not alone'.

Nurturing growth

Mayeroff (1971, p. 1) writes, 'To care for another person, in the most significant sense, is to help him grow and actualise himself.' There is no mystery or mysticism to this idea. It does not need to be wrapped up in a web of scientific jargon or elaborate artistic strokes. It is fundamental to life itself and as such must be expressed in its exquisite simplicity. To actualise self is to fulfil one's human potential whatever that might mean for the person (Maslow 1968). Newman (1994) illuminates how suffering creates the opportunity to stand back and take stock of self, especially when suffering becomes life-threatening. Then, one's taken for granted mortality is shaken, forcing self to contemplate life as impermanent. Forced out of our complacency we may question the very essence of our existence and the things that are really important to us. Illness confronts the sufferer with the taken-for-granted nature of health and much of life, prompting crisis – a breakdown where things no longer go smoothly, where things spiral out of control creating anxiety. The breakdown is experienced as a period of disorganisation and uncertainty. Old patterns of organisation no longer work. The person feels threatened on a deep existential level and is thrown into crisis. To overcome the 'crisis' the person needs to learn new ways of organising self conducive with health. As Remen (1996, p. 156) suggests, 'In the struggle to survive our wounds, we may adapt a strategy for living which gets us through. Life threatening illness may cause us to re-examine the very premises on which we have based our lives, perhaps freeing ourselves to live more fully for the first time.'

This can be very difficult as the person is locked into ways of living that are not so easily changed. The practitioner's role is to help the person 'see himself' and to guide the person to reorganise their life pattern in ways that the crisis is resolved.

It is one thing to write words like suffering and growth, yet what do they mean as something lived? How can practitioners best respond to ease it? Such questions lie at the heart of caring practice and my reflective self-inquiry.

Knowing caring

Nurses have tended to view themselves in terms of what they do rather than in terms of what they believe or who they are. It is a functional as opposed to a philosophical/ontological understanding of self. However, does this lack of attention limit nursing's therapeutic potential?

A vision of caring is informed by caring philosophers or theorists who challenge practitioners to reflect on caring. For example, Jean Watson, in her transpersonal model of nursing (1988, p. 49), states the goal of nursing is to help persons gain a higher degree of harmony within the mind, body, and soul which generates self-knowledge, self-reverence, self-healing, and self-care processes while allowing increasing diversity. This goal is pursued through the human–human encounter caring process and caring transactions that respond to the subjective inner world of the person in such a way that the nurse helps individuals find meaning in their existence, disharmony, suffering, and turmoil, and promote self-control, choice, and self-determination with the health–illness decisions.

Savour Watson's words and sense the meaning. Can nursing be defined in this way? Would it suit all practice areas, health visiting, psychiatry, midwifery? Watson spirals nursing out of the realm or shadow of the medical model into a world of existential suffering where the uniqueness and mystery of what it means to be human is fundamental to healing and fulfilment of human potential. Disease and illness are part of that pattern, although the part that often creates crisis for the person.

Watson's words are offered as a moment for reflection, as a challenge to widen the readers' vision of what caring might mean, not as a prescription of how the nurse should think about nursing. I know that such statements may seem far removed from the messy everyday world of practice.

I wonder to what extent Watson's vision resonates with the Burford model?

Nursing as functional gained prominence during the 1960s with the rise of technology and the medical model. Within the medical model, the ill person is reduced to the status of a patient with a set of symptoms that requires investigation, diagnosis and subsequent treatment. Little significance is attributed to emotional, psychological, spiritual and social aspects of being ill or causes of illness. The nursing response is primarily to support the medical task. I am sure many readers will remember being told not to sit on the bed and talk to the patient – there is *work* to be done! The implication being is that talking to patients is not work.

Within this culture nurses suspended their own (caring) beliefs as relatively unimportant to the medical task. Even today, caring has been increasingly subordinated to unqualified staff as nurses continue to embrace medical technology work despite its obvious contradictions with a person-centred approach.

As nurses have endeavoured to define nursing and construct nursing models, nursing as caring has become a sub-culture furtively taking place alongside the 'real work' of supporting the medical model. Whilst it is imperative to assume that all healthcare practitioners value caring, when the head is locked into the medical sphere and the medical sphere is most valued within organisations, then practitioners may lose sight of the caring ideal and fail to realise caring. I know many readers will have experienced this state of affairs when visiting family or friends, or experienced their own health care. It is important to bring this conflict to the surface because only then can nurses take action to resolve the contradiction to realise caring as a lived reality rather than as some nice ideal. Yet in a world where the health agenda is dominated by productivity, and a culture of 'more for less', times are hard for caring. Practitioners may switch off their caring, simply because it is too painful to witness suffering and the failure to ease suffering. Indeed, as Halldórsdóttir (1991) suggests, suffering is caused by the lack of caring (see Tom's and Joan's stories in Chapter 3). The focus of quality agendas on the 'patient's experience' offers a glimmer of light into this black mechanical void, if nurses can be political enough to grasp the opportunity. The emergence of story as a quality marker is also a helpful positive movement away from the starkness of number crunching approach to quality that simply reinforced the fact that patients are numbers to crunch.

From this exploration we can see that caring is the *balance* between *doing nursing* – reflecting theories and necessary skills, and *being nursing*, reflecting ontological ideas about what it means to be a nurse in terms of selfhood and relationships. This balance is *craft* – skilful, purposeful, ethical, compassionate and informed action, or *praxis* for short.

The internal environment of practice

The internal environment of practice is primarily concerned with the relationships between healthcare practitioners who work together – the healthcare team. The team exists to serve the patient with each professional bringing specific abilities to the table. As such, the team needs to develop collaborative ways of working together based on shared purpose, respect and responsibility. However, collaboration of the multidisciplinary team has been exposed as a myth due to the traditional domination of the team by doctors (Rowe 1996). Classically doctors have asserted team domination.

Ask yourself, does the pattern of relationship between colleagues reciprocate the *working with* pattern of relationship with patients and families? Relationships between colleagues must be invested in dialogue around shared purpose, that acknowledges and values each person's view, that is mutually and genuinely supportive. Fine words, but they need to be lived as a reality. It requires each practitioner to have an assertive voice; a voice that is connected to the patient's and their own experience, informed, ethical, passionate, respected and heard. As evidenced in the narratives throughout this book, a predominant focus for reflection is creating an environment to support clinical practice, notably dealing with conflict.

Social utility

Social utility (Johnson 1974) is concerned with the role of the unit within society, that is, what does the unit exist to do? It is responding to and influencing societal expectations, and wider professional issues such as research and teaching, challenging practitioners to look beyond the immediate context of the practice setting towards the wider social and professional communities. From this perspective a vision can be a public statement that challenges society to 'see' nursing differently, as making a significant contribution to the lives of its members and more generally to the health care of community. This is important, considering that so many people in society view nursing as some subordinate role to medicine, and nurses as the ubiquitous 'doctor's handmaiden'. Make no mistake, the general practitioners who had admission rights to Burford hospital would have been happy to patronise nursing. To reorientate society to value nursing requires positive action, yet such positive action is also required to ensure that society's 'new perception' of nursing is constantly reinforced by nurses living out the person-centred vision through their everyday dialogue and actions.

The context of Burford's practice was a community hospital. We felt strongly that the hospital was an extension of the community it served and provided in-patient services for those members of the local community who required medical care, but not admission to the local general hospital 20 miles away in Oxford. The hospital also took local people following major illness or surgery for rehabilitation, respite care and people with terminal illness.

As long ago as 1988, Watson (1988, p. 33) urged nurses to action. She writes,

> Caring values of nurses and nursing have been submerged. Nursing and society are, therefore, in a critical situation today in sustaining human care ideals and a caring ideology in practice. The human care role is threatened by increasing medical technology, bureaucratic-managerial institutional constraints in a nuclear age society. At the same time there has been a proliferation of curing and radical treatment cure techniques often without regard to costs.

Watson's words emphasise the significance of social viability. Practitioners may think that these *political* issues are above them but unless they accept a responsibility for caring on a societal plane as well as within their everyday practice, then there is little chance for nursing to become more valued or assert any political clout to realise its therapeutic potential. The caring ideal as love may be scorned when we as nurses are so damaged or wounded that we cannot care or love. Watson says that it is this love that provides the driving force to care. It is love or compassion for the other that makes the practitioner more available to the other. Simply, without love for the other person, we cannot care because care is love. Without doubt, nurses, midwives, health visitors and all healthcare practitioners are aching to care. Such ache is like a flower that has not bloomed, like a sun lost behind a cloud; if caring is unfulfilled then it turns to acid to scar and burnout. Without doubt, patients and families need to be loved by nurses. They ache for this love, and when they do not receive it, they suffer.

Words convey meaning. The word 'hospice' means 'a place to die' for many people. Improved symptom control and respite care allows a lot of patients to go home and continue living. With this in mind we feel a less disturbing title would be more appropriate. But then why should 'a place to die' be disturbing unless people fear death and dying. Saunders (1975) raison d'être for hospice was to engender more positive societal attitudes to death and dying. So what words would be more appropriate? Specialist symptom management unit? But what message would that convey?

From vision to reality

To ease suffering and enable growth is only known when experienced and reflected on, and only then does dialogue with the words of others becomes meaningful. In my experience visions of practice do not profoundly influence practice. These visions are often written in vague rhetoric, often by a practice leader many years ago, pinned on office walls covered by layers of organisational memos or worse buried away in a policy file. The rhetoric is often grounded in caring clichés such as 'we believe in holistic care' that has no meaning for practitioners and is clearly contradicted by even the most casual observation. It is one thing to say I believe in holism; it is another thing to realise that as a lived reality. I shall assume that the failure to realise our vision is deeply felt and frustrating, eating away at our integrity. Reflection enables practitioners to use their frustration and resolve the contradictions so visions can be realised.

Rawnsley (1990, p. 42) writes,

> Caring may be a desirable image for nursing, but is it meaningful? Is there congruence between the lived experience of nursing practice and the intellectual pursuit of caring as nursing's

professional crest? When living the reality of their practice, nurses need ways through which they can connect the conceptual concerns of the discipline with the raw data of experience.

Reflective practice is the way.

A structural view of a reflective framework for clinical practice

To enable Burford practitioners to live their vision as a lived reality, I designed four *reflective systems* set against a background of *organisational culture*.

A system to ensure the vision is realised within each clinical moment

Imagine I am being admitted to your care service. The basic question you must ask is, 'what information do I need to nurse this person?' Hall (1964) challenges that nurses can only nurse what the person reveals of themselves. As such, the nurse's skill is to create the conditions whereby the person can reveal himself. This may seem obvious in terms of the medical conditions, but more subtle in terms of being a person and the impact of their medical condition on their life patterns and well-being.

Burford hospital used the Roper, Logan and Tierney (1980) activities of living model. My audit of its value indicated the model was an inadequate representation of the hospital's new vision. The model was inherently reductionist, breaking the person into bits of activity that encouraged the practitioner to fit the patient to the model, rather than using the model creatively to see the person.

The audit revealed that practitioners viewed assessment as a task undertaken on the patient's admission. The constant failure to adequately complete the boxes was apparent.

For example:
Nutrition – 'likes a cup of tea in the morning'
Sexuality – 'likes to wear lipstick'
Dying – (most often left blank).

These observations acknowledged the difficulty in seeing such 'activities' as part of everyday functional living. Sexuality reflects who people are. It is synonymous with the person's identity. Even responding to sexuality in terms of the 'sexual act' could not be addressed because of its social taboo. It is difficult to talk to a stranger about sex. It is even more difficult when one's sexuality may seem irrelevant to the healthcare experience. Then assessment can be insensitive and intrusive. Being assessed was felt by patients to be a ritual of depersonalisation – a transition from person to patient. The problem with assessment schedules is that they demand to be completed, especially when audit systems are linked to completion. Hence when an activity of living box was not completed, it indicates the practitioner had not assessed adequately. The effort was to complete the assessment sheet rather than to know the person.

Undoubtedly, the functional approach to nursing has encouraged practitioners to perceive models of nursing from a utility value, often taking or modifying bits from models, breaking up the integrity of the model. For example, *self-care* may have an attractive appeal because it suggests that a target for nursing care is to enable people to regain their independence and return to their level of functioning before the illness event. Yet on a philosophical level, self-care must mean self-determination, being able to take control of one's life in a positive frame of mind. If this is true, then the focus of self-care on functional issues would be misplaced because the functional would always need to be viewed within the meanings the illness or disease had for the person. The focus on functional self-care may lead practitioners to fail to see the person at a crisis point in their lives. Self-care at a functional level is a deficit model rather than a growth model, with its emphasis to return the person to as normal levels of activity. The patient becomes a series of deficits that need fixing rather than a person whose illness pattern is understood within the whole pattern of their life.

The Roper *et al* model is easily understood from a functional perspective because it seems to represent what nurses already do. Hence adopting the model required minimal accommodation. Neither is it written in an obscure intellectual language that characterises so many American models of nursing. Pearson (1983, p. 53), in justifying the use of the Roper *et al* model at Burford, noted the way the model 'speaks to nurses in a language which is familiar and related to nursing in this country and hence its greatest advantage then is its ability to convey meaning to clinical nurses.'

Whilst practitioner's identification with the model's language might seem an advantage, it is also its weakness because, if it fits in with what nurses already do, then its impact on changing practice will be limited. Pearson seems to imply that models *should* convey meaning to nurses, but this goes against the grain that the nurse must first find meaning for herself and then collectively with her colleagues. Only then are practitioners in a position to consider the value of external prescriptions of nursing to inform their practice. But if practitioners have developed their own vision for nursing, why would they want to use someone else's?

The outcome of the audit was to quit using the Roper *et al* model and to construct a reflective approach to appreciate the person's life pattern that emphasised the therapeutic relationship.

Such an approach must simultaneously

● tune the practitioner adequately into the person within the hospital's vision so that the vision can be lived moment to moment
● tune the practitioner into herself, so the practitioner is mindful of self moment to moment within the unfolding therapeutic relationship.

My tuning fork was to construct the core cue and nine reflective cues that guide the practitioner to appreciate the pattern of the person's lifestyle and needs (Box 13.2). The

Box 13.2   The Burford NDU reflective cues

> *Core cue*
> What information do I need to be able to nurse this person?
>
> *The nine reflective cues*
> • Who is this person?
> • What meaning does this illness/meaning have for the person?
> • How is this person feeling?
> • How has this event affected this person's usual life pattern and roles?
> • How do I feel about this person?
> • How can I help this person?
> • What is important for this person to make his or her stay in the hospice comfortable?
> • What support does this person have in life?
> • How does this person view the future for himself or herself and others?

term *pattern appreciation* (Cowling 2000) is more helpful than assessment. It better represents the complex interplay of the signs practitioners need to pay attention to in order to know the other person; reading the person's life pattern as a complex whole – a pattern continually shifting moment to moment along the person's health–illness journey. This is achieved by reading the signs on the person's surface, for example, pain, anxiety, high blood pressure, sadness in the eyes, and pursuing these signs into the deeper self as appropriate. Pattern is always shifting in light of unfolding events. Only when the practitioner is in tune with the person can he or she understand and respond appropriately to the person's unfolding needs.

Newman (1994, p. 13) writes, 'The new paradigm of health, essential to nursing, embraces a unitary pattern of changing relationships. It is developmental. The task is not to try to change another person's pattern but to recognise it as information that depicts the whole and relate to it as it unfolds.'

Wavelength theory

The practitioner intends to tune into the person's wavelength. The practitioner must then flow with the person's wavelength as it unfolds. Newman (1994) describes this as synchronicity, a rhythm of relating in a paradigm of wholeness. This movement along the wavelength can be viewed as a dance (Johns 2001b, Younger 1995); each dance step is a caring movement sometimes led by the practitioner and at other times led by the other as appropriate.

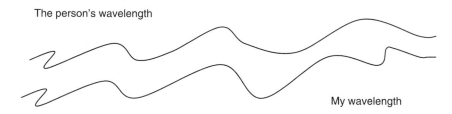
The person's wavelength

My wavelength

When people experience crisis in their lives, their wave patterns are likely to become chaotic. When practitioners are not person-centred, they expect the person to fit into the wavelength of the stereotyped 'good patient' – a symbolic straight line that literally flattens humanness. The patient (or diminished person) tries to 'fit in' to be accepted and cared for. Failure to 'fit in' often leads to censure as characterised by the image of the 'unpopular patient'.[2]

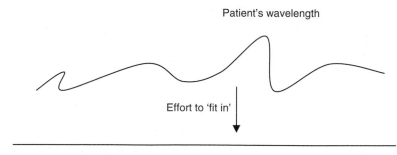
Patient's wavelength

Effort to 'fit in'

Practitioner's wavelength

Jones and Jones (1996, p. 185) capture the sense of wavelength for people in their portrayal of an eagle:

> Look up and see Eagle ride the invisible. Up and down, coasting, then back up and down again. With deliberate intent, she manoeuvres her wings in order to catch the next current, rising to a new height. Levelling and riding a straight course, she gains new sights. Then, accepting the inevitable downward drift, she surrenders to each experience. Invisibly changing and unpredictable, the air currents carry Eagle to the places she must go. Eagle understands the dance of life and accepts the downward as naturally as she accepts the upward.

Understanding the person's experience opens up the possibility to tune into and synchronise with the person's wavelength and to flow with him on the ebb and flow of his health–illness experience, helping him find a new, more harmonious, wavelength in tune with well-being. To stay on the other's wavelength the practitioner must be mindful of the pitch and roll and manage any resistance they may have towards the patient. Sometimes this can be difficult when the person is resistant, angry or uncooperative. A bit like surfing!

The Burford NDU reflective cues

Each cue is significant to pattern the response to the person. The practitioner internalises the cues as a *natural* reflective lens to appreciate the unfolding clinical situation moment by moment. As such, pattern appreciation and pattern response are ongoing as a dynamic unfolding process. The cues are *not* intended as a formulaic response to assess the patient, whereby each cue demands an answer; they cue the practitioner to pay attention to key processes within pattern appreciation. I emphasise the point because the practitioner who has embodied a reductionist systems approach may miss the reflective point and view the cues as another set of boxes to complete.

Sutherland (1994, p. 68) noted, 'Although at first I did find myself going back to the Roper *et al*'s headings to make sure that I had not missed anything, omitting what was physically important, I did not need to do this for very long.'

Sutherland further noted the impact of the reflective cues in changing her mindset:

> Because the emphasis is centred on feelings and the total picture of that person's situation rather than on their ongoing physical needs, it forced me to move away from a need to find things out, fill things in and get things done as soon as possible in an orderly fashion. It forced me to start listening to what patients themselves were saying was important to them and then to plan care with them from this basis . . . it gradually became a welcome release for me. (p. 68)

There is something astonishing in Sutherland's words about the way she thought the Burford cues *forced* her to listen to the person, as if she hadn't really listened to the person before. I think it is true, as she suggests, that the 'old model' became the task – hence the effort was to complete it rather than really listen to what the patient or family were saying. As Sutherland suggests, the key is listening and connecting; and then working with the person towards meeting their health–illness needs.

The apparent simplicity and profundity of the cues disarm people conditioned by complex systems models. If practitioners want to be reflective practitioners, then clearly they need to frame practice through reflective approaches. Models are merely tools to enable something to be accomplished. As such they must be fit for purpose. Does a carpenter use a spoon to chisel wood?

To help appreciate the cues, I invite the reader to engage with my narrative of working with Tony one morning at a hospice that utilises the Burford NDU model.

Tony

Susan asks me to help Tony get up for lunch. I have not met him before. I was informed by the morning handover report that he is 53 years old. He has primary lung cancer with liver metastases. He is in the hospice for respite care. He has been here 4 days. He is unhappy here and wants to go home. He finds it difficult to co-ordinate himself but doesn't want help. I ask Susan, 'Anything in particular I should be mindful of?'

'He's bit moody,' she says.

I knock on the closed door. No reply. I knock again and enter the room. The hand-drawn cards fixed to the bedroom wall immediately catch my attention.

I say, 'Hi Mr Birchall, I'm Chris. I'm here to help. How are you this morning?'

He looks at me but doesn't answer. Tuning into his wavelength I immediately sense his irritation. I sense it must be difficult for him having to deal with another new person. My assumption – he doesn't say that, at least not in words. Another assumption – he would rather have Susan.

I gaze at the cards pinned to the wall. Seeking connection, I ask, 'Who made the cards?'

'My granddaughter'.

'She has talent. Tell me about her.'

'Her name is Michelle. She is 4 years old. . . .'

He becomes animated talking about her. She is very special to him, adding to his sadness and restlessness. As Benner and Wrubel (1989) note, the things we care about are the things that make us vulnerable. Things that make us happy also make us sad.

I have opened a door to connect with Tony, talking about the thing that he cares most deeply for and grieves its forthcoming loss. We talk about schooling, about my two children. We talk about his work – he had been a plumber; he knows he is not going to work anymore and accepts this. All the while I sense his anger simmering. Do I let him know I sense this? Such catharsis might prick the tension and yet it might embarrass him.

I take the risk, 'You seem irritated being here?'

In doing so, I release some of my own anxiety. As if I have pressed a button, he pointedly says, 'I want to be at home. Not that it's unpleasant in here but. . . .'

His words drift off. Patiently I wait, he adds, 'I want to be at home.'

I respond, 'I sense that . . . so why are you here?'

'I have no choice about going home because my daughter is away for the week and I need her support.'

He relaxes. He has expressed his irritation – a potent cocktail of anger at the hospice, at me, at himself, at the cancer, at his daughter, that he may die, at the world at large. In my experience some patients like to tell their story over and over, and others prefer their own solitude. Tony is one of the latter.

He moves out of the shadow of his despair more willing to engage with me.

He asks, 'Tell me about yourself.'

Now he needs to know me in order to accept my presence. I explain I often work at the hospice to maintain my palliative care skills to ensure credibility as a palliative care teacher. He is intrigued.

He stands and takes off his pyjamas. His nakedness exposed. I hold him steady as he moves into and out of the shower. Slowly he dresses. I help him with his socks and shoes. I have been with him over an hour.

I ask, 'Do you have any pain?'

'No.'

We eventually get to lunch in the communal dining room. It is empty. We are late. Everybody else has gone. He invites me to join him for lunch. I stay with him until he has finished. There is something normalising about having a meal with someone. He tells me he was a keen cyclist. Something concrete to connect with. I tell him I am a morris dancer. By the time we finish I am on his wavelength and sense his ease. I too am easier, having worked through my lack of poise. I sense the way feelings are reciprocated. It highlights for me the fundamental need to know people in order to respond appropriately to them on a level that is meaningful.

As long as Tony resisted me, no therapeutic relationship was possible. We got there, but it took an effort. Did I hang in there for my benefit or his? Perhaps I should have said to him, 'I'll get Susan to help you,' acknowledging his initial discomfort with me. Do patients have the right to choose their nurses in hospice? It is a profound question because I cannot impose my idea of relationship on patients. The very nature of suffering and facing dying must always make relationship precarious. In getting to know someone who is suffering I trip along a fine edge of raw emotion.

I could have simply (simply?) connected superficially with him by helping him to wash, dress, escort him to lunch, administer and monitor his pain medication and other symptom relief; this was not the level of help he really needed. On a deeper level I knew he was in crisis. I could read that, but that was my difficulty. I could not respond easily to the superficial caring issues outside that deeper context. Hence helping him wash and dress became difficult once I had held his eyes and touched his suffering. He also knew that and perhaps resisted me because he needed to protect himself from this intruding stranger. On the other hand, he might have preferred my superficial attention. As it was, I did feel intrusive, as if my caring ethic had trapped me. Although he eventually accommodated me, I felt as if I had pushed his limits and challenged his control of the situation.

Later, holding this dilemma, I share this experience with Susan. She affirms my experience, acknowledging Tony's struggle in facing death. She also acknowledges my difficulty in tuning into him. She feels I shouldn't worry unduly as Tony is 'difficult'. In other words, my experience is normal. Sensitivity flattened in order to cope with the stress of the day. Yet, Susan's concern for me is genuine. But I am struck (yet again) that it is the patient who has the problem rather than the nurse.

Before I leave the hospice I go and shake hands with Tony and thank him for accommodating me. He reciprocates my thanks, for having the patience to stay with him. I sense he is lonely here without his daughter and granddaughter visiting. A week can seem a long time when time is running out and when such relationships are precious. As Schön (1987) notes, practice is often messy and indeterminate without clear solutions. These are only found within the moment in response to the unfolding drama.

Who is this person?

This cue challenges me to see Tony as a unique 'whole' person in the context of his world. His family and culture are brought into focus and scope of care. The cue encourages me to see *him* and counters any tendency to see him primarily in terms of his symptoms and diagnosis, as significant as these things are. Of course, humanness is a reciprocal thing. If Tony sees my humanness he is more likely to see and respond from his own. The cue also intends to remind me to be mindful and curious – who *is* this person that I endeavour to connect with?

What meaning does this health event have for the person?

This cue focuses me to listen and be empathic to Tony's experience: what does this health–illness event *really* mean for him? I emphasise *really* because so often I have read the surface signs and assume what it means. The reflective practitioner holds the space to inquire, digs a little deeper below the skin where the real issues lie. Tuning into Tony opens these doors to knowing him and for him to know himself, so he can make sense of his bewildering experience. Empathic inquiry is compassionate and intentional listening to connect with what the other is experiencing. Yet I can never really know Tony' experience. I must guard against jumping to hasty assumptions, being patient in dwelling with Tony, mindful to check out any assumptions. It is the practitioner's greatest skill for it sets up possibility.

It is tuning in and flowing with the unfolding pattern of the person's experience, opening a therapeutic space for the patient to reveal himself or herself as the basis for care, enabling me to appreciate the meanings he or she gives to their health–illness experience.

How is this person feeling?

This cue guides me to inquire into Tony's particular concerns and anxieties. As noted in the text, Tony experiences a cocktail of distressing emotions that ripple through him, bubbling to the surface in his manner. I trip along this cue cautiously, not wanting to intrude inappropriately into his private world but opening a space whereby these emotions can be safely expressed and discharged. Until these emotions are released, it is impossible to talk through his experience in any meaningful way.

How has this event affected their usual life pattern and roles?

This cue prompts me to appreciate Tony's lifestyle pattern. I guide him and his family, as appropriate, to review their lifestyle, reading the pattern for deeper underlying factors that may have influenced the current situation. Often, serious illness can prompt a radical reassessment of lifestyle and what values people consider significant within their lives. It focuses caring as both a health promotion and illness prevention activity. I could utilise a checklist to consider aspects of lifestyle, rather like the Roper *et al* activities of living, or any other reductionist scheme. If you were to construct a check list, what would it include? Obvious issues include work, leisure, daily living and religious activities. Related to this are issues which affect these activities, such as mobility, fatigue, sleep, personal self-care, nutrition, pain, mood, bowels and so on, and social factors, such as support, attitudes, finance and so on. These aspects of daily living might be self-assessed as appropriate. In the narrative I mentioned pain, but it seemed irrelevant to pursue other issues at that particular time.

How do I feel about this person?

This cue prompts me to pay attention to my own feelings, thoughts, concerns and prejudices that inevitably influence the way I see and respond to Tony, especially as he arouses strong feelings in me due to the expression of his suffering. Without doubt I felt uncomfortable. I wanted to fix his despair and hence absorbed it – so I suffered alongside him – what I term *sympathetic resonance*. I recognised my own lack of poise and my difficulty recovering this poise so I could be more available to him. It is a situation I often find myself. Reading the text, it reads as if I dig myself out of an emotional hole.

Morse *et al* (1992) differentiate sympathy with empathy, whereby sympathy is an emotional response to the experience of the other as a result of absorbing the other's suffering to some extent. In contrast empathy is an objective view – a dispassionate glance yet motivated by deep concern for the other. And yet, sympathy has a therapeutic impact because it reveals to Tony my own humanness, or put another way, that I am not an object doing care to him.

It is vital that practitioners like myself acknowledge how we feel. Otherwise we defend, avoid emotion and assert control to manage our anxiety, impasses to therapeutic relationships (Ramos 1992) that stem the flow of compassion. Whereas my concern opens a clearing, my compassion fills it with a loving presence.

Roach (1992, p. 58) describes compassion as

> . . . a way of living born out of an awareness of one's relationship to all living creatures; engendering a response of participation in the experience of another; a sensitivity to the pain and brokenness of the other; a quality of presence which allows one to share with and make room for the other.

Compassion is a nebulous concept, difficult to grasp and certainly difficult to talk about and teach. It is heartfelt. It isn't a technique to apply. I know Tony would sense if my compassion was false. Ask yourself, how would I know if I am compassionate? How would I know when my compassion is diluted? These are vital inquiries if compassion *is* caring. And yet, at every turn, my compassion is under threat in a world where compassion is strained. Do we who purport to care have a responsibility to develop our compassion if compassion is a vital ingredient of caring? Do we fail our patients and ourselves if we lack compassion? I play out the tension between a trace of pity for Tony's plight and compassion (Levine 1986). As with all my reflections, I nurture compassion and dispel any aversion or pity to the other's suffering. It is a constant play. A chipping away at deeply embodied forces that limit my ability to be most available to him. Compassion is not something easily attained. It is a spiritual dimension of being.

How can I help this person?

This cue prompts me to pause and analyse the information I have gained as the basis for negotiating a care plan with the person (to the extent they are able) in collaboration with other healthcare practitioners. It is the most practical cue in the sense of the nitty-gritty of what healthcare practitioners do. The extent I help ease his suffering is minimal. He endures me as he endures his suffering. Perhaps I take a slight edge of his suffering for a passing moment so the enduring is eased, but I have no illusion that I helped more than this. It is important that practitioners recognise the limits of the ability to ease suffering yet without any sense of failing the person (Randall and Downie 1999).

In helping him, I pick up his care plan to date, working with it, evaluating it, amending it as necessary to fit the moment-by-moment shift. The care plan is not a static thing but a living narrative I tune into.

What is important for this person to make his stay in the hospice comfortable?

This cue prompts me to acknowledge that admission into the hospice is a disturbance to Tony's normal lifestyle that exacerbates his suffering yet is necessary for his greater well-being so his daughter has respite. Realising this tension enables him to endure this misery at being here. The cue raises issues of comfort and control, especially those 'little things' that make a significant difference to the person's comfort and perception of being cared for (Macleod 1994). For example, talking about cycling.

What support does this person have in life?

This cue draws my attention to Tony's ongoing care outside the immediate care environment. I draw any family, friends, community into the caring gaze to explore the meaning of this event in terms of the future. At the time, I did not explore the support Tony had in life except to note that his stay in the hospice was for his daughter's holiday. I did not know the daughter. Perhaps I might have asked Tony about his support at home and whether this was working out OK, and giving feedback to those practitioners, such as psychologists, social workers, Macmillan nurses and chaplains, who are more involved in this aspect of work. Contemplating this cue raises issues of role, boundaries and the way that roles are often demarcated. For example, in my role as a therapist, I feel I am all these roles woven into one.

How does this person view the future?

This cue prompts me to dialogue with the person/family to explore what the future might hold, especially fears of dying and death and what support resources exist within the person's life and towards mobilising and developing resources to support the person's future. As with the previous cue, such dialogue may raise many difficult issues and feelings, such as the possibility of dying, disability, losing one's home and so on. Both cues are vital to focus care towards successful exit of the care relationship or transition of care across healthcare boundaries. I did not pursue this cue in any overt way with Tony – perhaps because his fear of loss rippled through the whole encounter. It is a significant point to emphasise that these cues are rarely used explicitly – 'Tony, how do you view the future?' – would seem an insensitive and intrusive question. Yet holding the cue in my mind alerts me to the possibility of exploring Tony's view of dying if appropriate at that moment in time. It reminds me that pattern appreciation is in constant motion.

> I bend with you to ease your suffering
> As the reed bends with the wind

In graceful dance and harmony
It bends but does no break
So I too must learn.

Reflection on being available to Tony

I hold my intention to be patient-centred. On reflection I gained deeper insight into the nature of being patient-centred especially when the person is less than enthusiastic about this relationship. Tony's resistance opened a space to reflect on the tension between compassion and poise, acknowledging my vulnerability in the face of rejection (see also my poetic poem concerning Rita Pyke in Chapter 21). I felt my response to Tony did open a therapeutic space albeit tentative and momentary. But I also accept the limits of my therapeutic ability in the face of such deep suffering. Perhaps I could have challenged Susan's analysis of Tony as 'difficult'. Labelling is such a perverse act and disrupts any therapeutic potential. It highlights yet again the way patients are expected to conform to be a good patient as a flatline even in a hospice. I recognise my failure to confront uncaring reflects a deeper need to avoid conflict – reflecting how practitioners also conform to a social norm or flatline of fitting in.

A system to ensure effective communication

My retrospective audit of nursing notes revealed the nursing process had no real value either as a comprehensive record of care or enabling the continuity of care. Indeed, the nursing process was considered a hindrance to effective practice because it required completion. Imagine what a waste of time doing something that is meaningless!

Communication is vital. It is the collagen that holds together practice to ensure the patient and family receive consistent, continuous, congruous, compassionate and collaborative care within and across practice settings.

Using reflective techniques, the reflective practitioner *communicates* to ensure

- *continuity* of care over time despite changes in personnel
- *consistency* of care between different care workers
- *congruence* of care between care workers in tune with shared vision and best practice
- *compassionate* talk that is positive and affirming
- *collaboration* between care workers to ensure the above points.

These might be described as the six 'Cs'. Communication is both verbal, through language, and non-verbal, through body posture, senses and intonation. Communication is both formal and informal. Formal verbal communication takes place through writing notes and reports, through shift reports, ward rounds and various care meetings that may include patients and families. Informal verbal communication takes place in the way practitioners relate to each other and with patients and families throughout the day: corridor conversations, passing remarks, the sluice room conference, coffee chat and so on. I am sure the reader can coin up many euphemisms for such informal verbal meetings – all accompanied by a vast range of non-verbal communication that convey positive and negative power messages. The reflective practitioner is always mindful of the presentation of self.

Narrative notes

Ideally notes are one set of patient notes rather than separate notes for different professions. The practitioner writes a story of meeting the person and family on admission governed by the reflective cues. In summarising the story, the practitioner clarifies how she intends to help the person and an evaluation of responding to the person's needs. This creates a rich background for all other professionals even though many will still cover the same ground. People like Tony, who resist care, must wonder about such demand to tell the story yet again. It counters any primary focus on disease process or a symptom management approach rife in hospices. The narrative is then continued, reflecting the shifting drama. This requires a parsimonious writing approach. The advent of standardised computer records does not have to mitigate against such an approach. Nurses must communicate effectively despite systems that would seem to limit or even censor such approach. Political action required!

Talk

The way practitioners talk with patients, families and with each other is a caring act. What we say is a reflection of our values. Therefore, if I espouse to be caring, compassionate and work in collaborative ways with my colleagues, you might expect my speech to reflect those values. Anything less would be a contradiction that the reflective practitioner would acknowledge and work towards resolving. Talk is both a process – an act in itself, and an outcome – it aims to achieve something. However, talk can also be uncaring; tongues can be sharp and venomous.

Dialogue is the core of reflective communication whereby practitioners listen to each other with respect towards realising best person-centred care without personal agendas and egos closing down the space.

Reflective handover

The function of the shift report is to communicate relevant information to ensure the smooth transition of care and responsibility to the next shift. At Burford, patient care had been communicated through an oral culture at the shift handover report. The nurse who gave care during the shift gives information to the nurses commencing the next shift. The practitioner might say 'read the patient's notes', but as discussed, these would not be an adequate account. Given the inadequacy of written notes, the verbal report is probably the most significant form of communication to ensure continuity of care because it is traditional and more accurately captures the current patient status.

The traditional scenario – conscious of confidentiality, the office door at shift report is closed to prevent breach. The emphasis is on the nurse reporting – the new shift nurses write notes on scraps of paper. Some exchange of views takes place, but this is usually in the form of opinions rather than dialogue around decision making or care dilemmas. Nurses rarely express their personal feelings – 'lets keep focused'. The report usually lasts for about 30 minutes, which for 10 patients is longer than most units engage in this activity.

I reflect on this routine with the nurses involved, suggesting we might move to a more reflective format with a greater emphasis on dialogue, creating the opportunity for people to reflect on the way we think, feel, and responding to care issues around the patients and their families. Most practitioners agree this might be helpful, but practice does not change, as if we are locked into a habit. I ask why do nurses write notes on scraps of paper when the patients' notes are available? In response I am told 'it's handy to have a list in the pocket rather than keep referring to the notes'. Writing such notes is a distraction from dialogue; indeed it is a means of avoiding dialogue. I challenge the senior nurses to role model dialogue by revealing their own thoughts and feelings and to challenge others to respond. A dialogical approach shifts the culture of the report from essentially 'handing over' information to reflection. This does not mean that information will not be given – but the emphasis has changed. The notes can be read either before or after the report, and considered in light of the shift report dialogue.

Bedside handover

I declare that this tradition of shift report is not good enough. Sitting closed in a room talking about patients is a contradiction with person-centred care (Ward 1988). A counterargument is do patients want to be involved in decision making and taking responsibility for their health? A considerable literature emerged in the 1990s that explored patient participation in decision making (Ashworth *et al* 1992, Biley 1992, Jewell 1994, Waterworth and Luker 1990).

I propose a shift to a bedside handover. Initially, nurses do not feel comfortable with this shift of routine. Yet they were willing to give it a go. Shift report now had meaning. It became a more mindful practice rather than simply routine. It fundamentally shifted the power relationship between nurses and patients. Resistance was wrapped up in fear of breaching patient confidentiality by disclosing information in public areas or that some patients would not be able to or even resist such talk.[3] Working with and negotiating decision making is fundamentally a manifestation of the hospital's vision. Whether patients are able to or want to be involved is another issue. The reflective practitioner appreciates this dynamic and judges whether to accept the other's dependency or confront it.

The approach to implementing bedside handover was written as a protocol that involved visiting each patient before moving into 'the office' to complete the report.

We anticipated that this approach would enable

- the nurses greet each patient (and family) at the commencement of shift, informing the patient who is available for care
- the nurses invite patients to reflect on their care and care decisions
- the patient gives his or her perspective first
- to make care values and processes more transparent
- the nurse to make better sense of any ensuing information, having seen and spoken with the patient beforehand.

The protocol emphasises the primacy of written notes as the means for continuing care, written as narratives rather than in nursing process format. We decided to store these notes with each patient simply because we viewed them as patient notes. The idea of patient-held records is well-known in community settings – again reflecting the philosophy of working with the patient in terms of their health. This practice really challenged practitioners to become mindful of what they wrote, knowing that what they wrote might be read by the patient or the patient's family.

Patient notes

In an observational study of the impact of primary nursing on the culture of a community hospital (Johns 1989), one practitioner commented: 'Much of it is just nursing, you don't have to write that down.' This comment reflects the pattern recognition and common sense knowing that this practitioner and her colleagues possessed, and their struggle to write down what was so obvious to them. Another practitioner commented – 'patients we know well don't need care planning' – a comment that again reflects all elements of intuitive knowing.

I asked one staff nurse on her return from holiday if she had read her patients' care plans. She commented, 'I haven't had time because it's so busy.' The comment reinforces the comments above, symbolising the way the nurses on the unit did not use care plans as part of their daily planning. However, I sensed that this apparent intuitive knowing was not based on appreciating the patient's life pattern, but from knowing the patient in terms of the report given to her at the shift report and normal routines. In other words, patients did not need care planning because we know them as a group of similar patients. This was reflected in the notes that had a strong focus on medical and physical care issues with very little focus on emotional, psychological and spiritual aspects of care.

As one of the primary nurse's said, 'When I deliberately change something on the care plan, I came back from my days off and it hasn't been carried out . . . is it because they disagree with what's been said or are they too busy to read the care plans?' Other nurses countered this comment by saying they resented less experienced nurses telling them what to do, or that they disagreed with what was written and therefore disregarded it; that is, if they had read it in the first place.

Completing patients' notes is often done as a task to be done at the end of the shift. Practitioners recognise this task as generally meaningless and yet feel anxious about writing something, possibly motivated by an internal censor that if nothing is written, then care has not been carried out. The fear becomes reinforced when audit systems are constructed around the completion of patient notes. Hence, what is written tends to be descriptive rather than evaluative, and meaningless in terms of communicating the essential nature of continuing care. If the nursing process is meaningless then, as Batehup and Evans (1992) have challenged, 'why do we keep this sacred cow?'

For most practitioners since the late 1970s, the nursing process has dominated the approach to thinking and writing about patient care. Essentially the nursing process is a linear problem-solving approach that structures thinking through four stages:

Goal setting	– an interpretation of assessment in terms of identifying specific actual or potential problems/patient needs and goals to be achieved in responding to the problem/need
Planning	– establishing the best response to solve the problem/need
Intervention	– carrying out the planned care
Evaluation	– determining whether the set goal has been met, including redefining the problem or goal as necessary in light of events

The care plan is designed as a table consisting of these four columns. In theory, a practitioner should be able to pick up the care plan and continue the patient's care as a seamless activity. However, most aspects of care cannot be prescribed in advance, at least not without reducing the patient to an object to be manipulated. Some aspects of care may be more amenable to prescription, for example, technical solutions to medical problems such as wound dressings and responses to pain and nausea. Yet these responses are better framed within a protocol based on evidence of best practice as guidelines to inform practitioners. Aspects of care concerned with the human–human encounter are almost possible to prescribe, given the uniqueness of each individual and each caring encounter.

The nursing process has attracted much adverse criticism in the 1990s (Howse and Bailey 1992, Latimer 1995, McElroy *et al* 1995, White 1993). Although the nursing process was intended to promote a culture of individualised and negotiated care (De La Cuesta 1983), ironically the opposite tended to happen when it was accommodated with the prevailing nursing culture in the UK characterised by allegiance to the reductionist medical model. Rather than change practice, the nursing process was accommodated to fit within this existing culture, resulting in a minimal or lip-service response to the ideology of individualised care (Latimer 1995). It is easy to see why – because the splitting up of the patient into problems mirrored the medical model. The nurse was now able to diagnose problems. The patient became a set of problems or needs (problems being viewed as too mechanistic) based on complex systems advocated within an accompanying array of nursing models. These models were almost exclusively from the USA. These models were theory driven and, as in the nature of any model, sought to find a comprehensive representation or conceptualisation of nursing.

The nursing diagnosis movement (North American Nursing Diagnosis Association) (NANDA)) has been a natural development from the nursing process within the USA, yet in my view, is a process fraught with difficulty because it imposes abstract meanings on 'nursing' concepts in the futile effort to ensure consistency of diagnosis. In this respect this movement mirrors medicine's approach to diagnosis. Practitioners might find some common understanding of what a grade 4 glioma is, but can practitioners find common meaning in using the word suffering, spirituality or agitation? Of course not. It is a positivist illusion to think otherwise.

Consider

- What does individualised care mean to you?
- Do patient's notes reflect the wholeness of care?

These are profound questions. Is it even necessary to put the adjective 'individual' in front of care? How could care be anything other than individual? The opposite might be termed institutionalised care. Ray (1989) coined the expression bureaucratic caring as a reflection of the way the individual might become obscured within the layers of bureaucracy. The human within the machine becomes a contradiction. As Wilber (1998) puts it, systems are the language of 'it' and 'it' is a stark colourless landscape of labels. The individual's cry can be difficult to hear amidst the din. To compensate we need to say 'individualised' to remind ourselves that we care for unique human beings and that we carers too are unique human beings. We can only find meaning in the unfolding moment and respond with our humanness, a humanness at risk of being buried beneath an avalanche of concepts and prescriptions. The nurse becomes a technician.

As practitioners begin to respond within a person-centred perspective, they realise the nursing process is a contradiction, making little allowance for holistic and intuitive processes that are acknowledged as significant in the way experts make decisions about complex caring situation (Cioffi 1997).

The Dreyfus and Dreyfus (1986) model of skill acquisition indicates that the expert practitioner intuitively makes clinical judgement based on grasping the whole situation

Box 13.3   The Dreyfus and Dreyfus model of skill acquisition

• Pattern recognition	– A perceptual ability to recognise relationships without pre-specifying the components of the situation
• Similarity recognition	– An amazing human ability to recognise 'fuzzy' resemblance despite marked differences
• Common sense	– A deep grasp of the language culture so that flexible understanding in diverse situations is possible
• Skilled 'know-how'	– The practitioner can respond without resorting to rule-governed behaviours
• Deliberate rationality	– The expert practitioner has a web of different perspectives that allows him or her to view a situation in terms of past situations

(Box 13.3). If this is true, then the mechanical linear approach of the nursing process does not fit with expert thinking. Indeed, it is a hindrance.

Logically, communication systems need to be based on the way the expert practitioner thinks. Anything less will be absurd. It constrains thinking simply because practitioners do not think that way. Most practitioners know this, and yet have been unable to move beyond this deeply embodied worldview because the nursing process has dominated the way nurses conceptualise their practice. Even when practitioners acknowledge the absurdity of the nursing process, they seem powerless to move to more meaningful and practical ways of communicating care.

So, what alternatives are there given that a person-centred approach eschews any reductionist and deterministic approach to nursing practice, yet values the idea of best practice?

Narrative

At Burford hospital, given the inadequacy of the nursing process, practitioners embraced the idea of reflexive narrative as a more congruent form of communication (see accounts by practitioners in *The Burford NDU Model: Caring in Practice*, edited by Johns (1994)).

Reflexive means that when one looks back over the narrative a concise account of patient care unfolds. Narrative intends to capture the unfolding experience of working with or journeying alongside the patient through their health–illness experience. In noting the shifting pattern, the practitioner appreciates what is unfolding with what has gone before. Has the analgesia made a difference? Is Mrs Jones more restful? Is the wound healing? Is Alison better able to breastfeed? Has the new bed for Mr Smith been delivered at his home? As such – assessment and evaluation are two sides of the same coin – what is unfolding now and what has happened before.

In writing, the reflective practitioner is mindful of being meaningful and pragmatic. As such, narrative should always be concise, reflective and evaluative, and capture the drama of the unfolding story. Writing a brief background story of who the patient is really helps to see the person in their humanness and not just a disease object. This makes such a difference to perception, especially in hospices with its primary focus on symptom management. Facing death is not a collection of symptoms but a human being and family experiencing the most dramatic point of their life.

Remember, the reflective cues are not concrete questions that require specific answers. They are merely cues to guide to tune the practitioner into her thoughts and feelings. If the person makes me feel anxious, as with Tony, I would acknowledge this by writing something like this:

Tony's irritation at being in the hospice is difficult to respond to. After helping him wash and dress we lunched together and shared many common factors that helped to lift his despair at least for the moment. He acknowledges he needs to be here as difficult as that is for him.

My emotional reaction might be 'Tony's anxiety manifests itself as demanding and abusive'. I may initially have felt abused and defensive as these darts of anxiety were fired at me, but hopefully, being mindful, I see my reaction is a defensive ego response. In other words, I write about what I have done with my concern rather than about the concern itself. I acknowledge Tony's feelings as valid – hoping to counter any negative labelling of him.

Narrative offers a more coherent reflective approach than the nursing process to communicating meaningful information about the person's care and treatment. Simply put, narrative is way of journeying with the person whereby significant issues of practice are clearly identified and recorded. Similarly, oral communication, such as shift reports, shift from being information giving towards dialogue where significant issues of journeying with the person were explored.

A reflective quality system to ensure effective practice

How do we know whether our care is effective or not? Indeed, how might best practice be known? We enter the world of clinical governance. A reflective approach to quality is to live quality as part of everyday practice where effective care is everyone's business and mutual responsibility.

Burford was using patient questionnaires such as QUALPACS and Phaneuf's nursing audit (Pearson 1983). All these approaches involved outside agencies looking in and judging against set criteria that allegedly equated with quality of care. When quality is measured against external criteria that does not involve practitioners, then quality becomes someone else's business and practitioners do have to take responsibility for their own performance. The bureaucratic advantage of such measurement is it enables benchmarking – comparing hospitals with other hospitals and the inevitable construction of league tables. But do these tools actually measure quality or simply what it looked for?

It seems to me that a measure of reflective practice is practitioners, both collectively and individually, take responsibility for their personal and collective performance, using double feedback systems that challenge not only care processes and outcomes but also the standard by which caring is judged. Things change constantly and so approaches to quality must be fluid in response.[4] In response, we established professional supervision (Chapter 17), clinical audit and standards of care (Chapter 16). These approaches all contribute to creating a dynamic reflective learning organisation whereby practice is constantly and systematically explored in the quest to realise the hospital's vision as a lived reality and deliver the most effective care.

A system to ensure staff are enabled to realise the vision as a lived reality

In 1990 I established a project at Burford hospital to explore the value of guided reflection to enable practitioners to become effective practitioners (Johns 1998a). The project was the foundation for developing my ideas about guided reflection. Initially, I appointed an associate nurse on an 18-month contract on the understanding she entered into a formal guided reflection relationship. We met approximately every 2–3 weeks for 1 hour in which she shared experiences of her practice. My leadership role was to guide her to learn through these experiences towards becoming an effective practitioner.[5] This set the ball rolling. It led to implementing guided reflection throughout the hospital and eventually within six other community settings within Oxfordshire. The analysis of this work led to the reflective ideas that underpin much of this text. There was no prescription towards this work, we just did it, and reflected constantly on its process and outcomes.

Organisational culture

What sort of organisational culture needs to exist to accommodate a reflective and person-centred approach to clinical practice? I know that existing transactional or bureaucratic cultures cannot accommodate reflective practice simply because they are by their very nature static, reactive and unreflective. Such organisations are overly concerned with risk at the expense of creativity and professional responsibility. What is required is a culture committed to creating and sustaining a learning environment and reflective leadership that serves and invests in people.[6] These are, in themselves vast subjects. Although Burford was part of the bigger National Health Service (NHS), as its leader I was able to create a bubble of autonomy, yet ever mindful of the bureaucratic demand on Burford to comply with the 'bigger picture'. I was fortunate that Burford was a nursing development unit and had legitimate license to play with ideas. I was also fortunate that Burford was a community hospital and I was its general manager. Perhaps, as a unit within a large hospital, I would have experienced more bureaucratic resistance. Perhaps. And yet, if healthcare services are committed to the patient's experience, then surely innovative practice is to be encouraged and welcomed? As a rational idea you would say 'of course!' However, the transactional bureaucratic culture of the NHS is wrapped up in its own self-serving agenda of smooth running, dangling to the puppet strings of government to ensure targets and the suchlike, paradoxically far removed from the quality of the patient's experience. Food for thought.

Conclusion

To be reflective does not happen in a vacuum or educational system. To be real, reflective practice is a state of being lived in everyday clinical and organisational practice. As such, it requires organisational structures that embrace reflection *seriously* through reflective systems and leadership. I emphasise *seriously* because so much rhetoric and lip service is paid to the idea of reflective practice and person-centred practice.

Notes

1   This framework has been revised from the original work where I had identified four cornerstones (see Johns 2000).
2   For example, see Johnson and Webb (1995), Kelly and May (1982), Stockwell (1972).
3   A specific standard of care on confidentiality was written. See Chapter 16.
4   I develop the issue of ensuring quality in Chapter 16.
5   The development of professional supervision as clinical supervision is explored in Chapter 17.
6   Reflective leadership and the learning organisation is explored in Chapter 14.

Chapter 14

Reflective leadership

Perhaps the most significant focus for healthcare development is leadership. Leadership is the driving force to create and sustain effective working practices and quality. Yet ideas on leadership vary considerably depending on your perspective. Healthcare organisations are transactional, where leadership is little more than management to ensure targets are met. The prevailing mantra is 'Command and control!' In this transactional world, people are pawns to be moved around the board. Wheatley (1999, p. 164) writes, 'management is getting work done through others. The important thing was the work; the "others" were distractions that needed to be managed into conformity and predictability.'

In contrast, the contemporary literature on leadership advocates a transformational style of leadership concerned with creating and sustaining a dynamic and moral learning organisation (LO). Burns (1978, p. 19) writes, 'transformational leadership is where one or more persons engage with others in such a way that leaders and followers raise one another to higher levels of motivation and morality.' I might add 'and achievement.'

It follows that leadership is more about being a certain type of person (being with) rather doing certain sorts of things (doing to). Jaworski (1998, pp. 57–8) writes, 'We're always talking about what leaders do – about leadership style and function, but we put very little emphasis on the being aspect of leadership.'

My assertion is that the core of leadership is being mindful – that leaders are mindful of self as a leader and of the creative tension between leadership vision and the realities of working in a transactional organisation.[1] To reiterate: being mindful is the ultimate consequence of determined reflective practice.

Theories of leadership are framed in fine words – yet what does it mean to live these words as a lived reality? Words such as transformational, authentic, servant, primal and the suchlike are found in the literature.

Since 2002, I have guided practitioners from diverse healthcare backgrounds working within National Health Service (NHS) organisations towards becoming the leaders they desire to be.[2] Guidance takes place within a *community of inquiry* where practitioners learn (gain insight) through their lived leadership experiences. Through meta-analysis of 80 leadership narratives,[3] I came to understand the tensions leaders faced in becoming a leader within the transactional healthcare organisations in which they worked. Understanding and resolving this tension was the focus of the practitioners' learning. These tensions can be viewed as a series of shifting norms – moving from one set of norms that characterise a transactional culture to a new set of norms that characterise a transformational culture (Table 14.1). From a reflective perspective, the contrast of norms offers

Table 14.1   The movement from transactional to transformational social norms (Johns 2012)

Transactional culture	Transformational culture
Vision (often postulated as a mission statement) set 'on high' influenced by external agendas.	Vision set collaboratively by practitioners within the organisation that accommodates external agendas.
Structured through a rigid set of hierarchical rungs that define role and authority. At each level, the pyramidal shape of the organisation is replicated.	Structured through a collaborative network based around a shared vision of clinical practice towards shared success.
High level of anxiety to meet its organisational objectives transmitted down through the strata of hierarchy. This leads to a strong sense of compliance.	Low level of anxiety due to genuine patterns of collaborative relationships working together towards shared success. This leads to a strong sense of commitment and motivation.
Views problems as threat to the organisation's primary goal of ensuring its own smooth running. (blame/shame culture)	Views problems as positive learning opportunities. (risks/experiments and learns)
Views people in terms of tasks to be done – in exchange for reward – extrinsic motivators of reward. Staff do not feel valued.	Invests in people to unleash talent and intellectually stimulate – intrinsic motivators of reward. Staff feel valued.
Emphasis on force (command and control) with an emphasis on authoritative power (French and Raven 1968) (thin trust/high fear or insecurity)	Emphasis on sharing power with an emphasis on facilitative power and being of service to support practitioners (French and Raven 1968) (thick trust/low fear or insecurity)
Relationships with subordinates characterised by parent–child patterns of relating (from a transactional analysis perspective) (views people as essentially irresponsible)	Relationships with colleagues characterised by adult–adult patterns of relating (from a transactional analysis perspective) (views people as essentially responsible)
Single feedback loops – to monitor objectives being met and maintain the status quo. This approach views the organisation as essentially mechanical where parts are viewed in isolation of the whole. Change tends to be reactive to fix the machine part. (Newtonian/reductionist perspective)	Double feedback loops – to monitor both process and outcome and the relationship between them. This approach views the organisation as a whole and the relationships within it as dynamic and evolving. (Chaos theory/holistic perspective)
Emphasis on management (either passive or active) that is reactive, oppressive and mindless.	Emphasis on leadership that is proactive, moral and mindful.
Staff are socialised to 'know your place' within the organisation's bureaucratic structures (self-regulation based on fear)	Staff are enabled to 'be in-place, for optimum performance and self-realisation. (self-liberation based on aspiration)

(Centre column, vertical text: Creative tension)

practitioners insight into the leadership journey. These tensions are illuminated through Sally's edited narrative written as an assignment on the Masters programme.

A little voice in a big arena[4]

I work as a deputy ward manager within an elective orthopaedic unit. It is an ever-demanding job! Policies and protocols, targets, deadlines and budgets are the everyday reality. Against this background, front-line staff like myself, struggle to provide patient-centred service in a system that seems intent on constraining rather than enabling effective practice and leadership.

I am ward based, which enables me to maintain patient-centred contact whilst experiencing management and leadership within the NHS. I work alongside my ward manager and aim to maintain high standards of care in a professional and organised environment. However, what is professional and what is organisational are often two sides of a coin. My role is often one of confusion and difficulty. I am viewed as a leader but not completely let off my reins to explore. When those reins are sometimes dropped, I find I'm pulled back with the understanding I wasn't ready to go it alone!

With new government initiatives being continually developed, there is increasing pressure placed on the organisation to meet targets and deadlines and deliver a cost-effective health care, contributing to a rapidly changing environment. The pressures placed on the NHS today are filtering down to ward level where the cracks are beginning to show and ward leadership is becoming an uphill struggle. As Klakovich (1994, p. 42) writes, 'to preserve the caring practice of the nursing profession in today's healthcare environment a new leadership theory is needed.'

Cope (2001, p. 1) notes,

> Within organisations we see managers struggling to come to terms with new demands on their managerial and leadership style. We have shifted from a position where control is managed by virtue of a formal badge of office (manager, patient, director, etc.) to one where we have to lead people through the use of more intangible and flexible forms of leadership.

I wish Cope was correct. The formal badge still rules OK! Yet more people are talking about leadership, but I suspect it is a leadership to drive forward change rather than the transformational style advocated by Burns (1978, p. 28) who expresses transforming leadership as 'being committed, having vision of what could be accomplished and empowering others with this vision so that all would accomplish more with less. The leader meshes with followers on deeply held values.' Klakovich (1994, p. 42) shares this view: 'for some time, nurses have been pressured to *do more with less*; that is, to maintain high productivity without sacrificing quality.' Leaders have to balance the reality of maintaining quality of care on a reduced budget with reduced resources. *Do more with less* – the klaxon call at the factory gate. Because of the pressures being placed on the health service and each department managing their own resources, issues of conflict inevitably arise. Barriers are erected, protocols and policies are barraged around, and common courtesy becomes a thing of the past.

Taylor and Singer (1983) suggest that through tension, companies' capacity could grow as long as the people involved can survive the stress. They discuss that without a certain amount of tension within the working environment, barriers for change would not be broken down. However, tension can cause upset and barriers to be extended, not broken down; then staff can become demotivated, demoralised and unsatisfied. Can I hold this tension creatively? I support others but who supports me?

This reflection exposes issues of conflict and how I am learning to respond to conflict congruent with my values as an emerging leader. One conflict situation involved the placement of a patient on the ward arising from pressure within the organisation. Since the government introduced the traffic light system for bed management, 'red alert' has become an everyday event in my hospital. Working within an elective ward environment we have a rapid turnaround of patients and on some occasions are left with an empty bed. We often assist the organisation by accepting non-orthopaedic elective admissions and minor trauma admissions to assist with the tight bed management of the hospital. We have strict guidelines on what we except due to our rapid pace of work, the experience of our team and the infection risk to our elective patients.

On the occasion in question, the bed manager approached me regarding a man who had been admitted to the accident and emergency department with severe head injuries. He had been brutally assaulted, and the police were treating it as attempted murder. His condition was unstable and he required a nurse to special him. As the assailant had not been caught, he was deemed at risk and would also have a police guard.

I was surprised at the bed manager's request to place this gentleman (whom I shall call George) within our ward environment. I felt the environment to be inappropriate, the staffing was already tight, and there was no room for movement to create a nurse special. The ward was busy, and there were several acute post-operative patients being monitored and there was also the very real issue due to the open ward environment of risk to the patients and staff. I expressed my concern and stated my case in a 'professional manner' to the bed manager, who accepted the situation and the admission was refused. Even as I use the words 'professional manner' I realise I am uncertain what I mean. It feels like defensive learnt behaviour I retreat behind. Enough to just note it.

Two hours later I receive another phone call from the bed manager. In an uptight and forthright manner he states, 'there is nowhere to place George and that pressure is now being placed on me to have George moved from accident and emergency. It has been discussed with the hospital manager and hospital administrator and George will be admitted to your ward!'

The wind is taken from my sails, I take a deep breath and restate my case detailing the ward policy and stating the ward would be unsafe in the event of George's admission. My outrage ripples through me; outrage that discussions have been held without my input and decisions made without one of the managers entering the ward to see the environment, the workload and the staffing levels. No respect for myself and my staff, no reasoning or compromise, just a dictatorial attitude.

An assembly of senior management appear on the ward: the bed manager, the hospital manager and the hospital administrator. They inform me that George will be brought to the ward shortly, and they are providing a nurse from another area to special George for the shift. I feel overpowered by the situation. I manage to question why the situation has been handled in this way and why there has been no discussion with myself and my team over the appropriateness of this patient's placement. My questions are not directly answered; the hospital administrator states the ward staffing has not been affected as they are providing cover for the next 12 hours, and the situation will be reviewed in the morning. Although I can see that to resist further is pointless, I express my unhappiness with the situation, the lack of communication involved. My lament falls on deaf ears. The managers leave the ward and George arrives with his nurse and police guard. My shoulders feel heavy.

An hour later, now late evening, the chief executive of the hospital appears on the ward. She approaches me and acknowledges the situation that has occurred with George's admission. She explains the difficulty in finding an appropriate placement for George and acknowledges the issues I have raised. She thanks me for the co-operation of my staff and myself and asks to be made aware of any problems.

I am left feeling bruised by the situation, but the chief executive has eased the swelling. Because she went out of her way to visit the ward and acknowledge a difficult situation, I do not feel so alone. It may have just been clever and kind words, but it gives me an inner strength to review the situation.

Reflection

Conflict situations surrounding bed management and appropriate placement of patients continue. The situation I experienced touches on issues of conflict manipulation, 'focusing on getting away from what we don't want rather than creating what we do want' (Senge 1990, p. 157). The hospital managers saw that George's admission to the accident and emergency department had caused disruption, and once George's condition had been stabilised their priority was to move him to a more isolated environment. George was a problem that needed to be fixed!

I perceived the need to provide George with a more secure environment but had real concerns that the area of elective orthopaedics was inappropriate and that little would be gained from this transfer except to enable the organisation to tick off a problem that disturbed their 'smooth running'(Friedson 1970). Cavanagh (1991) discussed that competitive style of conflict management usually occurs when a person follows his or her own gain to the detriment of others. This can lead to frustration, anger and arguments, creating damage to relationships and not viewing the situation as a whole but with tunnel vision.

In the community of inquiry, Chris challenged me as to whether I could have resisted the bed manager's demand from an ethical perspective and suggested using ethical mapping to help me see the situation from different perspective.

From my perspective, I had the right to be involved in the decision concerning bed use on the ward. Ward staffing was stretched, and the ward environment was not suitable for the patient's care. From the bed manager's perspective, representing the organisation, the bed was needed.

In considering ethical principles, my autonomy had been disregarded. I was also anxious about 'doing harm' to the other ward patients, but I sense this was an emotional rather than rational response. I was responding to a bruised ego! Their ethical claim was a utility claim of needing a bed so the organisation could run smoothly. I was simply a thorn in their side.

Johns (1999, p. 289) writes, 'Ethical mapping helps the practitioner see different and often contradictory perspectives of any situation and to examine the factors that determine which perspectives prevail.' It quickly became apparent to myself that the only gain of George being admitted to the ward was that the organisation managed to place their problem patient. I feel that George would have received better short-term gain from being placed within a more secure environment. The high-dependency nursing environment that was required for George was unacceptable and inappropriate within a busy ward.

Abiding by the Nursing and Midwifery Council Scope of Professional Practice, as a nurse I need to have competence and confidence with the care I provide to my patient: 'Acknowledge any limitations in your knowledge and competence and decline any duties or responsibilities unless able to perform them in a safe and skilled manner.' Perhaps this is my 'professional manner'?

As the Deputy Manager, I failed *in my duty* to act as an advocate for the nursing team; to express our limitations and knowledge to care for such a highly dependant patient. I felt overpowered by the organisation, having been told what I was to do, like a naughty school girl rebelling against her teacher.

This transactional manner left me feeling angry and frustrated. The managers involved were working from a negative short-term vision and not considering all the components involved within their decision. Cope (2001) discussed this as map conflict – conflict occurring when two people viewed the same situation from different perspectives. Map conflict can lead to tense situation, and lines of communication can break down, leading to little or no resolution.

Theorists in the past have believed that conflict situations have a positive effect on ourselves and the organisation. Deutsch (1971), cited by Cavanagh (1991), discussed how conflict could be 'highly enjoyable' as you gain experience of your own capabilities. I feel we have to be aware that a conflict situation does not turn into a game for one or both parties' enjoyment and self-development, and we keep the problem in the forefront of our minds; otherwise, it could develop out of control. Cope (2001) discussed the 'fantasy ladder' where a factual problem becomes modified and distorted, turning into fantasy, which then has a potential for conflict. Both parties can end up being on the fantasy rung of their ladder, causing a gap to develop between them (fantasy canyon). 'The fantasy is built on both sides until the conflict is no longer about anything substantial – it is simply about ego, beliefs, political position and power' (Cope 2001, p. 116). Conflict then becomes a battle of wills, and casualties develop. The opportunity to solve the problem becomes reduced and only concludes because one party intimidates or shouts the loudest.

Chris challenged me: 'Am I always fighting a losing battle that leaves me demoralised?' Maybe seeing the bigger picture I might have seen that and yielded. But I wanted to make the point. I didn't want to yield! I wanted to resist the autocracy that mangers can always do what they want to do, to run rough-shod over everyone. I wanted my voice heard, even if it was a rebellious angry childish voice! But I see Chris's point.

Chris asks, 'How would a transformational leader respond?' I say with integrity, assertively, seeking collaboration, treading the fine line between pushing the point and yielding. The theory spins from me. The difference was staying in adult mode rather than reacting and slipping into child mode. But yes, I was right to resist, simply on the basis that I had not been involved in the decision. Transactional analysis (TA) (Stewart and Joines 1987) helps me position myself in relationship with the managers; unfortunately, I quickly became the child within the situation with the parent telling me what I was going to do.

Within TA, the ideal pattern of communication is 'adult–adult', based on rationality and responsibility. However, when someone becomes anxious, he or she tends to flip into parent or child mode as a way of managing his or her anxiety, leading to crossed lines of communication and communication breakdown unless the other person adjusts to accommodate. As Johns's (2004) analysis of transactional systems illuminates, managers tend to be anxious and parental, and staff passive and compliant like children.

Although parent–child situations can at times be comforting, this situation became one of a critical response to a rebellious non-conforming child. Taylor and Singer (1983, p. 71) touched on this view when they discussed a bureaucratic organisation; they expressed a feature of such an organisation 'is that people should obey rules and should know their place.' However, they went on to say, 'contacts with staff in other departments are limited and these people are often seen as competitors for resources or even enemies who do not understand the difficulties and needs.'

However, I do not feel staff are always viewed as competitors, and I do not believe this was the case in this situation. I *do* feel I was viewed as not understanding the organisation's needs as a whole, which went on to incite the parent-like attitude of the hospital administrator. If I had been approached in a collaborative way, then I feel certain a compromise would have been reached. I was trying to maintain 'professional' or adult approach, but the response was parental. My 'outrage' reflects my shift into a rebellious child digging her heels against an overbearing parental attitude.

Once George had been placed on the ward, my focus was on the staff as I felt I had let them down and allowed the ward to be placed in an unacceptable position. I saw myself as the parent, comforting and nurturing the staff around me, ensuring the staff remained focused on George and his needs and not the negative energy felt towards the situation that had occurred.

Dunham and Klafehn (1990) expressed the dilemma leaders can feel trying to show alliance to two separate groups who expect them to take two different forms of action. Although I had a feeling of guilt for not 'fixing' the situation, I feel that the staff around me showed me allegiance. They were disappointed, but didn't take the view that my action should have been any different. However, my self-esteem took a big knock. I became accountable for the situation that had developed, trying to ensure no harm was to come to George and aiming to provide a good quality of care. I had an inner fear regarding the situation and the way my position had been viewed. I felt anxious and unconfident in my abilities; I had become a shell of the Deputy Ward Manager who had started her shift. I was trying to save face with my staff and function as if the situation had never arisen. Dickson (1982, p. 147) writes, 'Anxiety is our biggest enemy, it holds us back, makes us doubt our worth and ability, makes us worry about losing approval.'

I found myself within a coat of armour, protecting myself from possible further conflict from the ward staff. I was afraid of criticism for accepting George's admission from my colleagues. Instead of being impulsive and strong, I became concerned I had placed us in an unacceptable position and the ward was at risk. All healthcare workers live out the daily tension of balancing what is therapeutic against what is safe. Perhaps practitioners err on the side of safety for the fear of criticism if the people in their care come to some harm.

Reflecting on the conflict surrounding George's admission and the involvement of the chief executive has opened my eyes to the leadership styles involved. The hospital administrator approached the situation with a transactional manner showing a dictatorial attitude oozing negative vision. This clashed with my emerging transformational leadership style in which I felt I had approached the situation. By visiting the ward late in the evening and not on an official timetable, the chief executive approached the situation (me?) using a connective leadership style. She expressed her understanding of my concerns and the needs of the organisation. She offered her support and acknowledged my dedication to my role, she expressed thanks to myself and my team for assisting in George's admission. She showed me warmth and empathy throughout our conversation. This created an uplift of my confidence and my self-esteem, maintaining and cultivating my caring attitude. She bridged the gap between the organisational leaders and myself. When I shared this experience in guided reflection, Chris proposed her action was like *putting a band-aid over a raw wound*. I hadn't seen that perspective because I was in hurt-child mode and needed comforting. Chris's response in guided reflection puts doubt in my mind as to whether the chief executive was indeed responding as a connective leader. Perhaps she is just a clever politician! I must reflect more deeply on that! Dickson (1982, p. 159) expressed,

As women develop more familiarity with the skills, they learn how to be more reflective in situations instead of reacting only to the other person. Thinking and consequently acting with more clarity improves self-confidence at a deep and fundamental level instead of muddling along, feeling generally burdened with worries and concerns, they learn to decide on priorities and to sort out who and what really does matter in their lives.

I found myself in the big muddy puddle that exists within big organisations created by power plays, different agendas, breakdown in communication, and unresolved conflict. The puddle gives off a bad atmosphere and creates a negative working environment.

What insights have I gained? Most significantly, to see the whole picture. As Senge (1990, p. 212) writes,

> If you can cut a photo in half, each half shows only part of the whole image. But if you divide a hologram, each part, no matter how small shows the whole image intact. Likewise when a group of people come to share a vision in an organisation, each person sees an individual picture of the organisation at its best . . . the component pieces are not identical. Each represents the whole image from a different view. . . . When you add up all the pieces of a hologram . . . the image becomes more intense. When more people come to share a vision, the vision becomes more real . . . people can truly imagine achieving (the vision).

Only by seeing the whole picture can I see things for what they truly are. Becoming emotional, I lost sight and became defensive. Then I either fight or flight. To flight is to accommodate the demand. To fight leaves me beaten up for the managers are more powerful. Neither is a good way. I must hold collaborative intent and hold my ground and then yield if I must because Rome wasn't built in a day. In this way I hold my poise and vision, and my integrity, and not need so many band-aides! My little voice in a big arena becomes more powerful, yet powerful in a new transformational language. The leader inside me is unleashed. See if I get my promotion or whether I am now tarred.

Transformational leadership

Sally's vision was to become a transformational leader. Her vision . . . yet what about the reality?

She reveals the contradiction between two different worlds. On the one hand is the dominant transactional world characterised by high anxiety transmitted through its bureaucratic hierarchy resulting in command and control tactics to ensure its targets are met. In such a culture, people are means towards reaching targets. The humanness factor lost in the machine reflected in Sally's metaphor of having only a 'little voice'. On the other hand is the transformational world that seeks to create the best environment for patients and staff. One is a machine world, where people are means to an end. The other is a world where humanness is valued. It is as stark as that.

Reflect on the norms set out in Table 14.1. Individual practitioners might chip away at such norms, but the transactional culture does not and cannot be expected to shift easily. The system may not be malleable to change, even demanding subordination with threat of sanction to ensure conformity. As such, being assertive and using voice may be problematic in a culture where it is safer to keep quiet and avoid trouble. It is an important appreciation because otherwise the idealism of leadership would hurtle the practitioners against walls of shattered dreams.

Power

Sally's reflection reveals the way power is exerted – notably the organisational *force* to have its way – dependent on its position up the ladder of command with the threat of sanction if Sally resists. French and Raven (1968) offer a useful framework to reflect on

Table 14.2   Leadership and sources of power (French and Raven 1968)

Authoritative sources of leadership power (emphasised within transactional organisations)		Facilitative sources of leadership power (emphasised in transformational organisations)	
Positional (legitimate)	Based on the subordinate's perception that the leader has a right and authority to exercise influence because of the leader's role and position in the organisation	Relational (referent)	Based on the subordinate's identification with the leader. The leader exercises influence because of perceived attractiveness, personal characteristics, reputation, or what is called 'charisma'.
Coercive (sanction)	Based on fear and the subordinate's perception that the leader has the ability to punish or bring about undesirable outcomes	Expert	Based on the subordinate's perception of the leader as someone who has special knowledge in a given area.
Reward	Based on the subordinate's perception that the leader has the ability and resources to obtain external rewards for those who comply with directives	Based on intrinsic rewards that ensue from shared success in realising one's vision of practice as a lived reality.	

the pattern of force/power within any experience. They identify five sources of leadership power; either authoritative or facilitative (Table 14.2). The authoritative sources bearing down on Sally are evident within her text. I can feel the threat of sanction in the air as she resists. She was simply brushed aside like an object. Yet her small, hurt voice was heard along distant corridors, prompting the chief executive's band-aid response. Sally's situation is not unusual. Indeed, it is a scenario played out daily across the healthcare arena, leaving nurse managers like Sally bruised and battered. The metaphor of 'band-aid' is very apposite. The chief executive is the nurturing parent coming to heal her child's wounds. When she was acknowledged and valued, it was immensely surprising and healing. Perhaps, it should not be surprising. That only reflects the way Sally was perceived as a spanner in the works disrupting the system. At the moment she needed to be supported, she was made to feel more stressed.

It is significant to distinguish between force and power – force being used against someone to ensure control and power being used to create something with facilitative sources of leadership power. Sally found herself more powerful as a leader when she invested in collaborative relationships with her staff.

Journal entry – realising our power

Imagine standing at the doorway of a room full of people you usually find intimidating.

How do you feel?

Now measure your personal power by positioning your hand at a point on your body between your feet and top of head. Feet represent minimal power whereas top of head represents full power.

I ask Keri, one of the leadership students, 'where is your power?' She places her hands at the level of her knees. She laughs slightly shamefully, judging herself. She senses how those administrators and doctors take her power away. She takes a deep breath and imagines projecting her full power into the room. With each inhalation she pumps up her power until the room is full of it. She is amazed that just imagining power can have an effect.

Two weeks later in the leadership class, Keri shared an experience that involved attending another unit meeting. She had used the technique. She now positions her hand at hip level: 'It worked!' she exclaims, 'I still felt a sense of fear ripple through me but I took courage and found my voice. The projection was astonishing, I couldn't believe how it made me feel so different. I am now more mindful of my power.'

Just imagining her power empowers her, as if I am an energy catalyst. We explore a parallel technique of giving someone back their intimidation. 'I think this is your stuff not mine – have it back.'

Keri laughs 'I can't do that!'

I laugh in response, 'Oh yes you can! Just imagine you hold the moral high ground and he is below you and cannot touch you.'

Two weeks later Keri looks different, more self-assured, as if her power is radiant. She says,

> I couldn't believe it! The medical director was sarcastic as usual. I asked him why he felt it necessary to put people down. The room went quiet. He was non-plussed. He apologised and said he hadn't realised he came across in that way. My power surged. I felt triumphant and thanked him. The meeting took a very different turn. It was so good. I think I can begin to put my hand on my shoulder at least . . . not the top of my head yet because I still felt fearful he could retaliate.

I respond, 'You are amazing. You helped him see another way, a more human way. We must celebrate with some tea![5]'

Perhaps this was the most significant part of Keri's leadership journey, plotting her personal power over many months, being mindful to remember her power especially when the going got tough. Slowly she inched towards the top of her head, where all great leaders must position their hands. Only then can she be truly dialogical with her colleagues.

Journal entry – self-deception

Many managers consider they are good leaders. During the MSc leadership programme, practitioners undertake a unit whereby they negotiate shadowing a 'leader' within their organisation. The intention of this work is to judge the leader against a set of leadership characteristics; for example, Schuster's 12 attributes of leadership (Box 14.1). Many practitioners ask the 'leader' to self-score their leadership. Over time, the result has become quite predictable. The manager will score themselves highly against all characteristics except 'You risk, experiment and learn. Information is never complete' and 'You can share power with others –you believe sharing power is the best way to tap talent, engage others and to get work done in optimal fashion'.

These two attributes are most concerned with control. The leaders justify the lower scores by stating that one has to be realistic rather than be idealistic. Or put another way, to fit within the norms of the transactional culture. The rhetoric of leadership is powerful

Box 14.1   Schuster's attributes of leadership

- You hold a vision for the organisation that is intellectually rich, stimulating and rings true;
- You are honest and empathetic. People feel emotionally safe and trust that you have their interests at heart;
- Your character is well-developed, without the prominent dark side of ego power – your behaviour aligns with your words.
- You set aside your own interests in looking good and getting strokes, instead making others look good and giving others power and credit;
- You evince a concern for the whole (not just your organisation) reflected in your passionate and ethical voice being heard when necessary;
- Your natural tendency is to develop others to become engaged, deepen perspectives and be effective;
- You can share power with others – you believe sharing power is the best way to tap talent, engage others, and to get work done in optimal fashion;
- You risk, experiment and learn. Information is never complete;
- You have a true passion for work and the vision. That's evident in commitment of time, attention to detail and ability to renew your energy;
- You effectively communicate, both listening and speaking;
- You understand and appreciate management and administration. They appreciate that – you move towards shared success without sacrifice;
- You celebrate the *now*. At meetings or wherever, you sincerely acknowledge accomplishment, staying in the moment before moving on;
- You persist in hard times. That means you have the courage to move ahead when you're tired, conflicted and getting mixed signals.

as exemplified through contemporary leadership literature (Barker and Young 1994, Soffarelli and Brown 1998), reflecting the way leaders must believe that they are indeed good leaders even though the evidence from these observations rarely supports that. The problem with distortion – look into the mirror what do you see? The ego threat is considerable. Such distortion or ignorance is a major barrier to individual change.

The practitioners then contrast their observation of the leader with themselves – strongly challenged to see through their own self-distortion. The exercise also intend to get practitioners to deeply understand the tension between vision and theory as words and what these words might mean as something lived in practice.

Reflective leadership

Different philosophies or theories of leadership can be reduced into reflective frameworks (developmental framing) to inform and frame insights. Examples include Schuster (1994) (see Box 14.1) and Bass (1985) (transformational leadership), Greenleaf (1975) (servant leadership), Goleman *et al* (2002) (primal leadership) and (Johns 2012, in press).

My preference is 'servant leadership' with its radical inversion of the power pyramid that views leadership as fundamentally being of community service to practitioners to enable their realisation of best individual and collective performance. Such an approach decentralises power into communities of practitioners. It most fits with reflective practice. Playing with these ideas, I reflected on my own leadership within clinical and educational practice and deduced eight key qualities (Box 14.2). It will be of no surprise that the first and defining quality of leadership is being reflective/mindful. Without this quality, the other qualities are simply meaningless. As with Schuster's list of attributes, it offers the leader a reflective framework in which to view self as a leader. Whilst such frameworks

Box 14.2   The characteristics of reflective or mindful leadership

- Leadership is reflective and mindful. This is the hallmark of leadership.
- Leadership is visionary; with shared values congruent with its purpose (effective person-centred clinical practice).
- Leadership is moral (Bass 1985); acting with integrity towards creating better worlds for others no matter what resistance is encountered, yet yielding graciously as appropriate.
- Leadership is having foresight (Greenleaf 1975); the ability to be on the front foot and anticipate the next move. Foresight is a reflection of wisdom in simply knowing what to do within a complex and largely indeterminate world.
- Leadership is being of service (Greenleaf 1975) through genuine collaborative relationships that invest in people to enable them to grow and fulfil their potential.
- Leadership is being poised and emotionally intelligent in the face of disturbance and uncertainty, with the ability to sustain self within mutually supportive networks.
- Leadership is authentic; necessarily transparent for deep trust, mindful of walking the talk of leadership, without being hooked on ego.
- Leadership is inspirational and energetic; it lifts people to higher levels of motivation and achievement within a learning community.

are compelling, it is vital to remember, as indeed Schuster reminds his readers, that leadership is not simply a set of characteristics. It is much more than that.

All practitioners, like Sally, on the MSc leadership programme, are guided to design and test their own visions of leadership rather than get wrapped up in established theories. At the time of writing this first-year assignment, Sally was exploring a transformational leadership (following Schuster). Her next stage is to transcend these ideas towards a more personal vision – and only then can she seek to become who she desires to be rather than fit within someone else's theory.

The learning organisation

Truly excellent organisations are those that know how to tap people's commitment and capacity to learn at *all* levels of the organisation. In her narrative Sally makes reference to the LO. Creating and sustaining the LO is undoubtedly the most significant task of leadership. Senge (1990, p. 3) describes LO as 'One where people continually expand their capacities to create the results they truly desire, where new and expansive patterns of thinking are nurtured, where collective aspiration is set free, and where people are continually learning how to learn together.'

Senge identified five disciplines that collectively constitute the LO; vision, personal mastery, mental models, team learning and systems thinking. Collectively, these offer a reflective model. Indeed, many of the systems are reflective:

Vision is a collaborative consensual statement of shared beliefs and beliefs that give meaning and purpose to clinical practice. It sets up creative tension.

Personal mastery is the discipline of holding and resolving creative tension so that the vision can be realised as a lived reality. It involves clarifying and deepening personal vision and seeing reality objectively. Senge (1990, p. 141) writes, 'It (personal mastery) goes beyond competence and skills, though it is grounded in competence and skills. It goes beyond spiritual unfolding or opening, although it requires spiritual growth. It means approaching one's life as a creative work, living life from a creative as opposed to reactive viewpoint.'

Mental models are deeply ingrained assumptions or images that influence how the practitioner understands the world and how they take action. The discipline of working with mental models starts with turning the mirror inward; learning to unearth our internal images and assumptions of the world, to bring them to the surface and hold them rigorously to scrutiny, and subsequently shifting them in alignment with desirable practice.

Systems thinking is appreciating and critiquing the pattern of underlying systems that govern practice and shifting to align these systems with desirable practice.

Team learning is collaborating with colleagues to realise a shared vision through dialogue – the capacity of members of a team to suspend their individual assumptions and engage in genuine thinking together, recognising and overcoming patterns of interaction that undermine learning.

Isaacs (1993, pp. 24/25) writes, 'Unfortunately, most forms of organizational conversation, particularly around tough, complex, or challenging issues lapse into debate (the root of which means "to beat down"). In debate one side wins and another loses; both parties maintain their certainties, and both suppress deeper inquiry.' Debate reflects patterns of power relationships and rivalry, where people jostle for control typified by people lining up to get their point across and win the argument. Very little genuine listening takes. People partially listen to what they want to hear, seeking feedback to reinforce their position rather than be open to new possibility through dialogue.

Few healthcare institutions can be described as LOs since, in a system largely dominated by highly structured, hierarchical and historically determined professional demarcations, it is an infrequent occurrence that norms or assumptions are challenged or that the required unlearning or relearning take place (Garside 1999). The task of managing these tensions and inspiring and motivating people to learn and contribute to the LO in such a difficult, highly pressurised arena is the primary leadership challenge.

LOs are created by small groups of empowered practitioners. It requires a decentralising of the organisation and an equalising of power. No easy task for the transactional organisation that seeks to direct and control from the top in order to manage its anxiety and ensure smooth running. Torbert (1978, p. 113) exposes the very real tension whereby 'The rhetoric of collaboration alone will not promise shared purpose and self-direction among members. On the other hand, to attempt to develop shared purpose and self-direction through coercion is self-contradictory.'

Leadership holds this tension through deliberate irony (Torbert 1978). The leadership must at one and the same time succeed in speaking the members' language whilst introducing them to a new language of the LO, and motivating exploration of basic assumptions about reality by constructing tasks wherein members feel the limitations and self-contradictions inherent in their old language and practices. Put another way, the Chief Executive's Board meeting must itself become an LO, acknowledging the transactional anxiety for what it is and liberating themselves from its tyranny. Imagine.

In looking at taking the NHS forward to greater quality in a time of limited resources, Nicholson (2009) writes, 'Great clinical leadership is fundamental to this. Sustainable health systems are created when clinical leaders are empowered to bring about transformational change supported by managers who back good ideas, remove blockages to progress and provide support.'

Fine words that support the idea of the LO. However, Nicholson fails to define great leadership. I suspect these leadership behaviours he seeks are those necessary to ensure 'more for less', or put another way, outcome focused that reduces practitioners and patients to pawns in the game.

Vision

Realising its vision is the fundamental reason the LO exists (I describe this as a community of inquiry). People take individual responsibility (personal mastery) and collective responsibility (team learning) to realise the vision as a lived reality. Organisations learn only through individuals who learn. Individual learning alone does not guarantee organisational learning but without it no organisational learning occurs (Senge 1990). In team learning, mental models and systems are aligned to realising this purpose through dialogue and subsequent action and reflection within double feedback loops – do we get the outcomes we desire? Are our vision and processes adequate?

Vision, what vision?

Mandy writes,

> One of the workshops on the reflective practice course was about being reflective in everyday practice, in which Chris provided an example of a philosophy that had been constructed through reflection. This was a sharp wake up call. I recalled that the department had its own philosophy but if I was challenged as to its contents I would have failed miserably. Once back in the department I eventually found the operational policy buried away in a filing cabinet. Included in its contents is the department's philosophy of care; however, it did not state who had devised it and when. I asked one of my colleagues who had worked in the department for many years as to the origin and author of the philosophy she looked at me blankly and said 'I am sorry, I did not know we had one duck.'

In my next management supervision I raised this issue with my manager who also was ignorant of these facts but thought it might have been based upon the acute services philosophy. I compared the department's philosophy with one of the acute inpatient wards, only to discover that it was exactly the same. Johns (2000) draws attention to the difficulties caused by having an imported philosophy imposed on a practice: it denies articulation of the practitioner's own beliefs and values and is easily forgotten. What then is the point in having a generic philosophy devised by someone else, locked away in a filing cabinet? None whatsoever. Reflecting upon this, I established that the team believes that we provide a high standard of individualised care for patients within the department. However, we lack evidence to validate this. By not having a philosophy of care constructed on our collective beliefs and objectives of our practice, how do we know where we are going and the rational for the journey?

Conclusion

Leadership is a broad and complex subject. Sally's narrative is not a hero's story. Indeed it is a sorry confessional tale of struggling to be a leader against overwhelming odds. It paints a vivid picture of real life governed by power interests. Table 14.1 is an example of how I construct 'theory' from reflection. Insights emerge that are patterned and subsequently continuously tested for its veracity informed by extant theories as appropriate. It is what might be described as 'organic theory', grown from the ground of everyday reflective practice.

Notes

1   I have written a new book, *Becoming a Reflective Leader*. The book is grounded in my analysis of leaders' experiences of becoming a leader working within transactional healthcare organisations.
2   The setting for this work is an MSc Healthcare leadership offered part-time over 28 months. See Figure 8.2 for an outline of this programme.
3   Each leader is required to construct a reflexive narrative of becoming a leader. To date, more than 80 narratives have been constructed, enabling me to undertake a significant meta-analysis of becoming a leader within NHS organisations.
4   This narrative is one exemplar of a narrative edited and included here with the author's permission.
5   The leadership community of inquiry had a ritual tea party each session.

Chapter 15

Teetering on the edge of chaos

Reflection paints a canvass. The more descriptive, the better the impression of the whole. The whole is the vast expanse of history that has led to this particular moment. Everything within the whole is related. As such, to understand things you have first to look at the whole and then the relationship of issues within it. The whole is complex and indeterminate, and yet there is an inherent order within it shaped around purpose and meaning. The parts do not add up to the whole. Neither is the whole greater than the sum of its parts in human systems. It might work that way for a machine. Wheatley (1999, p. 139) writes, 'A system is composed of parts, but we cannot understand a system by looking only at its parts. We need to work with the whole of a system, even as we work with individual parts or isolated problems.'

From a chaos theory perspective, the world is essentially self-organising. In other words, it organises around values and purposes (what are described as strange attractors) without the need to impose rigid routines and specific outcomes. Yet it requires conviction to let go of the need to predict and control events – the legacy of a Newtonian age that continues to shape healthcare organisational culture. The image of the machine that demands smooth running (Friedson 1970).

Reflective practice sits uneasily within such organisations, whether healthcare organisations or universities. Hence, the difficulty with a reflective curriculum that goes against the grain of a deterministic and systems- oriented curriculum with its focus on learning outcomes rather than learning processes. Practitioners are not cogs in a machine or numbers to be crunched. Practice is inherently uncertain whereby things cannot be predicted or controlled.

Chaos theory is constantly creating the world. It is finding the creative edge between stability and instability. It is teetering on the edge of chaos (Mycek 1999). As Mycek summarises, 'giving up control and embracing uncertainty can lead to a surprising creativity' (p. 10).

In the following narrative, Lazell frames her practice within chaos theory. She exposes the prevailing tension between risk management and therapeutic midwifery and the way this tension is mediated by the bureaucratic demand to minimise risk at all cost. The consequence is to fail the woman and the idea of woman-centred care and compromise one's integrity and that of a whole profession.

Becoming a Reflective Practitioner, Fourth Edition. Christopher Johns.
© 2013 John Wiley & Sons, Ltd. Published 2013 by John Wiley & Sons, Ltd.

Lazell writes[1]

This narrative concerns a scenario at work which came to my attention as a supervisor of midwives. A woman who had a risk factor for birth was asked to exercise her choice in the way she wanted to deliver her baby.

Some months ago, I was approached by Sally, a supervisory colleague, to discuss how best to support Harriet who was 30 weeks pregnant. This woman wished for a water birth in hospital. She did not want continuous foetal monitoring, because she wanted to avoid restricted mobility in labour, and she felt the water would be relaxing and reduce the need for epidural or opiate analgesic. Harriet was expecting her second child. She was motivated, because her first birth had culminated in a Caesarean section due to 'failure to progress'. Her previous Caesarean section placed her in a risk (small at 0.5–1%) position of a possible scar dehiscence in a subsequent labour. Some units round the UK offer water birth as an option after a Caesarean section (Garland 2004), yet in our unit, water birth would not be allowed.

Currently, there is little available evidence for or against water birth after a Caesarean section (Garland 2004, 2006). Under our maternity unit protocol for management of birth after a Caesarean section, continuous monitoring is advocated, although National Institute for Health and Clinical Excellence (NICE) (2004) recommends that water birth should be 'offered'.

Harriet's community midwife had directed her to speak to the labour ward manager, also a supervisor of midwives, because her request for her forthcoming labour placed her outside hospital policy for management of birth after Caesarean section.

When I see the words 'failure to progress', this language depicts a machine that has failed. The words have little connection to a woman. In these words, she is disconnected from her body, a machine failing to move the baby through. There are numerous clinical examples of how a woman's body 'fails': the use of oxytocin accelerates *dysfunctioning* labour, prostaglandin stimulates the woman's body *failing* to go into labour, epidural *numbs* the sensations of labour. Obstetrics is littered with examples where the body is seen as a machine that is inherently imperfect and untrustworthy, needing to be managed or fixed (Davis-Floyd 2001).

Newtonian knowing: The machine in parts

In my work as a community midwife, pregnancy and birth is now a measurable process of separate parts that would be controlled or made linear by increasingly familiar and routine medical procedures and screenings. Disconnection of the woman from her body parts begins early in pregnancy. The booking visit identifies many possible risks, in order to process the woman's pregnancy and to exclude or monitor deviances. I find myself apologising for the interview, appearing so depressingly focused on what can go wrong with her body and baby rather than sharing with her a celebration of new life. After my visit, the woman is soon aware both body and baby are capable of going seriously wrong (but my detective work and interventions just might keep it all from falling apart)!

Obstetric language defines the compartmentalised notion of the act of birthing. We speak of stages of birth – first, second, third – stages that are defined and measured by graphs depicting time and progress. Defining stages fragments and disconnects the flow, the continuum, of the way things might naturally need to be in birth. Wheatley (1999,

p. 120) says 'the process of linearizing nature's non-linear character blinds scientists to life's processes.'

Women in managed technologised hospital births are *disconnected* from their own intuitive life/birth processes and knowing their body. They are away from their familiar surroundings of home, yet *connected and tethered* to technology, the hospital and the obstetrical domain.

I reflect upon a recent experience of a woman transferred into hospital from a home-birth, having pushed hard for 2 hours at home. Totally exhausted, she yielded to augmentation of her labour contractions and a Ventouse extraction of the baby. The doctor's words ring in my ears: 'Now you are here, we will get you some decent contractions and get you pushing properly'.

I wonder how much of a failure she felt then.

Davis-Floyd (2001) paints a graphic image of the intravenous line as symbolic of the woman's tethered dependency to the medical institution, like the baby's umbilical dependence on the mother in the uterus. Davis-Floyd describes technocratic society's metaphorical fusion with technology, with women no longer believing in their own human capability to birth.

I wrote the following words, sometime ago, after I was struck by the similarity of the way my clients do not believe in their body's capability; the words offer my impression of the effect of technological dependence, in this case women's dependence, on ultrasound scanning to 'know' all is well and to 'believe' in themselves.

> What will make it 'feel real' Anita?
> Seeing your baby on a screen,
> black and white, squirming, throbbing bud?
> Didn't it 'feel real',
> when that little clump of cells became one with you,
> and made you sick, and made you spit?
> Couldn't it, didn't it, 'sink in' then?
>
> Could you just for once, imagine, and feel,
> that private dark place,
> of water and blood sound,
> pulsating with life,
> where your baby grows and knows
> in a safe cocoon
> of your body and love?
>
> When did the world
> take that sense from you Anita?
> with its' prying eyes,
> needing to know,
> and show the world everything,
> to fix the bits that didn't work,
> and throw the bits it didn't want.
>
> When did we stop 'feeling real?'

Newton's scientific discoveries resulted in a world where explanation, prediction and control were proposed possible, and his understanding of physical mechanics was the basis for the industrial revolution. Davis-Floyd (2001) writes of the idea of body-as-machine as an echo of these industrialising periods of history. Newton explored nature with the abstract tools of mathematics and made possible the triumph of the machine. Whittemore (1999), writing of the historical background to natural science, says of the effect of Newton's discoveries: 'The mechanistic deterministic reductionist spiritually void perspective of the world was born.' In short, Newtonian thinking means that by studying the component parts of things we can understand, know and control. Wheatley (1999) writes that viewing the world using the imagery of a machine results in things being fragmented into component parts.

In this way, within this domain of obstetrical compartmentalised knowing, Harriet is no longer seen as a whole person; she becomes a malfunctioning uterus. In short, an 'it'.

Yet understanding and knowing Harriet 'whole' rather than her uterus as a component or 'it', as described, brings to mind Wilber's fours quadrants of knowing (Johns 2010a). Wilber (1998) identified sources of knowledge offering only partial views of the truth, of that which is known.

Objective knowledge is one such paradigm of knowledge and has been adopted by medical science as the dominant way of knowing. It is a linear, and seemingly measurable, way of knowing. For example, objective knowledge measures and 'knows' that a standard cervix will open 1 cm per hour in labour if we measure it every 4 hours. Torbert (1978, p. 110) writes,

> For the past several centuries, Western society has been enchanted by its supposed value-free exploration of the power of methodologies in the world of knowledge and technologies in the world of action. Unfettered these powers enhance man's manipulative capacity and diminish moral capacity. The twentieth century illustrates increasingly vividly the ecological political ethical and ontological horrors and dilemmas to which such a narrow preoccupation with efficient impersonal causes and effects leads.

Subjective knowledge would be that which I or 'we' know. Intuitively I know labour, or indeed the person as whole, as essentially complex and chaotic. The way of labour defies explanation at times: intuitive midwifery knowledge about birth as an unpredictable non-linear process. Belenky *et al* (1986, p. 63) write, 'truth is personal and private and intuited,' The subjective voice positioned against an objective voice that would discount my own voice as authoritative. In my practice, truth is often based on 'gut feeling', or gained through experiences of seeing, hearing, touching or encountering something familiar or similar. It often has no basis in books or other received knowledge. Sometimes I just do not understand what I feel, yet I know. The throaty noises of a woman approaching the point of birth, or the baby that 'just doesn't look right' come to mind.

Complexity learning and knowledge cycles

The birth process is not linear; it is frequently not predictable and often immeasurable. As Harriet's previous birth demonstrated, a cervix does not always dilate at a standardised rate, and neither do contractions always frequent or strengthen in a measurable way.

Complexity theory acknowledges the unknowable, the links and webs of connections, impacting and influencing the whole birth process, the woman, as far as we can see 'the whole'. Complexity theory acknowledges midwifery intuition; the knowledge of the effect of co-creation of 'what is', even in minute acts of observation, knowing and presence.

Each time we measure or observe something, we interfere. Wheatley (1999, p. 67) writes, 'There is no objective reality; the environment we experience does not exist "out there". It is co-created through acts of observation, what we chose to notice and worry about . . . conflicts about what is true and false would disappear in the exploration of multiple perceptions.'

Thinking about Harriet's situation, and how empirical knowledge influences much risk management decision making, as a supervisor and community midwife, aiming to lead best practice for mothers and babies, I wonder if it is possible to integrate learning that birth is a complex phenomenon with an empirical science demand that Harriet's birth might also be understood and known in some measurable way?

Of complexity and chaos theory in relation to the unpredictability of birth, Downe (2004, p. 15) asserts that labour *can* be 'understood', using multiple paradigms of knowing. By building on the complexity theory of labour as a *connective* phenomenon, Downe (2004, p. 17) asserts that the usefulness to childbirth of understanding this connectivity is knowing that complexity is underpinned by simple rules and cyclical processes working within parameters; that is, complex feedback mechanisms and bounded instability. This requires a shift in thinking as there being 'one way of knowing' but using empirical evidence as a partial aspect of 'evidence' within a wider complex cyclical system of knowing. This understanding not only implies the complexity and super-sensitivity of the of birth process; as a leader it invites me to embed the idea of the small interconnected effects of transformational leadership as a force for change. An awareness of the magnifying butterfly effect of small imperceptible actions and ways of being not only on pregnant and labouring women but the effects and impact of the way I lead on my working environment.

Sally and the labour ward manager met with Harriet and explained the hospital protocol and the small known risk of scar dehiscence. Harriet was informed her choice would place her care outside usual hospital protocol. The Nursing and Midwifery Council (NMC 2002) states that when a woman rejects the advise that the type of care she requests may cause harm to her or her baby, the supervisor of midwives should provide guidance to the midwife caring for the woman, ensure correct documentation has taken place and then the best possible care should continue to be given to the mother. Indeed, a recent government document, 'Maternity Matters', states women *should* be given choices about the place of birth. This Department of Health document (Department of Health 2007) places *choice of place of birth* as a key component of its recommendations for maternity services by 2009.

Choice

As a supervisor, I felt Sally had given Harriet adequate information and acted appropriately to give the client opportunity for informed choice. I felt we should now continue to care for her as best as we could in her wish for normal birth in water. Along with several of the other supervisors, including myself, the Head of Midwifery responded to the circulated email regarding Harriet. She stated that Harriet would *not* be allowed into the birthing pool, as it was outside hospital policy. Midwives would be unable to enforce continuous monitoring, but the midwife *must not* turn the taps of the pool on. If they did, they would not be covered by the trust vicarious liability were there to be an untoward event. The midwife would be seen to be colluding with the mother's outside-of-policy choice. If the woman chose to birth at home, she could birth in water.

More emails circulated. Supervisors and consultants were divided on this point. Some feel Harriet's request placed her in danger; it was an unknown. Some felt her request should be supported.

The following week, I attended a standard review meeting with the community midwife manager and the head of midwifery. Carol, the head of midwifery, thanked me for my many articulate emails concerning Harriet, which she had considered carefully. I wondered if she considered me mad, bad and dangerous for my views. I suggested that Harriet might unwisely *choose* a water birth *at home* if we refused to offer her one in hospital. Did we want to encourage that? I expressed my passion that we must support this woman to birth naturally in hospital. Carol's stance was, 'if we agree to one, the floodgates will be open.' She wants to give a clear message – in here and conform, or out and do what you want!

I remember one of my clients some years previously, so distraught by the prospect of being tied to a bed by monitors, having had a Caesarean section with her first child; she remained at home labouring, without planning a homebirth. She delivered, her labour unattended, as the midwife arrived at the house. It was unsafe, although all was well in the end, and I reminded my head of midwifery of this incident.

I asked Carol if she might approach the hospital lawyers or the risk management team. Yet again, she put her manager's hat on, behaved authoritatively, and wasn't going to budge. She stated, 'I'm risk adverse and *the case* would be indefensible if things went wrong.' The word 'case' grated. She was much more than that. Not deterred, I suggested that if we gave Harriet no option but to deliver at home to birth in the way she wanted, she might take action against the trust if there was an untoward event at home. It seemed the trust was saying, 'do what you want at home, but in here you *conform*'. The threshold of the hospital doors, where medical knowing and power reign, was where Harriet's choice ended.

The dominat paradigm of medicine sets up a situation where the healthcare worker can coerce and control by use of rewards and punishment (Hewitt-Taylor 2004).

In this way, Harriet was presented with a stark choice: stay at home and do what you want or come into hospital, and do it our way. Stark choice. Stay at home is an inveigled threat of punishment wrapped up in concern for her safety. Come into hospital has an inveigled concern for her welfare: 'you will be safe'.

My head banging on a brick wall, I yielded. I asked myself, what does patient choice mean? I wondered if patient choice could ever exist as a reality. I didn't feel I could make any difference.

Freire (1972), cited in Hewitt-Taylor (2004), states individuals or organisations with significant power do not readily give it up. Hewitt-Taylor argues that whilst government directives suggest power should shift from healthcare staff to patients, the reality of power equations are complex.

Arguably true patient choice might mean patients asking for treatments or investigations detrimental to health, or merely for reassurance or 'soft' qualitative purposes. Harriet asked for choice encompassing the quality aspect of her birth, perhaps not a quantifiable or valued aspect of the obstetric domain. Once again the complex issue of what constitutes *valued knowledge* is apparent. As I have explored earlier, the dominating empirical scientific knowledge of best practice means the most important outcome seems to be a physical measurable benefit that becomes 'the truth'. A contrasting holistic approach to knowing 'what's best' would, in this case, be Harriet hoping for an outcome that is more emotionally and spiritually beneficial. This is *her* truth rather than a generalised empirical truth.

Maps, strange attractors and learning through leadership

Advocating patient choice is a highly complex cultural matter. Canter (2001), cited in Hewitt-Taylor (2004), says statements relating to shifting balances of power from health-care staff to patients are generally made in a manner which suggests power (in this case power held with those who sanction or decline patient choice) is an object that can easily be shifted. A neat transfer of power is not easily achievable, and therefore, a culture of honesty about basis of knowledge reality, limitations, differing views and acknowledging boundaries of power is the first step in achieving a shift. Conflict of values, knowledge base and ideals, all of which might be *known to be the truth* by each of the individuals involved, presents challenges when the system is faced with complexity of patient choice. In this situation, Harriet, the supervisor, the midwife, the manager, the doctor, the trust, the nursing and midwifery council, might all express differing stances and viewpoint on this dilemma.

As referred to earlier, complexity suggests the effect of observation and presence always affects the 'whole'. Leadership in organisations is responsive to similar quantum effects (Wheatley 1999). Wheatley (1999, p. 67) writes,

> Data are recognised as a wave, rich in potential interpretations, and completely dependent on observers to evoke different meanings. If such data is free to move, it will meet up with many diverse observers. As each observer interacts with the data, he/she develops own interpretation. We can expect these interpretations to be different, because people are. Instead of losing so many of the potentials contained in the data, multiple observers elicit multiple and varying responses, giving genuine richness to the observations. An organisation rich with many interpretations develops a wider sense of what is going on and what needs to be done.

Cope (2001, p. 108) describes the potential for creativity within situations when there are differing viewpoints, attitudes and conflict over of what constitutes the best way or truth.

In leading midwifery practice, Mycek (1999) states, 'I see an edge between two eras' two cultural mind-sets, two ways of doing things.' I suspect we have more than two.

Reflecting Mycek's stance of 'teetering on the edge of chaos' and finding creativity within this space, Cope (2001, p. 104) recommends comparative mapping in understanding differences, through recognising the acceptable and unacceptable, and the driving forces creating the maps. Mapping exercises mirror complexity as a model for working transformationally in relationship with clients and colleagues, creating a learning organisation when faced with multiple ways of 'knowing'. Somewhere between all the diverse and rich map terrains here, mutual values can be revealed. These values might be the strange attractors that bring meaning and order from such diversity. Or the rich interpretation and awareness of what needs to happen (Wheatley 1999).

In response to Harriet's request, midwives, doctors and supervisors, and the patient did *not* think collectively. Through dialogue, a group who has shared terrains and access to a pool of common meaning can explore complex issues and reveal incoherence of thought (Bohm 1996). Dialogue lifts assumption and allows free flow of meaning to occur. Envisaging this with a fresh lens, I can see a clearing for transformational leadership to align the often scratchy, professionally divisive edges of the clashes of empirical and subjective birthing knowledge and how to share success with clients. This challenges all levels of leadership working within maternity services to dialogue about alternative ways of knowing/understanding birth, values, limitations, fears and shared purpose.

Looking back, I am extremely frustrated by Carol's stance. The decision to prevent Harriet getting in the water to birth was not, in my view, a very intelligent one, because it sent out a negative butterfly effect to the ever-present, fear, risk-adverse culture and does not enhance organisational learning.

A week later, there was a supervisors' meeting. Again Harriet's situation is discussed. Carol listens to the views of the few midwives who quietly support Harriet's wishes, but she's made her mind up. I am disappointed in the supervisors that risk had become the overwhelming focus. The system must run smoothly. Risk is not to the mother but to the machine. Carol controlled and commanded in this situation. In her demand to keep Harriet's care controlled within the hospital, Carol demonstrated her fear of midwifery spinning into uncontrollable anarchy governed by the whims of professionals. Her manner is a reflection of the transactional organisation[2].

Carol visited Harriet at home and persuaded her to come into the hospital and give birth on dry land. Harriet went into spontaneous labour some weeks later and delivered normally without continuous monitoring.

Conclusions: Where chaos and leadership fuse

My frustrations as a transformational leader, trying to work with women, and lead best, woman-centred practice, has emerged in this work, up against a 'system' dominated by a risk-adverse stance towards offering women choice in labour. Given the scenario again, I wonder if I could have responded more in tune with my values of being with woman? It isn't easy to know given the organisational brick wall. How could that wall be effectively scaled?

Other midwives in the group-guided reflection sympathise and share their own versions of this story, and I am left wondering how can we be such a docile subordinate group anxious to conform in the face of potential sanction; the image of docile bodies (Foucault 1979) like sheep herded into a pen frightened to bleat in case the guarding dog bites. What would have happened if I or the labour ward manager had turned the taps on?

Our vision of 'being with woman' is in tatters. The contradiction hurts, and yet I can assure myself I did my best to raise a collective voice to challenge the system. I remember my own birthing and know how significant the birthing experience is for women and the potential for both physical and psychological morbidity. To reiterate, birthing is fundamentally a celebration, not a risk-adverse exercise.

Mycek (1999) speaks of the natural human instinct to retain control in an ever changing and rapidly changing healthcare system. Yet as an organisation we claim to want to increase normal birth and empower women to make choices about birth. Torbert (1978, p. 114) adds perspective:

> The organisation requires the vigilance of all its members to determine whether its purposes are hazy and whether its specific structure implementing behaviours and the products of its services are congruent with its purposes. But members' charges of organisational incongruities may well be untrustworthy as long as members are unaccustomed to searching for incongruities among their own presuppositions, strategies, practices and effects . . . charges of incongruity may mask an unwillingness to face personal incongruity.

Carol's thinking was not congruent with what midwives, and as a maternity unit, espouse to believe. In keeping with the idea of connectivity and quantum effects, Senge

(1990, p. 241) says once people accept a stereotypical way of thinking, the 'thought' becomes active in shaping the person's interactions with others and the individual they have the view on. Could this be a cause of the growing global culture of monitoring and trying to exclude every possible risk in many other society arenas? A butterfly effect of thinking and acting out of a shadow map, or as Torbert would assert, the 'organisational incongruity', left unchallenged, means clogged learning and cultivates fear amongst the group. Bohm (1996) writes, 'People become trapped in the theatre of their thoughts (the words theatre and theory have the same root, *theoria*, "to look at"). This is when thought starts to become incoherent. Reality may change but the theatre continues.' The reality is patients *are* increasingly asking for choice, and yet our theatre is the puppets and slaves we have become, controlled and dominated by policy and procedure and risk management. But we *did* teeter on the edge of chaos. Mycek (1999, p. 13) writes, 'Some people approach the edge become fearful and retreat to the safety of an old and familiar surface. Other people get reckless and fall off the edge into despair and ruin. A few brave travellers use the edge as a launch platform to leap into new possibilities.'

Litigation when things go wrong in maternity care is a costly reality. I understood Carol's map in this way, and yet I sense we might have leapt into new possibilities, rather than sticking with the knitting, playing it safe and staying inside the comfort zone, had we shared our maps, engaged in dialogue and worked as leaders together as a group (Cope 2001).

I am presently taking small steps as a transformational leader to make learning come out of complex situations such as these. I want to lead midwifery practice in a meaningful way in tune with my personal vision. So although I yielded to Carol's command, I still hang onto my vision and values and have gained a clearer picture of reality.

Choice is prominent on the new 'Maternity Matters' document (Department of Health 2007). My prediction is that we will encounter increasing requests for alternative styles of birth that challenge the hospital's policy. Is it acceptable that these women might be coerced by default into homebirths when this may not be the best place for them to deliver? This situation demonstrates a need for midwives to resist a culture of control and command, and 'do it our way'. Resistance is like the butterfly effect, and, for Carol, the floodgates may eventually open!

Chaos theory offers a clearing on a hazy horizon of uncertain terrains. For me, as a transformational leader, it involves working *with* the reality of risk, finding the creative edge between risk and what is therapeutic. Senge (1990, p. 234) speaks of harmonised energies when alignment and commonality of direction occurs in teams. I am currently working with other supervisors to bring shared vision to our group.

As I finish this assignment, as if emerging from sleep, sensations filtering through, I am aware again of the spring and my bursting, untended jungle-of-a-garden outside. I have been shut away writing for so many days! I have resisted the urge to go out there and be in it, amongst it, rather than do what I must for this course. Throughout this writing, I sense a theme of a need for nurturing relationship and connectivity with clients, colleagues, systems we work in, the world, indeed the cosmos that we do not fully understand. My garden and nature are examples of order emerging from complexity and chaos, the beauty and creativity when working *with* systems in harmony. By appreciating connections and relationships rather than trying to control or upsetting the gentle balance, it flourishes. Often, the less I *try* to do and control in the garden, the lovelier it gets, and the less problems I have with bugs and weeds.

Commentary

In group-guided reflection, I invite the group to identify the assumptions that govern Lazel's practice and, in doing so, to introduce the group to Brookfield's typology of assumptions in critical reflection: paradigmatic, prescriptive and causal assumptions (Brookfield 1995, pp. 2–3). It isn't easy to make the distinctions between these. We (the group) sense that we have to stand a long way back from the text to widen our perceptual fields. This is a new dimension to reflective practice that seems important, deeper than identifying influencing factors. Brookfield suggests practitioners commence with causal assumptions and work backwards.

Causal assumptions:
- Good arguments influences the risk-therapeutic tension
- Organisations increasingly lean towards risk management

Prescriptive assumptions:
- Yielding to power demands is not failure
- Best practice is enabling the mother to have control of her own birth

Paradigmatic assumptions:
- Clinical practice is political
- Health care is bureaucratic structured through layers of power

The group is not convinced as to the veracity of these assumptions. It is forcing the issue. However, in terms of critical reflection, the group acknowledges that practice is mediated by power concerns that the individual and even collective midwives and nurses are unable to influence and yet, is that true? A paradigmatic assumption put to the test. Back to the challenge – 'what if the labour ward manager had turned on the taps with the support of the other practitioners and doctors?' The group spends an hour speculating on the consequences. The outcome is not predictable. So many variables to feed into the equation.

It seems that health care should be mediated by what is the best thing to do rather than avoid risk at all cost. Every decision is ethical. Health is essentially moral, not political, but perhaps that assumption is naïve in the real world where the running of the machine seeks to smooth over any turbulence.

Lazell reveals reflection as essentially empowering, that in working through an oppressive issue, she finds meaning and resolve to take action. Her eloquent, if sometimes complex writing, is a call for action to other midwives to take action to maintain the integrity of midwifery vision of being with woman.

Her reflective account reflects the development of her reflective writing style. She breaks up paragraphs as if they are separate yet connected pieces. She is no longer interested in a conventional academic style flow . . . she seeks to find her own style, weaving in quotes, images, poetry to weave her narrative into a coherent and reflexive whole.

Three pointers for developing this narrative:

- She could have been more critical in her dialogue with an informing literature.
- She could have explored more deeply the ethical and influencing factors on her practice.

- She could have summarised her tentative insights – indeed she might have woven these insights more overtly into her narrative.

Conclusion

Reflection opens a door into the messy world of everyday practice that apparently seems chaotic. Organisational life is hell-bent to control things, imposing order but only creating more chaos, because imposing order doesn't work. Order follows its own patterns around meaningful attractors. Chaos theory teaches us we can 'let go' and go with the flow and order will emerge as a self-organising force. Chaos theory also informs us that we must always pay attention to the whole to see the pattern of relationships and the way things are shaped through conditions. Reflection is 'messy playfulness' – as Wheatley and Kellner-Rogers (1996, pp. 18, 39) write – 'All this messy playfulness creates relationships that make available more: more expressions, more variety, more stability, more support . . . patterns emerge as we connect to one another.'

Reflection is, by its nature, the application of chaos theory by

- Its focus on the whole whereby foci for reflection are pulled out against the whole background – enabling a dialogue between the whole and its parts.
- Acknowledging practice is inherently uncertain, and practitioners can work intuitively around strange attractors knowing that order will evolve as they progress.
- Practice is largely organic and self-organising with little need for prescription and control – in fact, any emphasis on prescription will usually be misguided and interfere with realising person-centred practice.
- Small differences have large impact, what is colloquially known as the 'butterfly effect'.

Notes

1 This narrative is edited from a written assignment for 'Leading in a chaotic world' unit on the MSc leadership in healthcare programme at the University of Bedfordshire.
2 The transactional organisation is explored in Chapter 14.

Chapter 16

Ensuring quality

The reflective practitioner is mindful of living quality moment by moment, sensitive to its markers. In doing so, she actively accepts responsibility for the quality of her own performance and for the quality of her whole organisation. No pressure then!

If I take myself seriously, I must ensure that I am the most effective I can be. As I never tire of saying – 'our patients deserve nothing less'.

So how is quality lived? In my view, it is only possible through individual and collective reflective practices across clinical and organisational practice.

Modern-day quality is wrapped in the cloak of clinical governance, defined as 'A framework through which Health Service organisations are accountable for continuously improving the *quality* of their services and safeguarding high standards of care by creating an environment in which clinical excellence will flourish' (Department of Health (DH) consultation paper – A first class service, 1998).

Who takes responsibility for creating this *environment in which excellence can flourish?* It requires a partnership between professionals and organisations. Quality is most ensured when organisations become learning organisations. Thus, the most paramount quality measure is establishing and sustaining the ethos of the learning organisation and that is rather dependent on leadership. Unfortunately, leadership is a rare phenomenon within healthcare organisations, wrapped up as they are in a suffocating transactional blanket despite espousing leadership rhetoric (see Chapter 14).

Irrespective of practitioners taking quality seriously, quality systems will be imposed, determined by external criteria, perhaps most significantly at the time of writing, the Care Quality Commission (CQC)[1] with draconian powers for failing organisations. The CQC bases its criteria around the patient's experience, patient safety and clinical effectiveness. The CQC emerged on the back of the DH report chaired by Lord Darzi (2008) that sets out a vision of the National Health Service that gives patients and the public more information and choices, works in partnership and has quality of care at its heart, quality defined as clinically effective, personal and safe' (*High Quality Care for All*, Department of Health 2008, p. 8).

The National Institute for Health and Clinical Excellence (NICE) also indicates and dictates the quality agenda. NICE has been integral to clinical governance, setting quality standards for clinical care towards which trusts work by approving treatments, equipment, interventions and procedures based on current best evidence. It would seem that by adopting such an evidence base, effective and consistent transfer of the lessons of

Becoming a Reflective Practitioner, Fourth Edition. Christopher Johns.
© 2013 John Wiley & Sons, Ltd. Published 2013 by John Wiley & Sons, Ltd.

research should be integrated into routine practice, rather than traditional and historical practice that do not improve patient outcome. However, much research and evidence base stems from a purely empirical scientific eye, and the quality of the patient experience is often invisible.

These quality systems impose conformity and compliance, and the creative opportunity of lived quality can be lost. The CQC emphasis on improving the patient's experience reflects the central purpose of clinical governance (Halligan and Donaldson 2001). As we develop person-centred clinical practice, the ensuing dialogues with people and their families will again sharpen the care response around meeting peoples' needs and improve quality.

Reflective approaches

Reflective approaches to quality include guided reflection/clinical supervision, standards of care and clinical audit that collectively provide a comprehensive response to realising an environment in which excellence can flourish. Each of these learning opportunities are grounded in reflection, highlighting the organisational value of reflection as a process of professional development and ensuring quality through double-loop feedback:

Loop 1 – Do practitioners' clinical judgement and skilled responses realise desirable practice?
  – Do the conditions of practice hinder realising desirable practice?
Loop 2 – Are the indicators for realising desirable practice adequate?

Clinical audit

Clinical audit is a clinically led initiative which seeks to improve the quality and outcome of patient care through structured peer review whereby clinicians examine their practices and results against agreed standards and modify their practice where indicated. The future development of audit, according to the *Clinical Audit in the NHS* (Department of Health 1996, pp. 3–4), would aim to achieve the following:

- A clear patient focus – through patient experiences that clinical quality and clinical outcomes become more meaningful
- Greater multi-professional working across the different clinical and managerial disciplines which contribute to the patient's episode of care
- An intersectoral approach where a patient's care is managed across primary, secondary and continuing care
- Professional self-development
- Better integration of effective information.

Clinical audit offers an opportunity for multi-professional group reflection around specific patients with the primary purpose to answer two fundamental questions:

- Did the patient/family receive best care?
- Do we know what best care is?

Clinical audit is a very practical reflective approach to assure quality by keeping the two clinical audit questions in focus. While clinical audit has a powerful impact on those who take part in it, many practitioners remain uninvolved. Consider this question for yourself. If you are involved – what factors influenced your involvement? If you are not involved, then, why not?

Practitioners are only likely to become involved where they retain a clear sense of ownership of the process of audit and feel it is a safe environment for discussing sensitive details about their professional practice without the fear of provoking management sanction or civil litigation (Department of Health 1996, p. 4).

Project

At one hospice where I led a project to establish clinical audit and standards of care, a practitioner prepares and presents an overview of the patient and family's care and treatment at the clinical audit meeting. The patient/family is usually chosen because their care has challenged the caring team in some significant way and highlighted areas of practice that are problematic. Following dialogue, the practitioner then summarises recommendations for future practice which are subsequently audited and presented to the clinical governance group.

Recent topics have included

- Appreciating the nature of agitation in terminal illness and knowing how best to respond
- Patients who are offhand and difficult to create 'good' relationships with
- Conflict with aggressive and demanding relatives
- Seemingly intractable pain
- Patients who did not 'die well'
- Very poignant or emotional deaths where staff have become (over) involved or felt they have 'failed' in some way.

What has been most interesting to note is that these issues have no definite solutions. They are complex and indeterminate, what Schön (1987) described as the swampy lowlands of practice. It is only through reflection that the nature of these topics can be grasped and alternative ways of responding surfaced. Of course each clinical situation is different, and learning cannot simply be transferred from one situation. But through reflection, a deepening of appreciation became evident.

Model for reflective inquiry (MRI)

I use the model for reflective inquiry (MRI) to structure the format of clinical audit (Figure 16.1). The MRI was developed as a more objective version of the model for structured reflection. Its primary focus is the aesthetic response written as a case study. The practitioner presenting the case tells the story, drawing out what she sees as significant moments in the 'patient's experience'. Indeed, the patient might be present to substantiate and expand the story. The ethical, empirical and personal influences can then be explored. More personal issues arise in relation to personal influences. This requires skilled facilitation to ensure the dialogue doesn't break into acrimony and recrimination when diverse

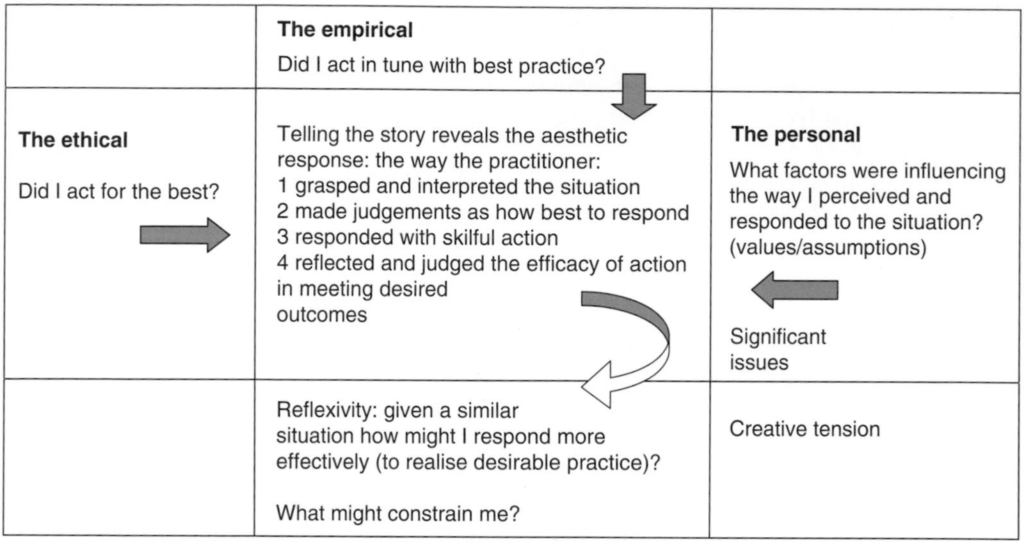

	The empirical Did I act in tune with best practice?	
The ethical Did I act for the best?	Telling the story reveals the aesthetic response: the way the practitioner: 1 grasped and interpreted the situation 2 made judgements as how best to respond 3 responded with skilful action 4 reflected and judged the efficacy of action in meeting desired outcomes	**The personal** What factors were influencing the way I perceived and responded to the situation? (values/assumptions) Significant issues
	Reflexivity: given a similar situation how might I respond more effectively (to realise desirable practice)? What might constrain me?	Creative tension

Figure 16.1   Model for reflective inquiry (Johns 2006).

views are confessed. It is vital that clinical audit rises above the blame-shame culture unfortunately characteristic of healthcare organisations. If not, very little is learnt, and clinical audit fails.

Having considered the event and drawn out significance, the clinical audit team can imagine the situation again and explore more different, and potentially more effective responses for future action.

At the next clinical audit session, the case is quickly reviewed to note its impact on subsequent practice.

Debriefing

At a recent clinical audit meeting at the hospice, it was felt that staff needed to be mindful of debriefing as a group at the end of each shift, in recognition of the emotional impact of caring for some patients and issues of misunderstanding. Staff had occasionally de-briefed following particular incidents, but debriefing as a daily ritual acknowledges that work can be stressful and that staff have a responsibility to be mutually supportive. Debriefing has a number of obvious benefits:

- It acknowledges that sometimes, for whatever reasons, practice can be tough.
- It acknowledges that it is okay to be distressed, angry, cutting across a culture where practitioners have hidden their feelings in the (misguided) belief that 'good nurses cope' or not to burden their colleagues.
- It is an avenue where practitioners can be legitimately heard and valued as persons with human needs and human frailties.
- It helps in constructing the therapeutic team by bringing staff together to create a new culture of mutual support in their caring quest, and of bringing vision into clear view.
- It helps in confronting inappropriate attitudes, behaviours, assumptions and defence mechanisms that disrupt therapeutic ways of working with patients and colleagues.

- It allows leaders to role-model the disclosure of feelings and to facilitate reflection with colleagues.
- It promotes the morale, self-esteem and motivation of colleagues, with organisational consequences of retaining staff, enhancing quality of care and reducing staff sickness.
- It helps in realising the learning organisation.

Standards of care

The notion of 'best care' suggests there is some standard against which 'best care' might be known.

Consider the midwifery mantra – *be with woman*. How might that be known? Perhaps to simply ask the woman the extent she felt the midwife was with her, what particular factors contributed to her judgement and what might have improved the quality of her experience?

From a more objective, observational perspective, we might collect a series of criteria to make such judgement. I say objective, but all criteria need to be interpreted by an observer and hence become subjective. Practitioner experience is often discounted as valid 'evidence' even though experience is the most significant determinant for clinical judgement and response (Read 1983). More technical aspects of care are usually formulated as protocols, pathways, guidelines, informed by 'evidence' (e.g., NICE), as much as such evidence exists.

Standards of care offer a reflective approach to managing quality by focusing on discrete aspects of practice. Although standards of care can be imported from a validated external body, a reflective approach is based on practitioners 'tailor making' their own standards. This approach, as adapted at Burford Community Hospital between 1989–1991, was based on the Royal College of Nursing Standards of Care project (Kitson 1989). This may seem old hat but as a reflective approach, it is overdue a renaissance.

A standard of care reflects a local practice situation that is professionally agreed, and is both desirable and achievable.

- *A local practice situation* is a statement of practice sited to the particular practice unit; for example, *patients are cared for in a safe and therapeutic environment*. A midwifery unit may interpret this standard in a very different way to a surgical unit, yet both will pay attention to research and policy that determine what is therapeutic and what is safe. Another example is *patients receive nutritious meals they enjoy*
- *Professionally agreed* involves all people involved in meeting the standard of care: nurses, doctors, paramedical staff, cleaners, cooks, pharmacists and so on. The idea of professionally agreed goes against the grain of setting patient-centred standards of care – can professionals and ancillary staff adequately set standards for patients and families? Do patients or patient representative groups need to be involved? At Burford, we invited Aged Concern to 'vet' our standards as most of our patients were elderly. At the hospice where I work, we involve volunteers who have experience of caring for dying relatives as part of the shadow clinical governance committee that oversees the quality initiative.
- There is a natural tension between what is *desirable and what is achievable* that captures the essence of quality. Quality is what is real, what is in front of you. You can feel the fabric of my shirt and sense its quality. However, quality is also something

relative or comparable with other shirts; that is, that quality has a desirable element to it. Clearly, standards of care have to be achievable; otherwise they would never be met, and the hospice would fail its annual review and be closed down. Yet standards also need to reflect desirability, as something to move towards.

A standard of care reduces the practice situation into structure, process and outcome criteria designed to be monitored:

- Structure is resource that needs to exist to enable the standard to be met.
- Process is action that practitioners need to take to meet the standard.
- Outcome is relevant indicators that inform the standard has been met.

Strucural criteria are very diverse – staffing levels, attitudes and skills of staff, for example, the complementary therapist ensures 12 hours of professional development yearly, number of syringe drivers, colours of walls, number of single rooms, maintenance contracts, and the suchlike. Practitioners often get confused between structure and process criteria, and to some extent they do overlap. For example, a policy is an example of structure, as is an organisation's mission statement. In contrast, a formulary or protocol is an example of process – actions that practitioners must take usually in a specified order of action, for example, mouth care.
   Process criteria might read,

   The practitioner greets each relative on arrival.
   The practitioner gives mouth care as per formulary.

The mouth care formulary would be appendixed to the standard. One might argue that the existence of the formulary is a structural issue, but it is a summary of various structure and process criteria.

Standards group

The hospital standards group met for 2 hours every 4 weeks to review existing standards and develop new ones. The group is open to all multidisciplinary staff and is chaired by the standards of care facilitator. In the spirit of the learning organisation, all nursing staff are expected to manage at least one standard of care around a topic of interest; to be the 'standard-keeper'. This person becomes the hospice resource person for that aspect of clinical practice, setting up and maintaining a resource file containing relevant information and research. The resource person is also responsible for ensuring the standard is monitored as designed and reports to the clinical governance group. Clearly, any member of staff whose actions contribute to meeting the standard statement must be involved in the writing of the standard. So, for a standard on nutrition, it was necessary to include domestic staff and cook.

Nutrition

Nutrition is a significant standard to consider in light of criticism that patients do not receive adequate nutrition in hospitals.

Standard statement: 'Patients can enjoy a nutritious meal'.

This statement recognises two elements of eating – nutrition and enjoyment. Meals are significant social events to structure the day. For people who are ill, nutrition is an important ingredient in getting well. Yet often when people are ill, their appetites are diminished; hence the significance of nutrition, although the quality of hospital food and service has often been criticised. I am sure most readers have first-hand experience of hospital food, either as a patient, friend or care worker.

So, what might be relevant indicators to inform practitioners that the standard statement, 'Patients can enjoy a nutritious meal', has been met?

Nutrition was raised as problematic by observing the size of portions served to patients and the amount of food left on the plate (in the days prior to plated meals). We concluded that some patients, when faced with too much food, simply pushed the plate away and said they can't eat it. Some patients ate everything, as if they had always been socialised to 'clean their plate', and some patients ate just what they wanted and left the rest. It was agreed that patients should receive the amount they needed. Common sense really, and yet the pressure to serve meals often meant we were careless at times.

The group brainstormed ideas about nutrition onto a flip chart. Different members of the group reflected on other situations where nutrition seemed to be a problem in some way. As the dialogue progressed, the group made connections between structural, process and outcome criteria. We designed a scan sheet that set out these criteria to monitor meal times (Table 16.1). We decided to ask student nurses on placement to monitor these criteria weekly and feedback the results to the standard-keeper. This is a good way to teach students to pay attention to detail around nutrition and other standards, and more generally, quality of care as something that mattered. A score of 30 is expected given the exigencies of everyday practice. A score of 24 is a *red light* that demands remedial action. No room for complacency with quality of care.

Table 16.1   Patients enjoy a nutritious meal scan sheet

The patient receives a meal	3 – Yes, 2 – so-so, 1 – no score + comment
1 That he/she has chosen within limits	
2 In an amount he/she can enjoy	
3 That suits his/her dietary requirements	
4 At the correct temperature	
5 In an environment conducive to eating	
6 On a clean table	
7 With a drink within reach	
8 That he/she is not rushed to complete	
9 With assistance as required	
10 That isn't unnecessarily interrupted	
11 He/she were prepared for	
12 Where any underlying symptom that might impair enjoyment has been adequately responded to (constipation, diarrhoea, nausea, fatigue, pain, etc.)	
13 Other factors – please state	

In constructing and monitoring standards of care, the relevant indicators are internalised by the practitioner as a reflective framework and so, at meal times, the practitioner is more likely to spot situations where the standard is not being met. Such observations can be recorded in the *standard file*. Scanning and spotting are observational techniques that are predominantly used because they are part of everyday practice.

Structural criteria included reviewing meal times, menus, introducing flexible breakfasts, involving the dietician more formally in patient nutrition and looking at more natural ways to ensure fibre in the diet. Process criteria emphasised better appreciation of patients' eating patterns and being more proactive as regards helping patients learn better eating habits.

Sleep

Another aspect of care that is often neglected is sleep. The trigger for this standard was a patient who exclaimed his dissatisfaction with sleep. Asked why, he explained that at home he slept in an armchair. This had not been picked up on admission and so, not liking to make a fuss, he put up with the bed. Such a little thing you might argue, and yet it made a significant difference to the quality of this man's care. Paying attention to 'the little things' is one of the reflective cues within the Burford Nursing Development Unit (NDU) model (see Chapter 13).

The standard statement: The patient is satisfied with sleep.

I designed a visual analogue scale (VAS) to enable the patient to mark his satisfaction with sleep along a 10-cm line and then to identify factors that influenced this score. It is helpful for the night staff to complete a baseline VAS on admission. An example is given in Box 16.1. As you can ascertain, his sleep improvement improved from an unhealthy 2 to a more healthy 4. It is not necessarily easy to sleep in hospitals even when influencing factors have been addressed. The use of hand massage was a significant development in the hospital's practice towards using less conventional modes of therapy.

Relatives

One idea that left an indelible impact on my practice was that relatives were an interference (Robinson and Thorne 1986). Was this true at Burford? The involvement and care of relatives is an important aspect of person-centred practice. The standards group at Burford penned the following standard statement: 'The family are informed, involved and supported within the caring process'.

How might this be known? I secured a small research grant to survey families' experiences attending the hospital. From the analysis, the standards group identified a number of process criteria alongside a number of monitoring questions. These questions are caring cues that can be unobtrusively slipped into dialogue between the practitioner and family member rather than as a formal questionnaire that demands the family's judgement (Box 16.2).

Writing this standard drew practitioner's attention to the Burford NDU model reflective cues, particularly the cues 'What support does the person have in life?' and 'How does the person view the future?'(see Box 13.2). The outcome of the standard showed that relatives did generally feel cared for prior to the standard being implemented, and

Box 16.1   Monitoring sleep

The sleep VAS was originally developed at Burford hospital as one of its standards of care: 'The patient is satisfied with their sleep.' If appropriate, the patient is asked about their usual sleep patterns and mark their normal satisfaction with his or her sleep. The intention is to improve his or her satisfaction with sleep.

Sleep VAS	Reg Simpson	6/11/02
Complete satisfaction with sleep	←————————*————————→	No satisfaction with sleep
Mark perception on scale What factors influence this mark? NB: pain, position, hunger, drink, temperature of room, environment, noise, bed, bedclothes, anxiety, emotion, usual sleep pattern, sleeping tablets, full bladder, other?	Reg says he sleeps worse than he does at home despite maintaining fairly normal sleep pattern. He feels being in the hospice was okay, although it is strange being in another bed – not so comfortable as his bed at home. Comforted by nurse spending time with him in the 'early hours'. No pain. Written up for night sedation if necessary.	

Sleep VAS	Reg Simpson	7/11/02
Complete satisfaction with sleep	←——————————*——————→	No satisfaction with sleep
Mark perception on scale What factors influence this mark? NB: pain, position, hunger, drink, temperature of room, environment, noise, bed, bedclothes, anxiety, emotion, usual sleep pattern, sleeping tablets, full bladder, other?	Reg is more dissatisfied with his sleep than last night. I sat with him, and he talked about his wife and the prospect of not being able to manage at home anymore. Even had half cup of tea. He seemed more settled afterwards. I offered night sedation, but he refused this.	

Sleep VAS	Reg Simpson	8/11/02
Complete satisfaction with sleep	←————————*——————————→	No satisfaction with sleep
Mark perception on scale What factors influence this mark? NB: pain, position, hunger, drink, temperature of room, environment, noise, bed, bedclothes, anxiety, emotion, usual sleep pattern, sleeping tablets, full bladder, other?	Reg is more satisfied with sleep although he was awake again – he said he enjoyed day care, that it took his mind off things. I gave him hand massage with some lavender, and he managed to doze for another hour.	

although 'results' did not dramatically improve as a consequence, staff became (in my opinion) considerably more attentive and sensitive to relatives. One reason I believe the 'results' did not improve considerably was that relatives did not like to be critical of 'their' hospital – thankful perhaps that the hospital actually existed in their community. Such understanding led me to consider involving outside agencies (such as Age Concern) in setting and monitoring standards of care as an objective representative of the community.

Box 16.2   Relatives standard process scan sheet

The caring team inform the family who they are and how they can be contacted
Q: *Do you know the caring team and how to contact them at any time?*

The nurse on duty initiates a 'concerned interaction' with the family each time they visit.
Q: *Do the nurses approach you when you visit and ask how things are or do you have to approach them?*

The nurse responds positively to the family's request for information and nurse informs the relative where he
    or she, for whatever reason, is unable to disclose information.
Q: *Are you adequately informed about the patient's condition and progress?*

The nurse is aware of how the family is thinking and feeling about the patient's care.
Q: *Do you feel the nurses knew how you think and feel about [the patient's] care?*
Q: *To what extent are you consulted and listened to in making decisions?*

The nurse has explored with the family their desired involvement with the patient's physical care and setting
    the limits of care giving.
Q: *To what extent do you feel welcomed and involved in caring for [the patient]?*

The nurse identifies and responds to the relatives' needs.
Q: *Could the care staff have supported you more? If so, how?*

Confidentiality

One morning, shortly after we had implemented bedside handover at Burford hospital, I observed the night associate nurse and primary nurse communicate at the bedside of one lady in the three-bed ward. They stood at the foot of the bed as the night nurse informed the primary nurse. The primary nurse was a little deaf – and so the night associate nurse spoke loudly – loud enough for me to hear at the end of the ward and loud enough for the other two patients to hear what was being said. The woman in the bed was also deaf. She was sitting up trying to listen to what was being spoken. However, she was not involved in the discussion. Clearly the protocol had failed, and confidentiality had been broken. We had a teaching session whereby each nurse was talked about in public as per the observed incident. The staff's reaction was a revelation – they felt very uncomfortable. As a consequence we wrote a standard of care: 'Patients do not have confidential information disclosed about them accidentally'.

The crux of appreciating confidentiality is to determine the meaning of 'public space' as set out in the UKCC code of professional conduct on confidentiality (UKCC 1987). Shared ward areas are public spaces, and hence the nurse could not say things about the patient or family without the patient's permission if others might overhear (Johns 1989). As such, any patient unwilling or unable to engage in the report were not talked about at the bedside. The nurse would cue the patient to self-disclose, for example, 'how are things this morning?', encouraging participation. In this way it was the patient who would disclose information about themselves. At least in principle.

Student nurses were asked to shadow the walk-round handover and feedback their observation using the scan sheet (Figure 16.2) to ensure we both involved patients in the handover as appropriate and did not breach confidentiality. As you might expect, such scrutiny of practice helped staff to become more mindful of patient involvement and confidentiality. It was also an excellent learning experience for students.

Standard statement – Patients do not have confidential information disclosed accidentally.

Scan sheet

Date............................ Handover observed by...

1	Patients are involved in the handover of their care.	Yes	So-so	No
2	Patients control the disclosure of information concerning themselves.	Yes	So-so	No
3	The nurses do not talk about the patient outside the patient's listening.	Yes	So-so	No
4	No accidental breach of confidentiality takes place.	Yes	So-so	No
5	Patient's notes are not left open in a public space.	Yes	So-so	No
6	Ask each patient, "Do you think your nurses have always treated what they know about your health/illness in a confidential manner?" (Sinha and Scherera 1987)	Yes	So-so	No

Score 3 for Yes/2 for So-so/1 for No

Figure 16.2 Confidentiality scan sheet.

From a person-centred perspective, the handover became an active act of care. Not to involve patients in the handover of their care was an obvious contradiction that reduced them to objects of care rather than active participants in their own health care. It may take more time, and may create some risk of public disclosure, but it did lead to greater trust that more than offsets bureaucratic concern of risk: the constant tension between managing risk and being therapeutic. Unfortunately, organisations, wary of litigation, tend to lean heavily towards risk management even when risk is minimal.

The value of standards of care

Standards of care are a true quality assurance tool because they do not just monitor quality but seek to develop quality. In summary, standards of care offer practitioners/the organisation

- A reflective and collaborative approach for developing specific aspects of clinical practice
- A change management model

- A way of realising vision within practice
- A resource management model – the focus on structure creates the opportunity to reflect on resources available and the way resources are utilised
- A means for practitioners to demonstrate professional accountability
- A proactive response to the quality agenda
- A reflective way to live quality as part of everyday practice.

To reiterate, quality needs to be lived as part of everyday practice whereby practitioners take responsibility for ensuring their own performance. The responsibility of organisations is to create the conditions whereby practitioners can realise this responsibility – the essential role of clinical governance. Perhaps healthcare practitioners have been passive about quality, seeing it as someone's else's business. As a result, quality measures have been top-down and imposed on practitioners rather than engaging practitioners in responding to the quality agenda.

The reflective practitioner takes responsibility for ensuring her own effectiveness and working collaboratively with others to ensure best practice. This is the bottom line. There can be no compromise with this expectation. Indeed, practitioners should welcome and embrace this challenge as the hallmark of professional practice.

In other words, quality is something that practitioners need to be mindful of within practice. As such, it is important that monitoring tools are designed to be integral with caring, as part of everyday practice – namely observational and interviewing tools. Of course, whether the tools are perceived as caring is a reflection of the person who uses them. Observational tools are basically either scanning and spotting. Scanning is a planned monitor of the standard of care using a designed scan sheet – usually a set of criteria that can be observed. Spotting is simply opportunistic observation of criteria during the course of the day; for example, noticing an immobile patient does not have a drink within easy reach at mealtime.

Setting a monitoring schedule is always tentative, especially in the first instance. Perhaps weekly or monthly depending on the particular standard and the extent it is 'spotted' as failing its criteria. Who should monitor? As I suggested with the relatives standard, monitoring techniques that involve asking patients or their families are best 'slipped into normal conversation as part of caring'. For example,

- 'Did you sleep OK last night?' (sleep standard)
- 'You seemed restless in your sleep last night?' (sleep standard)
- 'How was the meal today?' (nutrition standard)
- 'What is this drug for?' (self-medication standard)
- [to a relative] 'How do you find Bill today?' (relatives standard)

Obviously, questions that suggest judgement on care processes require sensitivity. Visitors may be especially reluctant to give negative feedback when still visiting (Nehring and Geach 1973). As such, questions are better designed as open questions than closed questions. In Box 16.3, I set out a checklist for writing a standard of care. The last point is rather hopeful because although practitioners are positive about quality as an ideal, in practice they struggle to accommodate this approach with issues of owning quality, time and technique. It sounds easy, but in practice standards are a difficult concept to embrace, difficult to write and even more difficult to monitor because of time. Hence the organisation must invest in a standards of care facilitator and create the space for this work to be accomplished. It is vital work.

Box 16.3   Checklist for writing standard of care

- Reflects agreement by all practitioners/workers involved in meeting the standard statement
- Reflects consumer rights and needs
- Reflects optimum quality – that is, the tension between what is desirable and what is achievable (within resources) (but always have a creative edge)
- Reflects organisational outcomes
- Reflects professional values and ethics
- Reflects relevant theory and research (evidence-based practice – ensure an index of literature explored)
- Resource file established
- Monitoring strategy designed and review date set (agenda for standards group)
- Avoidance of ambiguous statements or unnecessary jargon
- Has identified pragmatic monitoring tools (usually observation or questions to ask) and set monitoring schedule and review dates (this will be tentative in the first instance)
- Subsumes relevant policies
- Has converted process criteria into protocols or care pathways for 'best practice'
- Has been fun!!

/c revised May 03.

Box 16.4   Key points in developing a standard of care

1 Identify an appropriate topic for writing a standard of care; for example, 'patients are comfortable with their pain' – this topic may be a reflection of a current issue or part of a comprehensive list of standards that need to be developed (e.g. to respond to the National Care Standards Commission's core and specialist standards of care).
2 Write the topic in the centre of a flip chart.
3 Engage the group to brainstorm ideas that relate to this aspect of practice and cluster on the flip chart.
4 Accept all contributions non-judgementally.
5 After approximately 10 minutes, discuss each brainstormed ideas led by initiator.
6 Reflect on the experiences of patients around the brainstormed ideas – grounding the activity in actual practice rather than as an abstract idea.
7 Consider all relevant sources of knowledge that might inform the standard (theory, research, policy, etc.) – this will almost certainly require a literature search and review at a later date.
8 Draw relationships between the brainstormed ideas.
9 Reformulate ideas as structure/process and outcome criteria.
10 Write the definitive standard statement.
11 Ticked of 'checklist for writing standards'.

/ revised June 03.

In summary, standards of care are a reflective and versatile approach to managing quality that contribute to developing the learning organisation by creating an opportunity for focused multi-professional group reflection around specific aspects of clinical practice, with the intention of understanding and realising best practice.

Key points in writing a standard of care are set out in Box 16.4.

Conclusion

Ensuring quality is the professional responsibility of every practitioner. As such, the reflective practitioner lives quality as part of their everyday practice. Reflective practice can be structured through clinical audit and standards of care that enable a focus on discrete aspects of clinical practice. However, in the transactional world filtered down from government, the approach is to dictate quality against arbitrary criteria, wielding a sanction stick. Practitioners become like puppets jumping to the other's tune.

Note

1   http://www.cqc.org.uk.

Chapter 17

Clinical supervision

In 1990, I implemented *professional supervision* at Burford Community Hospital (Johns 1993). My intention was to use this approach to fulfil my self-defined leadership role of enabling practitioners to develop expert performance in tune with the hospital's newly developed philosophy or vision for practice. Key to this approach was practitioners taking responsibility for their own and collective practice. My leadership role was to support and challenge practitioners, not to prescribe or control practice.

In 1993, clinical supervision burst upon the general nursing agenda, prompted by the government's concern for greater professional accountability and surveillance to give the public confidence that nurses and health visitors' practice would be adequately monitored in the aftermath of the Beverly Allitt tragedy.

In *Vision for the Future* (National Health Service Management Executive (NHSME) 1993, p. 3), clinical supervision was defined as

> a formal process of professional support and learning which enables individual practitioners to develop knowledge and competence, assume responsibility for their own practice and enhance consumer protection and safety of care in complex situations. It is central to the process of learning and to the expansion of the scope of practice and should be seen as a means of encouraging self-assessment and analytical and reflective skills.

This definition was influenced by a psychotherapy and counselling model of supervision reflecting the backgrounds of the authors of a government-commissioned background paper (Faugier and Butterworth, undated).

The definition of clinical supervision suggests six key aims:

- To develop practitioner competence
- To sustain practitioner competence
- To safeguard standards of care
- To promote practitioner responsibility for ensuring effective performance
- To promote self-assessment of one's own performance
- To develop reflective skills.

On the surface, these aims may appear contradictory. On the one hand, the intention of clinical supervision is to open a learning space for practitioners to develop and sustain competence. On the other hand, a surveillance system to safeguard the public against

Becoming a Reflective Practitioner, Fourth Edition. Christopher Johns.
© 2013 John Wiley & Sons, Ltd. Published 2013 by John Wiley & Sons, Ltd.

standards of care. An immediate difficulty with the supervision agenda is 'what are these standards?'

If clinical supervision is a learning opportunity, then practitioners would need to feel safe to reveal their practice. If the clinical supervisor's agenda is to judge performance, then practitioners might be cautious of revealing their practice. The contradiction is mediated by the intention of clinical supervision to enable practitioners to develop responsibility to monitor their own performance.

It is worth noting the idea that clinical supervision opens a legitimate space within clinical practice for practitioner development. Given the diverse aims of supervision, I might assume this space could be structured through different developmental approaches. However, the aim to develop reflective skills suggests it is filled with reflective practice. This is not straightforward as many practitioners and supervisors lack reflective skills and guidance skills, thus limiting the potential of clinical supervision. It begs, what are these skills and how can they be best learnt? With effective guidance practitioners can develop reflective skills within the supervision process. This appreciation demands an injection of organisational resources to develop and sustain effective supervisors – perhaps one reason why supervision has faded from many organisational agendas.

Sustaining practitioners

The aim of sustaining practitioners to achieve a high level of performance is important, given the stressful nature of everyday practice. Nicklin (1987) observed that 85% of managers considered stress to be only a moderate problem with which they had no specific policy to deal with. The Briggs Report (DHSS 1972) identified that services supporting nurses are rare, inadequate, fragmented and not targeted to those most in need. There is no evidence to suggest this situation has improved since 1972. In fact, the situation may have deteriorated due to the persistent stripping of nursing resources since the development of the business culture prompted by the National Health Service (NHS) trusts. To say the least, it is profoundly ironic that a caring service should care so little about those who care. The emergence of clinical supervision is an acknowledgement of the need for formal structures and the failure of informal support systems. The cynic amongst you might consider that support is not the real agenda of supervision but a means of surveillance, however it is wrapped up. Whatever the truth of that, clinical supervision is no substitute for the therapeutic team.

Clinical supervision is a performance model of professional development in contrast with update and competence models (Mott 2000). A performance model asks the question, 'what is the professional all about?' Update model is interested in what the practitioner knows, and competence model is what the practitioner does in terms of specific skills and techniques. Given the complexity and indeterminate nature of clinical practice, a performance looks at the whole situation. Aspects of practice within the whole can be highlighted, enabling a deeper exploration and impact of systems on performance.

Clinical supervision, as with other reflective approaches to quality, practice and practitioner development, is significant in creating and sustaining the learning organisation. The aims of clinical supervision match with the aims of the learning organisation:

- To develop personal mastery through holding creative tension between a vision of best practice and an understanding of current practice
- To clarify and deepen personal and collective visions of best practice

- To scrutinise one's mental models and shift these towards realising best practice
- To review and revise systems towards creating the optimum conditions to support best practice
- To work collaboratively with colleagues through dialogue to ensure best practice.

Personal mastery is reflection. It is a commitment to lifelong learning to be the best the practitioner can be.

Bumping heads

I am always reminded of the story in *Winnie-the-Pooh* (Milne 1926, p. 1) when Edward bear, being pulled along by Christopher Robin, bumps his head all the way down the stairs. Milne suggests that this is the only way Edward bear knows to come downstairs, but if he could only stop bumping for a moment to consider it, he might just find a better way of coming downstairs. In this story we find the essence of reflective practice – creating space to pause and think about what is happening, why it is happening and ways it might change for the better, and yet realising that both creating space and affecting change may be difficult because we are locked into patterns of behaviour and relationships. But then he might not find a better way, the recognition that things are not so easily changed. Perhaps it is easier to conform and take painkillers for the sore head!

Clinical supervision offers a legitimate space within clinical practice to pause from bumping and consider other, more effective and desirable ways to practice, *including* our relationships with the Christopher Robins of this world; that is, unless Christopher Robin decides to supervise us – then we have some difficulty.

Revealing woozles

A different, altogether more positive image of Christopher Robin is found later in the book when Pooh and Piglet go hunting and nearly catch a woozle. Piglet joins Winnie-the-Pooh as he was walking around the tree 'thinking of something else'. As they do, they become aware of their own tracks but misinterpret the tracks, thinking that it might be woozles. Round and round the tree they go, becoming increasingly anxious until Christopher Robin, who is sitting up the tree observing, points out to Pooh his behaviour. Pooh realises what he has been doing and exclaims he has been foolish and deluded.

In this story, Christopher Robin might be a guide, helping Pooh to see things as they really are and to reassure Pooh. He doesn't tell Pooh what to think or do, but points out Pooh's flawed thinking. Often we get so caught up in things 'on the ground' that we miss the bigger picture, and lose track and panic. We feel stupid, get fearful and beat ourselves up. We all get things wrong from time to time. A guide helps the practitioner gain perspective. Woozles represent anything uncertain, unknown, cause concern and the suchlike.

Four variables of clinical supervision

- Voluntary or mandatory?
- Group versus individual supervision?

- Single or multi-professional?
- Who should be the supervisor?

Voluntary or mandatory

Should supervision be mandatory or voluntary? It is a vexing question. As yet, it is not mandatory for nursing, with the exception of safeguarding and midwifery, although it is pertinent to ask why it isn't mandatory, given the nature of nursing work. The Care Quality Commission (CQC) now includes a tick box regarding adequate supervision arrangements, which has led to a significant demand for supervision training over the past 2 years (2010–2012).

Of course, a mandatory approach requires resources and firmly places the agenda as an organisational issue.

Clinical supervision was promoted as a professional activity rather than a managerial activity (UKCC 1996), and yet clinical supervision is always (in my experience) a top-down organisational approach with very little resource attached to it. How is time created within practice to accommodate supervision when nurses are already stretched? What is intended to ease stress may well contribute to it. Nurses seem reluctant to use their 'own time' as if work is confined to shifts, reflecting a lack of responsibility to ensure their own effective performance. This itself reflects a lack of value in nursing – that it isn't worth investing in.

I lean towards a voluntary arrangement because practitioners, who have generally been socialised into subordinate work roles, are likely to view mandatory supervision as a form of social control and surveillance (Gilbert 2001) and not as a developmental opportunity, especially if the supervisor is the line manager. If nurses took themselves seriously as professionals to ensure and sustain their performance, then clinical supervision is a wonderful peer-led opportunity, especially if the outcomes of supervision are recorded as professional development evidence. When nurses are eventually held to account for ensuring their professional development, then perhaps nurses will take clinical supervision more seriously. Perhaps then nurses will arrange their own peer supervision within practice as a professional activity to help them stay 'fit for practice'.

Group versus individual supervision

When I established supervision at Burford Hospital, I naturally contracted individual supervision arrangements with staff. I had no rationale for this approach, even though I used group-guided reflection with nursing students as a curriculum model. In a subsequent research project with ward sisters (Johns 2003), I again used individual supervision as a developmental model. My reflections on this project led me to the conclusion that group supervision would have been more enabling because the ward sisters were isolated within their clinical and organisational practice and would have benefitted from developing strong peer relationships and to learn from each other, especially considering that they shared such similar experiences. This would have enabled them, in my view, to become politically stronger as a group. As it was, individual supervision reinforced their isolation.

I teach clinical supervision as group supervision to enable practitioners to experience supervision. It is fascinating to watch the group learn to gel and work together, breaking down their own vulnerability to self-revelation, even for the more reserved practitioners. Without doubt, the synergy of peer learning is powerful. This realisation is a significant insight.

In contrast with individual supervision, practitioners in group supervision have less 'air' time to share their own experiences. However, this is more than compensated by relating to the experiences shared by other group practitioners. Many practitioners say they learn more by listening and relating to others' experiences than they do by sharing their own. This may benefit less vocal or reticent practitioners who feel threatened by individual supervision. In groups, there is more diverse views and more support for practitioners, especially if others do relate to their experiences. However, people can feel more vulnerable sharing their experiences in groups. As such, groups may take longer to gel and create a safe environment – moving through forming norms. Establishing groups are fraught with pragmatic difficulty; for example, who should be in the group, managing time for the group that can come together. These are essentially contracting issues (see later discussion).

Needless to say, the guide's expertise is vital for the effective performance of any type of guidance or supervision.[1] Despite the forming difficulties of work-based group supervision, group supervision fosters collaborative teamwork, shared vision, team learning, mutual support, role responsibility and quality – all advantages over individual supervision.

Single or multi-professional

Working within multi-professional healthcare teams, it might seem logical to promote multi-professional group supervision. This would enable collaborative ways of working that could only foster mutual understanding and more effective patterns of collective performance, particularly if group supervision represented the clinical team.

Whilst this may seem the ideal, such groups rarely work well as a clinical supervision group. Normal power structures, for example between nurses and doctors, get played out within supervision, thus reinforcing professional norms that subordinate nurses. It is a model more suited for clinical audit with its more objective focus on a 'case' rather than on the individual practitioners. As such, multi-professional supervision may disadvantage less dominant groups.

Who should the supervisor be?

There are a number of positions to take on supervision: line-managed, non-line-managed and peer led are the three obvious permutations. My preference is for peer-led supervision because it is the most professional and democratic model and enables the development of supervision skills within the group or between individuals. I describe this as a community of learning whereby each individual within the group takes responsibility for his or her own performance within the group and the performance of the group as a whole.

In principle, within a peer-led group, each member of the group takes turns to be the supervisor. Practitioners new to supervision may require a period of time to become confident with this role and will certainly benefit from supervision training.[2] Without such training, bad habits can be learnt and transmitted as group norms.

Establishing supervision at Burford, I naturally took the role of supervisor. To reiterate, I viewed supervision as an approach to clinical leadership. Analysing patterns of recorded dialogue,[3] I recognised that practitioners never discussed any experiences concerning myself, illuminating that, even with collaborative intent and collaborative role modelling, practitioners still viewed me with caution. This insight was a revelation, evidencing the way practitioners had been socialised into subordinate and oppressive transactional type relationships that are not easily overthrown.

I know through supervising other line manager supervisors that this was a common phenomena (Johns 1998a, 2001a). Ironically, when I supervised practitioners as a non-line manager, the most common topic was conflict with the organisation. Such insight raises the question: should supervisors be line managers, given that it is likely to constrain a specific area of practice? Analysis of supervision dialogue (Johns 1998a, Johns and McCormack 1998) revealed a number of significant advantages and disadvantages with both line and non-line management supervision as summarised in Table 17.1. Similar advantages and disadvantages are liable to apply within other authoritative supervision relationships such as teacher–student relationships. At the core of the disadvantages of line management supervision is the prevailing transactional nature of healthcare organisations that is essentially concerned with its own smooth running, focused on outcomes and ensuring conformity to political correctness. Put another way, the transactional attitude dampens professional accountability in the demand for organisational accountability. From this perspective, it is perhaps easy to appreciate the organisational approach to clinical supervision and the potential threat of a liberated workforce from a more professional type supervision.

When the supervisor is not the practitioner's line manager, it may give the practitioner a greater sense of control or it may reduce fear of anxiety and judgement that seems endemic within transactional organisations. The non-line manager supervisor is likely to be more objective; to see things more broadly when outside the situation, and is less likely to have her own practice agenda than a line manager supervisor. Hence, supervision is

Table 17.1a   The relative potential advantages and disadvantages of line-management supervision

Potential advantages
The supervisor knows the practitioner's practice and therefore:
- Has a better understanding of issues the practitioner reveals
- Can tackle situations together
- Spill over of supervision into everyday practice
- Work towards a collaborative relationship in practice
- Opportunity to acknowledge and value practitioners
- Opportunity for mutual reflection and supervisor learning
- Opportunity for supervisor to fulfill clinical leadership role

Potential disadvantages
- Supervisor lacks vision to see other ways of doing things (tainted with the same brush)
- Takes action on behalf of the practitioner
- Manipulates supervision agenda to suit own needs/anxiety
- Supervises as manages – risk of reinforcing dependency and hierarchy
- Critical parent – overly critical and judgmental – need to 'fix-it' syndrome
- Nurturing parent – takes on board practitioner's distress as her own
- Molding the practitioner or being remedial
- Practitioner may avoid sharing certain types of situations especially linked to the line-manager (conflict avoidance)

Table 17.1b   Non-line management supervision

Potential advantages
- Supervisor chosen by practitioner gives greater sense of control/reduces anxiety and fear of judgment
- Greater expert input and issues less take for granted
- More professional model in line with ethos of professional responsibility
- Clearly differentiated from practice contamination (i.e. issues that should be dealt with in everyday practice)
- Clearly differentiated from appraisal

Potential disadvantages
- Many issues may involve manager (that might have been dealt with if supervised by manager but might not have been shared)
- Supervisor does not know the practitioner's practice/lacks expert knowledge that might lead to 'avoidance of issues' games
- Availability and cost of appropriate supervisors
- Potentially less developmental for supervisors as supervisee's experiences may not so easily related to the supervisor's own practice

likely to be less outcome focused or remedial with less risk of manager/supervisor impos-ing an agenda, although the risk of the non-line manager being transactional remains. In contrast, the line manager may view the practitioner's practice from the perspective of her own agenda, potentially demanding conformity to such views. This is likely where the line manager supervisor is anxious about performance.

Many issues the practitioner is likely to share in supervision involves the manager and hence might have been dealt with at the time if supervised by the manager. However, it is likely such issues would not be revealed by the practitioner because of the transactional culture.

Reflecting on my role as supervisor at Burford, the advantages of being a line manager supervisor were significant particularly in fulfilling my self-defined clinical leadership role of enabling effective practitioner performance. I do wonder if I would have trusted an *outside* supervisor to do a good enough job! Such fear reflects a need to 'let go' of the need to control the practice environment one of the most difficult things for managers to do in becoming leaders. Another advantage is that supervising staff models collaborative relationships, breaking down power inequalities and establishing more dialogical patterns of talk as normal within everyday practice. It breaks development out of the *supervision bubble* into everyday practice. The availability and potential resource cost of non-line manager is another factor to consider especially when it is unlikely supervision will have a budget.

Hence, there are advantages and disadvantages of line manager and non-line manager supervision. On balance I would support neither one or the other but promote peer supervision.

Peer supervision

Peer supervision is a collaborative and democratic approach to clinical supervision. It sets up a community of learning where each practitioner accepts mutual responsibility for ensuring effective supervision. A key benefit of this approach is that supervisors learn on the job, although I would strongly recommend supervision training for all supervisors and supervisees. Within peer supervision, each person takes turns to be the group supervisor as contracted. Where practitioners are new to supervision, a period of enculturation (say 10 sessions) is necessary to 'learn the ways' although reflection on the process of supervision should be reviewed each session – possibly along the lines of what people liked best and liked least about today's session. This opens a legitimate space for reviewing the session, enabling double-loop feedback that constantly challenges the process in terms of its adequacy.

Contracting

As I explored in Chapter 6, all guided reflection relationships, including clinical supervision, must be contracted as a formal relationship. Proctor ((1988), cited by Hawkins and Shohet 1989, p. 29) writes,

> if supervision is to become and remain a co-operative experience which allows for real rather than token accountability, a clear, even tough, working agreement needs to be negotiated. The agreement needs to provide sufficient safety and clarity for the student/worker to know where she stands; and it needs sufficient teeth for the supervisor to feel free and responsible for making the challenges.

In establishing a clinical supervision relationship, the supervisor and practitioner(s) agree to work positively within a set of mutual expectations, responsibilities and boundaries. Such issues include differentiating supervision from therapy work, group composition, maintaining confidentiality (especially in relation to reporting of unsafe practice), writing and storing notes, termination and pattern of supervision sessions, and preparing for each session should be discussed and agreed.

Some key points:

- Distinguish between clinical supervision work and therapy. For example, a practitioner in exploring her feelings about the death of a patient might explore her feelings about her mother's death. Perhaps, in responding to her anger towards her manager, the practitioner notes that 'he acts like my father'. The astute supervisor will point out the association and transference but should keep the dialogue focused on the practice event. Clearly a lot more can be said about such dynamics, such as transference and counter-transference, which are beyond the scope of this text. My view is that the practitioner can set the agenda as long it is related to her practice. The supervisor is mindful of such tensions and sets boundaries on what can be discussed and can refer appropriately as necessary. There is no room for amateur psychoanalysis.
- The utmost need to maintain confidentiality; whatever is discussed within supervision should stay in supervision. This is the basis for safety and trust. Trust may take some time to establish because of the vulnerability in self-revelation but quickly shattered if talk is taken out of the session and gets back to the practitioner. There may be times when confidentiality must be breached in terms of patient safety, although in my experience this is very rare. One example shared with me was a newly qualified staff nurse working in intensive care who witnessed a more senior staff nurse hit a patient in the next bed. The nurse did not know what to do. She was fearful of reporting it in case of retribution. We decided she needed help so I supported her reporting it to the senior nurse. The staff nurse involved was appropriately confronted.

- Session notes should be written by the practitioner and not by the supervisor. Notes should have a number of headings:
  - Pick up from last session – emphasising the reflexive developmental nature of supervision
  - What was talked about
  - What was significant about what was talked about
  - What actions to take as a consequence. It is these actions that are picked up in the next session.
  - Summarising these points helps the practitioner to focus on the significance of the sessions. I generally allow 5 minutes at the end of the session to complete the notes. This encourages the practitioner to actually complete them. Session notes build the practitioner's continuing professional development (CPD) file.
- Constitution of groups; group size should vary between 4 and 8 people to enable effective group dynamics. One disadvantage of groups is their vulnerability to irregular attendance for whatever reason, which makes group norming more difficult, especially when supervision takes place within normal hours of clinical practice when supervision time, no matter if allocated, becomes a victim of the exigencies of the clinical moment. One contentious solution would be to suggest that clinical supervision takes place outside clinical hours. I do not think this unreasonable in terms of professional responsibility to be 'fit for practice'. Resistance to this idea stems from a traditional 'shift culture' of doing work.
- Evaluating the impact of clinical supervision. The practitioner can evaluate the supervision process for its efficacy in facilitating practitioner development using the Supervision Evaluation Questionnaire (SEQ/a) (see Appendix – Clinical supervision evaluation tool). The effectiveness of the supervision process should never be taken for granted and be constantly scrutinised. Evaluation is itself a significant developmental exercise for the practitioner to analyse the supervision process and to give critical feedback.

Emancipatory or technical supervision

In my work of supervising other supervisors I identified a tension between an *emancipatory* and *technical* approach to clinical supervision, depending on the intent and emphasis of the supervisor (Johns 2001a). The terms emancipatory and technical are two types of knowledge-constituted interests (Habermas 1984). The *emancipatory* is knowledge that seeks to liberate people to fulfil their best interests whereas the *technical* is knowledge that seeks to shape people towards performing specific activities competently.

Ideally, guidance relationships are negotiated where the guide (supervisor) and learner (supervisee) surface their agendas and agree a mutual path that serves the interests of both parties. Habermas terms this as *communicative* knowledge that mediates between the emancipatory and technical knowledge interests.

The tension between the emancipatory and technical is lived within each practitioner – on the one hand seeking liberation to practice as desired and on the other hand a compelling need to conform due to transactional pressure. The supervisor too lives this tension and, in so doing, may emphasise either the emancipatory or technical depending on their transactional perspective. There is a real tension between supervision being promoted as a professional activity to benefit individual practitioners yet being implemented as an organisational quality tool – a tension played out along the continuum drawn in the intent–emphasis grid. (Figure 17.1).

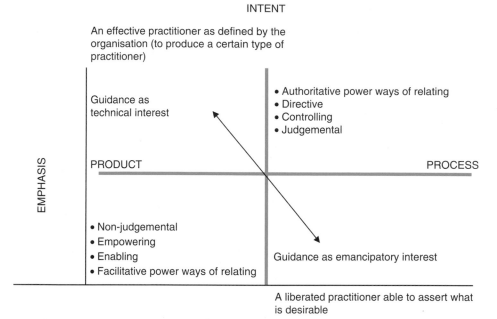

INTENT

An effective practitioner as defined by the
organisation (to produce a certain type of
practitioner)

Guidance as
technical interest

- Authoritative power ways of relating
- Directive
- Controlling
- Judgemental

PRODUCT   PROCESS

EMPHASIS

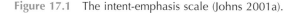

- Non-judgemental
- Empowering
- Enabling
- Facilitative power ways of relating

Guidance as emancipatory interest

A liberated practitioner able to assert what
is desirable

INTENT

Figure 17.1   The intent-emphasis scale (Johns 2001a).

The technical-oriented supervisor manipulates the agenda to produce their perspective of an effective practitioner. The emancipatory-oriented supervisor enables the practitioner to set and fulfil her own agenda. My research supervising line manager supervisors strongly indicated a technical approach even when the supervisor espoused an emancipatory intent (Johns 2001a). It follows that depending on the emphasis within the guidance relationship, supervision can be a very different experience. It is perhaps obvious that guides who lean towards the technical are more outcome focused and tend to use more authoritative patterns of communication, whereas guides who lean towards the emancipatory are more process focused and tend to use more facilitative patterns of communication.

Supervisors will never perform effectively if they are anxious about the practitioner's performance. Anxious people need to control their environments in order to manage their anxiety. Anxiety about performance tends to be transmitted down through the system level by level infecting the workforce. Line managers know that they are held to account for what takes place within their units rather than individual practitioners. In the attempt to control this anxiety, unit leaders attempt to control their environments by responding in parental patterns. The effect is to impose conformity and stifle responsibility. This would be ironic as supervision has the specific aim of nurturing responsibility. The risk is that supervision is viewed in the old sense of the word 'supervision' to ensure a competent yet docile workforce (Foucault 1979).

Previously, I have espoused that clinical supervision should be emancipatory. In a more pragmatic vein, I must question how realistic that stance is within transactional organisations that resist practitioner autonomy to act on new insights. If practitioners sense any supervisor manipulation I suspect they will only reveal 'safe' experiences. If so, both the spirit and intent of supervision will be lost. It will be a sham, a game being played out

Table 17.2   Six-category intervention analysis

Authoritative-type responses	Facilitative-type responses
Giving information • enabling the other to make a rational decision *Giving advice* • helping another see other, better ways of seeing and doing things *Confrontation* • challenging the other's restrictive attitudes, beliefs or behaviour	*Being cathartic* • enabling the other to express some emotion *Being catalytic* • enabling the other to talk through an issue *Being supportive* • communicating a sense of 'being there' for the other

that consumes time and fosters suspicion. It is the worse image of the 'confessional' (Gilbert 2001) where the practitioner is expected to confess her faults in return for guidance and absolution. Under conditions of trust, the confession is a positive opportunity to reveal and learn through difficult experiences towards realising desirable practice.

John Heron

One acknowledged approach to structuring clinical supervision is Six Category Intervention Analysis (Heron 1975, Sloan and Watson 2001). Heron proposes six basic therapeutic interventions (Table 17.2).

Heron distinguishes therapeutic with manipulative and perverse-type interventions where the practitioner abuses the responses to meet his or her own agendas. Of course, this would also apply within clinical supervision. The skilled practitioner chooses the most appropriate response to suit the situation, moving easily between each response as appropriate.

In using these interventions, both within clinical practice and clinical supervision, I follow a therapeutic pattern:

1 When an underlying emotion is sensed – use a cathartic response – 'you seem angry at your manager?' The intention is to surface and release the underlying emotion so it can be dealt with. At this level practitioners may fear releasing the emotion because they do not know how to respond to it.
2 Then, use a catalytic response to help the practitioners talk through the issue with the intention of helping them find meaning in their feelings, and through talking through it, to understand deeper underlying reasons and assumptions for these feelings. In this way the supervisees are helped to convert the released negative energy into positive energy for taking action.
3 Confrontation can then be used to challenge, yet always within a supportive framework. Confrontation is a subtle rather than direct intervention; for example, 'can you see other ways of responding?', implicitly suggests that the practitioner's response was not effective, yet without direct judgement. Confrontation is easier when a trusting relationship has been developed because the practitioner is naturally more open to challenge, especially when challenge is balanced with support.
4 Information can be given, but I am always wary of giving advice because it is taking responsibility for the other person. Much better to say, 'What options do you have'

rather than 'I would do this', even for novice practitioners who seek direction. When I do think it is appropriate to give advice I say, 'I am going to give you advice. . .' and imagine I have a neon sign over my head that says 'Giving advice', to remind me that this is a power intervention and to remind the supervisee to take it with caution.

Evidence exists suggesting that practitioners avoid using confrontational, cathartic and catalytic responses, preferring to use giving information, giving advice and being supportive (Burnard and Morrison 1991). These researchers noted that using confrontational, cathartic and catalytic responses involved an investment of self which may be emotionally draining for the practitioner. Practitioners are generally not prepared for this type of work or emotional labour (James 1989). James concluded that this type of work was not valued and therefore not taught, being a natural extension of women's work. Without doubt, working with patients and families is emotional work and, as James (1989) revealed, it is highly skilled. To be an effective practitioner requires the ability and confidence to engage in emotional work, even if it is personally threatening. As such, the supervisor's deliberate use of these responses within supervision, particularly in relation to emotional disclosure by the supervisee, opens a space to learn emotional and conflict work.

The nine-step model

The nine-step model offers a logical and sequential path through clinical supervision (Box 17.1).[4]

The first step is 'preparation'. The rules or engagement should have been established within contracting. This requires the practitioner to reflect on an experience to share in the supervision session. As you might imagine, the practitioner often turns up ill-prepared, resulting in sharing an experience off the cuff and using precious time to explore the model for structured reflection (MSR) cues (Box 3.1), which the supervisee could have done in preparation. Whilst the clinical supervision is the supervisee's space, they must learn to use it most effectively. For the supervisor, preparation is ensuring a safe, undisturbed venue, keeping time, ensuring confidentiality, being available, being informed around the issues emerging from the supervisee's reflections.

Box 17.1   Supervision process: The nine-step model

1 Preparation	Creating the best possible environment for successful supervision.
2 Pick up	Ensuring continuity of supervision from session to session.
3 Listening	Listening with intent to draw out significance from the supervisee's story.
4 Clarifying	Ensuring the supervisor has heard correctly from the supervisee's perspective, guiding the supervisee to draw out significant issues, and picking up and feeding back cues.
5 Understanding	Enabling the supervisee to gain insights into why he or she feels, thinks and responds as they do within situations.
6 Options	Enabling the supervisee to see and explore other, perhaps more effective ways to respond in future situations.
7 Taking action	Guiding the supervisee to draw conclusions as to how he or she would probably respond in a future, similar situation and its consequences.
8 Empowering	Enabling the supervisee to identify and understand barriers to taking envisaged action and working towards resolving these factors.
9 Wrap up	Ensuring the supervisee has summarised the session and feels OK.

The second step is 'pick up' – picking up issues from the previous session. This is helped if notes were taken from the previous session that clearly identified what action the supervisee should take before the next session (towards realising desirable practice). This step enables continuity through sessions. If I haven't met the supervisee for 4 weeks or more, it might be difficult to remember the issues – so the notes are helpful to remind us. Writing notes helps the supervisee to reflect deeper on issues explored and reminds the supervisee of significant issues that have emerged from the sessions and what actions he or she has chosen to take. If the supervisee chooses not to act, that's not judgment day, that's simply as it is. If the supervisee has not taken action as anticipated then that itself becomes a focus for the next session – at least from an emancipatory approach.

The third step is 'listening'; carefully listening to what the supervisee is saying and moving into dialogue. As discussed previously, dialogue is setting aside one's assumptions and judgements to be open to what the supervisee is saying.

The fourth step is 'clarifying'; picking up cues and reflecting them back to the supervisee, informing the supervisee that she has been heard correctly.

The fifth step is 'understanding'; checking out any interpretations and developing practitioner insights.

The sixth step is 'options'; guiding the practitioner towards identifying options for responding differently given a similar situation. This is often difficult for the practitioner locked into normal and habitual patterns of responding. Often the supervisor might generate a range of options for the practitioner from his or her wider perspective.

The seventh step is 'taking action'; this involves determining what particular response the practitioner would choose and what the consequences might be.

The eighth step is 'empowering'; considering what factors might constrain the practitioner from taking action and working towards understanding and shifting these factors. In this step, the supervisor may role-model or rehearse with the practitioner.

The ninth step is 'wrap up'; ensuring the session is summarised, that the supervisee is ok, that emotional issues have been adequately worked through and that the practitioner is not an emotional heap in the corner. Perhaps the supervisee can spend the last 5 minutes writing the notes.

The observant reader will note the way the *nine steps* resonate with the MSR (Box 3.1). The supervisor can use the MSR to structure the supervision session. This may be a very helpful approach for the novice supervisee unused to reflective practice.

Pragmatics of clinical supervision

Clinical supervision is not magic dust. It requires considerable effort and resource to 'do what it says on the tin'. As an ideal model, it is compelling. As a professionally driven process, it has generally failed because it fits uncomfortably within the prevailing transactional culture. Everywhere I look I see practitioners who are tired and demoralised – the mantra 'more for less' wears thin in unsupportive environments. There is no time to accommodate yet another new idea within the crammed clinical space. Supervision can actually increase stress rather than ease it. Practitioners, socialised into shift patterns and transactional thinking, scoff the idea of doing supervision in their own time. Work stays in work! Professional development, at least for nurses, seems to be the lowest priority – it is the easiest thing to give up with pressure of time and competing priorities, made easier because many practitioners do not like supervision because of its threatening nature – the fear of the confessional (Gilbert 2001). As noted, lack of investment in quality supervisors does little to improve a gloomy picture. It has become a quality measure, but this will itself become a transactional sham – a tick box that says yes, we have supervision in place but with no impression of the quality of what's in place.

Besides the organisational fit, there is the practice fit – how often, with whom, how long and so on. Pragmatic nuts and bolts questions. You may detect a pessimistic flavour in my words. I am certain there are places of excellent supervision. Like everything reflective, it takes commitment and investment. Otherwise, it will be a damp squid.

Karen

Karen was an associate nurse at Burford. She reflected on her supervision 'breakthrough':

> Sessions 1–6 were very much led by my supervisor, but in session 7 we had a sudden breakthrough and I took control. From then on I felt I was growing through supervision – I remember telling Chris, my supervisor, that I felt like a seedling in spring which has felt the sun and is now growing big and strong into a tree. I knew how much I benefited, but I also knew how much energy it took and I often felt drained afterwards. (Johns 1998a, unpublished PhD notes)

Karen's words are typical of a practitioner striving to learn through supervision or guided reflection. It takes time and the growth of commitment to value and work well within guided reflection. In other words, its value may not be evident for a number of sessions. Indeed, guided reflection is likely to be resisted because of its personal, revealing nature. Previous educational experience does not prepare the student for such a learning experience.

Karen revealed her initial ambivalence towards guided reflection; it was effort, she felt threatened that her lack of competence would be exposed and that she would be judged as a poor nurse. She was anxious to demonstrate her competence after qualifying with a nursing degree. As such, at the time when she most needed support, she resisted it because she wanted to show she was competent. An ironic twist, yet seemingly a common response from newly qualified practitioners (Cherniss 1980).

If reflection was meaningfully accommodated within professional pre-registration programmes, then it would be second nature for the newly qualified professional. The threats of being exposed and judged are real issues for students.

Once Karen had accepted responsibility for her performance and grasped the nature of guided reflection, she valued guidance because it gave her such positive feedback about practice and helped her resolve difficult situations and emotions.[5]

Practitioners like Karen need consistent and patient guidance to 'get going' so they can actually sense the point for themselves. It is no good saying research says reflection is good for you. The practitioner must experience this value for herself. It takes time to sense the point.

Trudy

Trudy Smith is a district nurse. She shared her experience of working with Catherine and Gary in clinical supervision with me over six consecutive clinical supervision sessions. Catherine has terminal cancer and Gary is her husband. The exemplar gives the reader an impression of the reflexive nature of guided reflection – the way each session picks up and develops the issues from the previous session.[6]

Session 1

Trudy read from her reflective diary:

> Catherine is a 47-year-old woman with cancer in her bowel and peritoneal secondaries. She has a colostomy. Her husband called the clinic at 17.45 requesting me to visit. The message was 'wife unwell/colostomy blocked!' It was taken by another nurse. My dilemma was, do I visit now or do I refer to the evening nurse? I left it to the evening nurse. I rationalised this by thinking that it would be good for her to make Catherine's acquaintance. On my way home I pass nearby this family's house. I was feeling guilty that I had not responded personally, so I popped in. The curtains were drawn upstairs. Catherine was blind, confused, she had 'gone off her legs'. She was lying in the bathroom. I helped to move her onto the bed and she then commenced fitting. Her two sons who were present could not cope with this. They fled. Her husband was shocked. She was fitting for about 15–20 minutes. I called the General practitioner [GP], who suggested I made a 999 emergency call. I resisted this; I was asking myself: 'do I want her to go to hospital?' I didn't know the preference of the family about managing Catherine's deterioration and eventual death. This had not become a topic of conversation. The GP arrived and gave Catherine some IV valium which worked although she continued to fit intermittently. Her husband decided on private hospital admission – we had to wait 2 hours for an ambulance to arrive. I stayed with her during this time. Catherine fitted again on the stretcher going into the ambulance. I felt bad because I hadn't spoken to the boys – was my decision to refer to the night nurse the best decision? I felt I didn't have the full facts of the situation and didn't know the situation well enough to make a good judgement.

CJ: Could you have rung the husband back to explore what was meant by 'unwell'?
TS: Yes, I should have done that as Catherine usually managed her colostomy well.

I pick up on Trudy's comment about eventual death and asked about her relationship with the family and talking about Catherine's impending death.

TS: I have known Catherine for seven months, she knows her condition is terminal.
CJ: Are you avoiding talking about this situation with the family?
TS: That maybe partly true . . . I need to manage hope and doubt whether I should confront Gary's denial at this time. . . . He is uncomfortable talking about these issues and for these reasons I haven't pushed it. I'm sensitive about a right time to discuss Catherine's death and that right time hasn't presented itself yet. . . . However, I do feel this event marks a crisis within Catherine's illness trajectory. . . . I will explore the meaning of this with Gary and discuss the different options for managing the situation when I visit him on Friday.
CJ: Trudy, do you avoid discussion with Gary and Catherine because it makes you feel uncomfortable?
TS: (squirms slightly): My relationship is largely with Catherine. Gary has always seemed in the margins, seemingly uncomfortable with the emotional issues and focusing more on managing the physical. As a result I don't know him very well. I blame myself for referring to the evening nurse when I know I should have made the decision to visit myself.
CJ: Maybe with hindsight we punish ourselves yet maybe at the time that was a reasonable decision . . . you couldn't have envisaged the way the situation unfolded?
TS: Yes, but did I want her at home for my own needs because I would prefer that?
CJ: If that was true, what would it say? . . .

TS is silent.

CJ: I sense that Gary and Catherine had different and potentially conflicting needs?
TS: Catherine's needs good symptomatic control right now but in a private hospital? I'm left with a sense that Gary just wanted her out of the way.
CJ: Taking Gary's perspective, perhaps he can't cope with what's happening with Catherine right now?
TS: Yes, that's likely. . . .

As it was nearing the end of our session I asked Trudy 'What has been significant about sharing this experience?'

TS: Recognising that my guilt is a reflection of the caring trap . . . thinking I should be there for my patients at all times. I seem to get entangled in these types of relationships. And secondly, my sense of unease with Gary that is against my belief of responding to the whole family.

Commentary

This was our first clinical supervision session. Trudy had prepared well writing a powerful story of her practice that identified dilemmas she faced. I helped Trudy put her feelings of guilt, distress and anger into the dialogic clearing where we could see them for what they were.

I had previously given Trudy Ann Dickson's book *A Woman in Your Own Right*. In the book, Ann Dickson (1982) describes the compassion trap as when the practitioner gets trapped by their caring ethic. Trudy has taken responsibility for Catherine's suffering; indeed she absorbed Catherine's suffering as her own. As a result she responded on this emotional level rather than rational level to her dilemma – should she visit or ask the evening nurse? The trap awaits the practitioner who lacks the ability to know and manage herself well enough in relationship with the patient or family member. Explanations like the 'caring trap' helped Trudy to see herself – she could see herself within the trap and she could see herself resisting Gary. Such visualisation helps understanding and shift the negative energy into positive energy for acting on her insights for the journey ahead with this family. Trudy felt the conflict of contradiction within her approach to Gary. She knows she is not available to him, that she resisted him as a threat to her relationship with Catherine. He makes her feel angry and defensive. Yet she knows within her vision of practice that she should be available to him, to feel compassionate towards him.

Throughout the session I was mindful of not absorbing Trudy's suffering as my own, modelling how she might, in turn, respond to Catherine's, Gary's and the boys' emotions in the future.

Session 2

Twenty days later. . . . Trudy and I met again. She shares her experience of visiting Gary:

He said Catherine couldn't possibly come home as she had a catheter, a syringe driver . . . a stream of problems. I struggled to respond positively to him. I needed to assess Catherine for myself so I phoned the hospital. They were reluctant to give me any information, but they said it was okay to visit. Catherine looked really well. If she had been at an NHS hospital they would have discharged her days ago. She had no memory of fitting. She was no longer fitting but had massive oedema of her abdomen and legs. I was questioning her treatment with the staff. She was not on any steroids. I thought the staff had a very limited understanding of Catherine's drugs; for example, they thought 'nozinam' in the syringe driver was for the epilepsy [in fact a broad spectrum anti-emetic]. It was making Catherine sleepy. Catherine said she wanted to go home. She said this in front of Gary when he arrived. I sensed the conflict between them.

CJ: Could you have responded in other ways?

TS: I'm unsure . . . perhaps ask the GP to speak with the hospital doctors?

CJ: I sense your anxiety that Catherine's desire to come home should be respected. Look at Gary's perspective and ask yourself whose needs are we responding to? Do you understand and respond to Gary on his emotional level or your own? Can he cope with Catherine's illness? Perhaps his difficulty with coping and emotional distress explains why arranging a support package to support Catherine at home was not enough to persuade him to have her home?

Trudy is uncomfortable. I sense my challenge has Trudy slightly on her back foot.

TS: I feel the hospital is colluding with Gary in terms of his own needs rather than Catherine's – as if Catherine had become some object to talk about and do things with.

We explore Trudy's options and potential consequences. One option was to involve Clare, the Macmillan nurse more actively in Catherine's care. It felt like bringing in reinforcements to battle Gary.

CJ: Do you want Clare to confront Gary?

TS: Clare doesn't know the family well whereas I do. I don't know how Catherine would feel if Clare came in.

CJ: What you're really saying is that you don't know how you will feel if Clare comes in – will you feel pushed out? Is that your fear? Is it time to confront Gary with the conflict of needs on an emotional level? Could you do that if you felt it appropriate?

TS: Say more.

CJ: For example, 'I can see this is tough for you Gary.' He might be feeling guilty about not having his wife at home, so such a response might help him face his guilt? It is not merely a stark choice of either hospital or home to die but to take each day as it comes, to leave the doors open. The cathartic response would make it easier to confront Gary: 'What does Catherine want?' 'Should you respect her wishes?'

TS: If she came home she could always go back into hospital or the hospice if things deteriorate badly. I haven't really talked with him. I feel concerned that I should be manipulating him towards my views. I accept my sympathies and interests have lain primarily with Catherine.

CJ: I sense a major issue for Catherine is being in control of her own dying, ensuring that those she leaves behind can cope without her. Issues about her two sons and why she needs to be at home.

At the end of the session,

TS: The session has helped me to see things differently, most notably paying attention to Gary's needs and how this is central to getting Catherine home. It has influenced my future actions and helped me anticipate what Gary may be thinking. I will arrange to meet him again! Thank you.

Commentary

Trudy continued to resist Gary yet struggled with this contradiction of her holistic beliefs. Holism is not a rational technique to be applied but an intuitive way for being. By empathising with Gary, I challenged Trudy to develop her own empathic understanding with Gary's perspective and understand his own suffering. This was vital if she was going to shift her perspective of Gary as adversary and become available to him. How do we sense what the other is feeling and thinking at such moments? Only when Trudy can work through her resistance to Gary can she truly empathise with him. Trudy's emotional entanglement with Catherine is revealed in her anxiety of Clare's involvement. It illustrates how judgement is blurred by her own concerns.

   Trudy moves on in her journey with this family. We have revisited issues that surfaced in the first session and yet, just because she could see things differently, does not mean she could easily shift her emotional responses or change her embodied responses. Learning through reflection is a holistic process of knowing and transforming self. Yet, we cannot imply shrug off who we are.

Session 3

Forty-one days later. . . . Trudy picked up the threads of her unfolding experience with Catherine and Gary:

> I did visit and confront him with the prospect of Catherine coming home. He was uptight. He said 'I know I am being selfish but I've got a life to lead, and the boys as well. . . . If Catherine is coming home then someone has to be here all the time.' He was adamant and said that he had to return imminently to work in Indonesia. I didn't pursue it because I could see it was making him more uptight. I contacted the hospital. They said Catherine could be kept on insurance funding because she had a syringe driver which counted as treatment. I offered to look after her if she came home. But after that I didn't hear from them or Gary. I became despondent about it. Then, this week, she was sent home for the day. Gary informed me and I went to visit her. She was downstairs sitting at the kitchen table. She looked well. No syringe driver, no catheter. She was eating and drinking. Walking up and down stairs. Her legs were less swollen although her ascites remained and made her look nine months pregnant. She said, 'I feel really well.' Gary interceded, 'You're not well, are you?' He was challenging what she could do, getting up and down stairs. I asked her when she was coming home? She said she was working on it, pulling a face at Gary. He said that she was not ready to come home. I asked her what I could do to help you when you do come home? And today? I heard she is coming home on Thursday . . . a phone message from Gary. The insurance funding has dried up. He has got to come to terms with it now she's returning home. I have arranged a package of care for her. She's really determined. She said that she had forced herself to eat to make herself better. There was no explanation for the epilepsy. They didn't do a brain scan and she isn't on any epileptic drugs. Perhaps it was a reaction from the nozinam? She was on dexamethasone, but now there is friction between them about coming home.

CJ: Trudy, how do you feel about your involvement with Catherine?

Trudy looks me in the eye:

TS: I know it's going to be tough when Catherine eventually dies. Gary's comments are off-putting for Catherine. I know I need to be supportive towards Gary rather than confronting him with his persistent negative attitude because he may be feeling guilty about not wanting her home. I do feel more in tune with Gary . . . sense how he's feeling more easily, and hence more available to him. After I last saw him, I let it go. I feel guilty about that. I saw him in the shops and I went off the other way rather than face him. I began to feel awkward pushing it for her. Often at home I would think how she was. I couldn't understand why they had kept the syringe driver going. Her body is covered with abscess sites from the driver – they had to change the site every day. She's on MST now. . . . I can see how I have been drawn into an emotional web, entangled and pulled between them. Talking it through with you I am less entangled. . . . I feel it differently now.'

CJ: That's a good image – visualise yourself in this web and pull yourself out. Here, let me help you. . . .

I pull on an imaginary rope, pulling her free. Trudy laughs. I help her frame her involvement with Catherine and Gary using the nurse–patient involvement theory of Morse (1991) and Ramos (1992). Trudy identified with the Morse 'type' of 'overinvolvement'.

TS: Yes, I've been there!

CJ: We all need to experience emotional entanglement, because only then can we recognise the place. Perhaps entanglement is an inevitable consequence of holistic relationship because it's so hard to resist the suffering of the other. It is like a tidal wave that we must learn to surf and control yet without relinquishing its exquisite intimacy and beauty. It's okay to be vulnerable, but like the expert surfer we can learn to ride it. Maybe we do get swept away sometimes but that's just another experience to learn from. That's where reflection can help us.

TS: It shows how unprepared we are for emotional work and then suddenly I find myself in an emotional quagmire. Seeing the best way forward is blurred by feelings.

Commentary

The idea of the imaginary rope is a technique I use to help pull practitioners free from emotional entanglement. Note how I also use theory (Morse, Ramos) to help Trudy see herself more clearly.

Session 4

Thirty days later. . . . Trudy is late: 'Sorry . . . I've been to a funeral and then an urgent visit.'

CJ: Not Catherine's funeral?

TS: No! She's up and well. I'm seeing her twice a week. She's been having some difficulty with her son. He has problems with drugs and also a recent court appearance because of stealing.

Picking up the cue I inquire:

CJ: Have you helped the sons talk about what's happening to their mother?

TS: No. Gary has not returned to Indonesia yet. He's saying he has got to go next month but he's also said that someone needs to be with Catherine the whole time.

CJ: Is this necessary?

TS: I don't think so, at least not 24 hours a day because if someone has 24-hour care she can't live a normal life, can she?

CJ: If you're waiting to die, can you live a 'normal life'?

TS: Well, she struggles to do the housework, but she can wash and dress herself, etc.

CJ: You're responding to her in terms of things she can physically do, what about her responses on an emotional level? Is she coping on this level?

TS: She doesn't seem want to talk on this level although she does give cues such as 'living on borrowed time' . . . it's difficult to talk to her because her husband and sons are often there and they don't want to talk about it.

CJ: Maybe they don't know how to talk about it?

TS: I have another Catherine, who is also dying yet very open to what was happening to her . . . she needs to resolve issues such as who was going to look after her five-year-old son. Of course, how people feel and what they think about their impending death can never be predicted. The wavelength becomes a roller coaster!

CJ: Perhaps Catherine is ambivalent? As you said, she is not in denial. She accepts she is going to die, but she also needs to cope and protect her boys. Perhaps she is trying to be brave? Imagine yourself in her shoes, what sort of things would you need to be doing?

TS: Well, sort out my children, put my house in order.

CJ: Do you remember the message from *Final Gifts* (Callanan and Kelley 1992) – that the primary task for the dying person was to ensure that those they left behind were able to cope?

TS: I do, that was very powerful . . . the other Catherine is 'coming to terms' . . . even things like changing internal doors in the house, things that she had wanted to do. She is now quite peaceful with everything sorted out.

Pursuing the point, I suggest,

CJ: Perhaps we can see that Catherine is trying to cope with chaos. Perhaps she does need confronting in order to help her sort things out? Perhaps you are avoiding this for your discomfort and uncertainty about her ambivalence?'

TS: I accept your point. . . . I just don't feel with this family that they are ready to talk about it. I don't feel her physical deterioration has become that marked where her dying has really become an issue. They are a 'difficult' family, I have a number of people who are dying where talking about death is not a problem.

I take Trudy back to the beginning of the session:

CJ: All this came out of me asking, was it Catherine's funeral?!

Trudy laughs and then seriously,

TS: We have had a lot of people dying – nine recently. It's stressful. It doesn't help having conflict with the doctors. One particular situation over drug dosage made me fume.

The doctor wasn't listening to me. I didn't back down and asserted my point of view. She was short with me but she didn't bawl me out of the office.

CJ: The intimidating factor – *being short*.

Trudy laughed:

TS: Some patients have commented on her manner – her new year's resolution is to be less short!'

CJ: It's promising she has insight! Maybe she's changing. It doesn't help when work is tough to have oppressive relationships within the team. Last session I challenged you to consider the balance of being challenging and being supportive with Gary and Catherine.

TS: My stance towards Gary has changed. I now see their relationship differently. I see that maybe he couldn't go to Indonesia because he couldn't leave Catherine at home and that being with her was an emotional rather than a physical thing. Could he focus on work knowing she was as she was?

Commentary

Trudy contrasts Catherine with other dying patients she visits in her effort to make sense of her struggle with Catherine and Gary whilst trying to position herself within the tension of confronting the family's reluctance to talk about Catherine's imminent death. What would be for the best? To know is to tune into the unfolding patterns of shifting wavelengths and sense it. My guidance is to make Trudy more mindful of this tension, indeed pushing the point. Other issues that impinge on Trudy's ability to be available emerge, such as the conflict with doctors.

Session 5

Twenty-one days later. . . . Trudy says,

Gary is letting me in now and that I'm responding to my intuition that it's now the right time to talk about dying. Catherine's in the terminal stage of her illness. . . . I went in following a phone call from Catherine that her colostomy was obstructed. Up to this time I had been going in twice weekly. She had been self-caring so I went in to discuss what had been happening to her. On this visit she was in bed. She said she had great abdominal pain. I sought the GP's advice. The GP had prescribed a suppository, but this hadn't worked and had since prescribed 'normacol'. Because of the pain I advised Catherine not to take this. I also referred her to the night nurse so she could get help if she needed it.

CJ: What treatment do you think might be best?

After considering palliative approaches to Catherine's bowel obstruction Trudy says,

TS: Gary was downstairs during this visit. I had informed him that the colostomy was obstructed and that this was a sign of things worsening and her imminent death. Gary said it wasn't fair to keep her alive. Why were we giving her all these drugs?

That we needed to put an end to all this! I asked him if Catherine was talking about dying? He said that he wanted to look after her at home and not to go back into hospital. I thought he might be strapped for cash, but he assured me that wasn't the reason. She didn't want to go back in and he had accepted that. The elder son didn't want to stray too far in case anything happened to mum. No talk of the younger son, he was still having his troubles. I'm now visiting every day.

CJ: Trudy why are *you* visiting every day?

TS: Because my enrolled nurse is no good at counselling. She 'whips in and out'. Both Catherine and Gary made this observation. She's a good nurse but prefers going in and doing something physical. I need to monitor the colostomy and to respond to her symptoms on a daily basis and to help the family through the crisis.

CJ: Being there for them?

TS: Yes, that's right. I had two other patients who were similar to Catherine with obstructed colostomies. One lived for 3 months after it had become blocked. She would vomit every day. In the end – faecal matter, not very pleasant. I have told them about such possibility. Catherine is struggling to eat just a little. She has requested some 'HiCal' drinks to keep her strength up. . . . I can tell by the look she gives me that she knows she has deteriorated, but she doesn't want to talk about that. She feels the lumps in her tummy . . . still hoping the tumour will still go away.

CJ: It must be hard for you to see her suffer like that, her grief all bottled up inside it . . . when you know it would help her to share it with you?

It was a poignant moment to dwell in that truth, in silence for a moment. I broke the spell by challenging Trudy over her team leader responsibilities – 'what do you need to do when you know that members of your team are not responding appropriately?'

TS: I find it hard to tackle such issues because I don't like conflict even when I know it compromises patient care. . . . I want to talk more about Gary? Gary is out of control, feeling helpless, very anxious and angry. He tested out the night nurse to gauge her response – which was okay! This is going to be tough, especially when she becomes more physically dependent, vomiting, etc. I feel ok, not overinvolved. I feel happy because Catherine is quite happy. Things are under control. I enjoy visiting them. Before, I wasn't in control.

Commentary

Trudy felt that the dynamics had changed with Gary because he now accepted that Catherine was going to die at home, although he clearly struggles with his feelings. The situation is very tense.

Focusing Trudy's attention on the situation with her enrolled nurse was misplaced in that her mind was wrapped up with Catherine and Gary. Yet her resistance to talk about her colleague reflects her avoidance of the issue in practice.

Session 6

Forty-six days later, Trudy noted how busy she was and the pressure she felt under just now. She picked up Catherine:

Catherine . . . her death. She was fighting to the end. She was on a massive dose of diamorphine – 500 mg in her syringe driver. She had another massive fit. I'll read from my diary – 'I visited Catherine Monday morning early; the Marie Curie nurse had rung me to say that Catherine had a very restless night and was not responding to oral commands, and there was a steady trickle of black fluid running from her mouth. I decided to assess the situation and rang the GP from Catherine's house. As I entered the bedroom I was shocked by what I saw. Catherine was groaning and rolling around the bed. Gary was trying to hold her onto the bed. She rolled from side to side, legs hanging over the edge of the bed, her catheter tube kinked and twisted around her leg, her tubing from the syringe driver had become detached. Clearly Gary was distressed. Catherine lay across the bed, her huge abdomen hard and contracting, her swollen legs looked heavy and shiny, her face, arms, and shoulders so thin that you see her bones protruding. I sat on the bed, reconnecting the syringe driver and checked the light was flashing. Gently I talked to Catherine, holding her hand. She was calm for a minute, and then she began to groan again, vomited and started to fit. Gary and I rolled Catherine onto her side in the recovery position. I called the GP to come straight away and rang the clinic, asking the reception staff to bleep my nursing auxiliary and ask her to come to Catherine's house urgently. While we waited Gary and I talked; I admitted to Gary that I had never witnessed anything like this before in all my nursing experience.

Catherine's strength was amazing, on occasions rolling onto to her enlarged abdomen. All kinds of emotions were spinning through my head. I felt sad for Gary witnessing this, Catherine's loss of dignity – what an awful death and I was helpless to do anything. I had no valium to stop the fit and no injection available to calm Catherine. I spoke to Gary and said the only good thing about this was that Catherine doesn't know what's going on. The GP arrived – he was visibly shocked and passed me a valium enema which I inserted into Catherine's colostomy. Within a few minutes Catherine was calm. I asked the GP for another in case she fitted again and asked him if he had any midazolam 20 mg that I could use to sedate Catherine as she was very agitated and restless. He wrote the medication and Stuart, Gary's son went to collect the prescription. Ann, my nursing auxiliary arrived, and we washed Catherine, talking gently to her, comforting her, cleansed her mouth and put a clean nightie on and clean sheets. By this time Stuart had returned and I could give the midazolam intramuscularly into her thigh. Within 10 minutes she was asleep. Gary, Ann and I sat around the bed emotionally drained just looking at Catherine. I knew I could not leave Gary alone. The situation was frightening for him. Gary thanked us both and felt reassured that he was not going to be left alone. He was happier that she was asleep.'

Trudy puts her diary aside and asks herself:

What was I trying to achieve? My main concern was for Gary who was visibly distressed. Catherine would have been horrified if she could see herself, nightie up around her breasts, legs and bottom exposed, rolling around her bed, groaning, complete loss of dignity. Gary was distraught, unable to restrain her almost falling out of bed. I was frustrated that there were no drugs prescribed that I could have given. When Catherine was asleep and calm, Gary could manage. He rarely touched Catherine – he always stood at the foot of the bed or sat in a chair. I never saw him hold her hand although he always talked fondly of her. I came to the conclusion that he was afraid, and it would be less stressful for him if Ann assisted me in all nursing duties. I've learnt so much from this, but I never did get to grips with Gary. I said to him, 'it won't be long' and queried whether he wanted her family present. He said that they can come at any time, but he didn't want them staying. He said, 'I don't think of her death, I think of the future.' He never shed a tear. I went to the funeral. Her father was heartbroken as his wife had died of cancer as well.

I acknowledged Trudy's feeling 'This must have been very traumatic for you . . . you moved a long way to accommodate Gary within your sphere of care.'

TS: That's been my real learning – to see and respond to the whole family. It's true, I do normally identify with the woman in the situation which often leaves me feeling angry at the spouses, as with Gary, because he seemed to interfere with helping me to help Catherine meet her needs.

Commentary

This dialogue is a story of Trudy coming to know herself. The contradiction between her holistic values and her practice were evident from the beginning. It was not a perfect ending, but such situations rarely are. Issues such as supporting the boys were left relatively untouched. She wanted to avoid her organisational difficulties to focus on her clinical practice.

As a general rule, I let practitioner speak until they pause. I then reflect back what I have heard or pick up any strong emotion as a cathartic response. My interpretations are offered tentatively not authoritatively – although sometimes provocatively to engender a response. Whilst Trudy may initially have been defensive to some of my interpretations, she did learn to trust that I was always on her side and never judgemental, although it is perhaps inevitable that supervisors cannot help but be judgemental to some extent especially when we disagree with the practitioner's perspective. The art of confrontation!

A quiet eddy

Imagine clinical practice as a fast-moving river. In the busyness of the day, many practitioners feel they are being swept along in the current, reacting to events as they unfold about them. Clinical supervision is like an eddy within the fast-moving water that enables the practitioner to pause in relative stillness, and reflect on what is going on in the fast-moving water. In this way, the practitioner, like Trudy, prepares herself to practice more effectively when she re-enters the current and not be so swept along. The eddy is still part of the dynamic harmony of events; it is not time out from the river itself. Yet the current of everyday practice is strong, and the effort to find the eddy requires vision, effort and resolve. The eddy must be seen as a desirable place because the current will not let you go too easily.

In Chapter 18 I offer three further exemplars of clinical supervision.

Notes

1 See Chapter 6 for exploration of guiding reflective practice.
2 At the University of Bedfordshire I lead a supervision programme consisting of 12 three-hour sessions spread over 30 weeks. Please contact me directly for further information.
3 Implementing guided reflection/supervision was established as a research project.
4 The descriptors within the nine-step model have been amended from the previous edition.
5 See exemplar of guided reflection involving Karen in Johns (2004) *Becoming a Reflective Practitioner* (second edition), pp. 131–144.
6 The dialogue was recorded and edited as part of an ongoing research project to enable development of expertise with district nurses (unpublished).

Chapter 18

Tales of clinical supervision

In the previous chapter I set out the nature of clinical supervision as a specific type of guided reflection within clinical practice. Analysing the content of shared experiences in clinical supervision, certain themes predominate, notably ethical dilemmas and conflict.

Ethics is the heart of healthcare practice. Being ethical is being mindful of doing what is right and good. It is being aware of the consequences of one's decisions and actions on the other. To realise effective healthcare practice the practitioner must necessarily develop ethical competence. Every clinical judgement and action is ethical; for example, whether to stop a treatment or avoiding eye contact with someone. Conflict is part of everyday practice, and yet practitioners are ill-equipped to respond positively to conflict situations.

The following exemplars shared in clinical supervision reflect on ethical dilemmas and conflict. The first exemplar concerns the practitioner's response to Mrs Denver's distress during a medication round. The second exemplar concerns the practitioner's response to medical demand to do something contrary to her values. The third exemplar explores a practitioner's dilemma in revealing uncaring practice. All the exemplars consider how the practitioner might respond differently given the experience again.

Michelle

Michelle is a mature staff nurse on a day surgical ward. She has been qualified 12 months. In clinical supervision she shared her experience concerning Mrs Denver, a woman admitted for a breast biopsy. Her supervisor is Janet, her line manager.[1]

Michelle: She was a nurse, a pleasant lady. Next morning I was on an early shift doing the drugs. I asked her whether there was anything she needed? She said 'No . . . oh I do feel weepy' and then she burst into tears. I pulled the drug trolley over and pulled the curtains around her bed. She said her friends had been saying how scared they would be if it was them having a breast biopsy. She hadn't appreciated these feelings until now. She said 'Oh my husband and my children!' It made me think – she's a nurse and she's so vulnerable. I don't know if I did any good.

Janet: Put yourself in her shoes. You spent half an hour with her. How would you have felt if a nurse did this for you? Nurses often underestimate the work they do with patients. Could you have done more?

Michelle: I made a conscious decision to blow the pills, no one will come to any harm. It made me feel so vulnerable – what do you say?

Janet: Did you have to say anything? Nurses aren't very good at sitting and listening . . . its okay giving out information and advice.

Michelle: The silence is difficult . . . it's keeping quiet I find the hardest. Did we give her the opportunity to chat? Did we keep away because she was a nurse? Are we frightened of being patronising? Should she be treated any differently?

Janet: Can you answer your own questions?

Michelle: I don't know (silence). . . . I was afraid of making things worse.

Janet: I understand that. It's not easy. However, you are the patient's named nurse, and therefore it was appropriate for you to spend time with her. Finding someone to take over the drug trolley or even finding the named nurse if you hadn't been the named nurse would have lost the spontaneous moment for this lady. Did you discuss this with other staff?

Michelle: Yes . . . we are not as sensitive to these ladies with breast lumps as we could be. Would a counselling course help? I'm at a loss to know what to say to them – am I helping or hindering? It's such a sensitive issue. They look jolly and jovial outside but inside it's like a bombshell!

Janet: Did you use touch?

Michelle: I put my hand on her arm when she apologised for crying. Not knowing her well enough stopped me from holding her hand.

Janet: Could you have done anything differently?

Michelle: I could have been more available to her pre-operatively. I couldn't have made it better for her, change what was wrong.

Janet: What would have happened if this had been a busier morning?

Michelle: I wouldn't have left her, but I wouldn't have been so calm. I'd have been thinking more about other work that needed to be done; premeds, eye drops, and things, thinking I wish you'd hurry up. That's really wrong – how do we get over that?

Janet: I don't really know. Perhaps as practitioners we need to be more prepared to defend our actions.

Michelle: It's true I am worried what others think of me being relatively new to the ward. I don't like conflict so I conform to expectations on me. But this experience challenges that – I would have felt guilty if I hadn't responded to Mrs Denver in the moment.

Janet: And if you faced the same dilemma tomorrow, how do you think you would respond?

Michelle: I think I would have got someone to take over the medication round.

Janet: And if no one was available?

Michelle: Umm . . . maybe stopped the round for a few minutes and then say to Mrs Denver I will come back later to talk with her – to let her know I have heard her cry and care for her. That's really important to me and can so easily be lost in the busyness of the day.

Janet: How do you feel now?

Michelle: So much better. I know I've got to be more confident with my communication skills. I shouldn't be so anxious about messing it up.

Janet: I've learnt that I can't assume staff have good cathartic and catalytic skills.[2] I think we should address these issues more in shift handover.

Commentary

Finding an upset patient whilst doing the drug round is a common occurrence on hospital wards yet in this dialogue it takes on profound significance. Mrs Denver is no longer a task to do but a suffering human being, a vulnerable and distressed woman having undergone a breast biopsy awaiting for her results.

In Figure 18.1, I apply ethical mapping. As you can see I do not entirely agree that Michelle acted for the best, even though her response was caring. She was 'mopping up a mess' that might have been lessened by anticipating Mrs Denver's distress beforehand.

Patient's/family's perspective/other patients	Who had authority to make the decision/act within the situation?	The doctor's perspective
Mrs Denver was visibly upset and needed care at that moment. Other patients may be watching and expect nurses to be caring yet also know they are busy. They may also expect Michelle to give them their drugs first and then see Mrs Denver – motivated by self-concern	Within-the-moment Michelle did have authority to respond as she felt best.	Most likely to see Michelle's primary role to ensure all patients received medication on time. Perhaps some sympathy for Michelle's plight – the doctor might have said – refer her to me.
If there is conflict of perspectives/values – how might these be resolved?	The situation/dilemma	What ethical principles inform this situation?
Michelle experienced intrapersonal conflict, uncertain in her own mind what's best. Options: 1 Michelle could have spent a lesser time with Mrs Denver. 2 She could have gone back to Mrs Denver after the drug round. 3 Get someone else to speak to her, or to take over the drug round.	Should Michelle stop the drug round or continue it?	Michelle had to weigh up the needs of Mrs Denver against the needs of the whole. Would other patients have come to harm? Virtue – what should a caring nurse do?
The nurse(s)' perspective	Consider the power relationships/factors that determined the way the decision/action was actually taken.	The organisation's perspective
Michelle was confronted with Mrs Denver's suffering. Her caring instinct ruled that she should stop the drug round and comfort Mrs Denver. However, she felt she should also continue the drug round – that her colleagues would criticise her for neglecting her task. Michelle also felt she lacked the skills to comfort Mrs Denver. This made her feel uncomfortable and fearful of not knowing how to respond. She had not experienced similar situations previously.	Michelle felt she should continue the drug round within the boundaries of normal practice. She did fear sanction from others if the medication was delayed.	Anxious to avoid complaint from patients not receiving their drugs on time or medical angst about 'irresponsible' nurse behaviour not giving out medication at prescribed times. Tasks are appealing because they reinforce the primary value of 'smooth running' of the organisation.

Figure 18.1   Ethical mapping: Should Michelle stop the drug round or continue it?

Michelle needed to be more mindful of the impact of breast biopsy on Mrs Denver and other similar patients. Michelle's comment, 'I could have been more available to her pre-operatively,' is insightful.

As Janet said, 'put yourself in her shoes.' What would you be thinking and feeling? Having a breast biopsy might only be a minor surgical procedure, but what does it mean to the woman faced with the possibility of being diagnosed with breast cancer? Mrs Denver's words – 'Oh my husband and my children!' – reveal her fear. The literature indicates that this is a very distressing time (Woodward and Webb 2001).

Woodward and Webb (2001) write:

> The quality of life a woman experiences during the process of investigation and treatment for breast disorders is linked with the communication and support provided by others, and includes family members, friends and clinic personnel. Knopf (1994) recommends that nurses working with breast cancer develop strategies to help patients clarify, interpret and process information. Greater attention should be given to the emotional experiences of all women during the diagnostic phase of breast disease. A breast biopsy is not a benign experience (citing Northouse *et al* 1995).

If Michelle had been cognisant of this literature she might have been more sensitive to Mrs Denver's potential anxiety and emotional reaction. Perhaps on a short-stay surgical unit that specialises in breast biopsy, such thinking should be second nature.

Michelle must be able to justify her decision to stop the drug round and confront other peoples' perceptions of priorities when these are misplaced. Did the other patients suffer by having their medication delayed? As Janet challenged, could someone else have taken over the medication round rather than just shutting the lid? The juggling of priorities is ethical action. Yet, choosing to spend time with Mrs Denver exposed Michelle's vulnerability, challenging Michelle's lack of confidence in communicating with such patients. She could see the way she avoided the situation, until the moment Mrs Denver's distress confronted her. It is a sobering thought to consider how many women suffer in silence and how many nurses are ill-equipped to respond to suffering and as a consequence avoid it. It gives credence to the idea that nurses may avoid certain types of patients for these reasons and hide behind a task approach. Not a recipe for person-centred practice. From a broader perspective, why do a drug round in the first place? Nurses could administer drugs on an individual basis. Reflection challenges normal practice.

Cathy and the GPs

Cathy is a district nursing sister. In one session[3] she shared her experience with Brenda:

Cathy: I want to talk about Brenda. She is an 84-year-old woman I have been visiting each week since last summer. I knew her from before when her husband had been ill. She has had stomach cancer for which she has had massive surgery. Initially, she made a good recovery but then had a blockage that resulted in a stent being inserted. She was a deeply religious lady. Three weeks ago I was talking to her. She seemed a bit 'lost'. There was something about her . . . I couldn't put my finger on it. Perhaps it was the up before the major down. We were chatting about things we normally talk about. I said something like 'See you next week Brenda.' She put a hand on my shoulder and said just as I as leaving, 'Yes, if

God's willing.' She gave me that look. She died later that week after being admitted to hospital. She wouldn't have wanted that.

Chris: Were there other signs you could pick up on?

Cathy: She was more relaxed. She had talked about two of her friends who had died recently. She was quite a brave lady, she didn't like tablets and she had pain in her back. We had tried different painkillers that had hardly touched her. I did notice that the lines she had around her eyes had gone . . . her eyes looked bright.

Chris: Intuitively you knew what she was saying to you? That she knew she was dying?

Cathy: Yes.

Chris: Could you have responded differently at that moment?

Cathy: I didn't because I didn't know what to say . . . I had a cry in the car for her.

Chris: Was she saying goodbye? I suspect she didn't want any fuss about that. Did you go to her funeral?

Cathy (tearfully): No . . . other things that needed to be done.

Chris: I can see this is tough for you. Perhaps these are tears you might have shed at the funeral?

Cathy: I know it's daft to get so emotional. I should be better at this side of my work, but when you know someone over time you can't just shut off your emotional side. I know I should be more poised.

Chris: Poise is not easy – we need to become better at understanding and then managing our feelings within the moment – a kind of mindfulness. Goleman (1996) describes this as *emotional intelligence*. I can give you a reference to explore that. How would you name your feelings in the situation?

Cathy: Guilt at failing Brenda and her family; anger at the GP for admitting Brenda to hospital against her wishes; sadness at Brenda's death.

Chris: A real cocktail of emotions.

Cathy: I know. . . .

Chris: What if you have responded to Brenda's cue?

Cathy: How do respond to someone like that? Maybe I could have asked Brenda if she thought she was dying and if so to hold her and say goodbye . . . it's such a difficult scenario to contemplate how I might have responded differently because I feel so emotional.

Chris: Is closing important for you?

Cathy: Yes. I didn't attend the funeral because of a management meeting I was expected to attend.

Chris: Could you have resisted this demand and prioritised differently?

Cathy: In what way?

Chris: Well, for example, to say to the GPs – 'Can you please reschedule this meeting as I am attending Brenda's funeral.' Another approach would have been simply to give your apologies for not attending the practice meeting. Did you miss the opportunity to help Brenda manage her death appropriately?

Cathy: Brenda definitely didn't want to go into the hospice. Her husband had died there. We had discussed this. She said 'The hospice is a lovely place, but I don't want to go in there because it brings back such memories.' She wanted to die at home, and she did have a strong family and friends network around her.

Chris: What were the conditions of her admission to hospital?

Cathy: The GP was a bit vague. He admitted her on the grounds of a range of deteriorating symptoms, notably breathlessness. I was thinking of what you previously said about the 'gap' – about accepting the inevitable as inevitable, and the way the GP had felt obliged to arrange her admission to hospital rather than accept she was dying.

Chris: Yes, the 'gap' exists when there is a mismatch of expectation between care staff in accepting the inevitability that the patient will die and that further treatment would be futile. The gap represents the potential for conflict.

Cathy: Yes . . . that's how it was. I acknowledged the inevitability of Brenda's dying before the medical team did. I intuitively felt this, and our role was to help Brenda die in comfort. The GP also knew the inevitability of Brenda's dying yet he still arranged her admission, as futile as that was, rather than arranging management of Brenda's death at home.

Chris: His learnt reaction. It does suggest how the 'cure' mindset works. Of course, he may have just taken the easiest way out. The consequence was that the patient's best interests were disregarded, and she died in circumstances she would not have chosen for herself. Were there other ways of dealing with this situation?

Cathy: Brenda was a strong character, but she would have complied with what the GP said.

Chris: How can you respond now?

Cathy: I don't know. The damage is done. What do you think?

Chris: Well, it might be useful to debrief with the GPs? Perhaps you can insist on being called if a similar situation arises so you and your team could have managed her at home? Issues of communication within the care team? I know in the emotional moment it was tough for you to respond to the cue she gave you, but we can see how circumstances unfolded that were not in Brenda's best interests, not in your best interests, and an expensive alternative for the NHS – the difference between being proactive and reactive?

Cathy: We are commencing a new series of meetings on Monday to improve our communication! The idea is to have 'team care plans' where everybody knows what the other is doing.

Chris: That shows how conflict can be used positively to create a better practice environment. Using ethical mapping,[4] let me face you with a dilemma – should you have attended Brenda's funeral or the GP's practice meeting?

Cathy: For me, the funeral was my priority. In future I would be assertive about going to the funeral and say I would come to the meeting afterwards.

Chris: Closing is important work for you. Can you find some literature to support that? Knowing the 'evidence' may help you assert your priorities with the GPs – talking the language of the rational mind rather than the emotional mind. Consider how might the GPs respond?

Exploring perspectives

Cathy felt that attending Brenda's funeral was the greater need but she wondered was this just an emotional reaction? She felt she had failed Brenda and Brenda's family, which distressed her; feelings she had yet to resolve. She felt the family would have wanted her and benefitted from her being at the funeral. She could appreciate the GPs' perspective but felt their response was both typical and arrogant. They assumed leadership of the team and expected compliance even though Cathy was not directly employed by them.

Cathy felt the organisation would expect her to conform to the GPs' demand so as not to rock the boat, reinforcing her subordination to medical dominance.

In considering Cathy's perspective we used the 'Influences grid' to reveal the factors that had influenced her decision making (summarised in Table 18.1). At the core of the

Table 18.1   Influences grid

Influence	Significance
Expectations from self about how I should act	To go to the funeral for closure and to support the family.
Conforming to normal practice	To attend the GP meeting and to go to Brenda's funeral.
Expectations from others to act in certain ways	The GPs expected Cathy to comply with their demand and know her place within the 'team'. Brenda's family would have liked Cathy to attend the funeral.
Need to be valued by others	Cathy felt she did not need to be valued by GPs. However, on deeper reflection, she admitted she did like positive feedback and wants to be valued and that this might be a subtle influence she didn't want to acknowledge.
Doing what was felt to be right	Attending the funeral would have been the right thing to do – more so than attending the GP meeting – even though both were 'right'.
Misplaced concernLoyalty to staff versus loyalty to patient/family	Cathy felt 'forced' to be loyal to the GPs rather than to Brenda and her family although in her heart her primary loyalty was to her patients.
Emotional entanglement/ over-identification Negative attitude towards the patient/family	Cathy had a strong involvement with Brenda who was strong. Indeed, she might be accused of being too emotionally involved which blurred her perception of what is best. In exploring this influence Cathy revealed her unresolved distress about her father's recent death. As a consequence felt she did become entangled in the suffering of dying patients although did not experience this as conflict. On the contrary she felt this made her more sensitive to the needs of patients and families whilst recognising she still had some grief work to do for herself.
Limited skills/discomfort to act in other waysLack of confidence	Cathy admitted she was not very assertive and felt she would have been humiliated if she had challenged the GPs more strongly. She recognised she was someone who avoided or accommodated conflict.
Time/priorities	Cathy's NHS trust had significantly reduced the number of district nursing sisters (G grade), forcing her into a team leader role to manage more junior staff. This had reduced her direct care role contact. Hence managing priorities and role conflict had become an increasing dilemma for her.
Anxious about ensuing conflictFear of sanction	Cathy's fear of sanction was the crux of her dilemma – what sanction might ensue if she defied the GP's demand? She recognised that she had internalised a sense of subordination and that any challenge to the GPs would be uncomfortable. She knew they would probably report her to her managers.
Information/theory/research to act in a certain sort of way	Cathy did not have a good argument to support her decision to attend the funeral rather than attend the GP meeting.
Need for control	Cathy liked to be in control of her workload, although this has become increasingly difficult with the GPs telling her what she should or shouldn't do. She recognised that her autonomy was a grey and shrinking area.

dilemma is the expectation from self and from others. Using 'the influences grid' was a revealing and powerful mirror for Cathy to look at herself. It reinforced many of the factors we had already explored and significantly expanded her own perspective.

Chris: We can see a tension between you and the GPs over your autonomy. What ethical principles inform this dilemma?
Cathy: The GPs would probably say I had a greater responsibility to all my patients rather than just Brenda.
Chris: The utilitarian tension between responding to the need of the individual patient versus attending the meeting that might result in benefit for the wider community. I think this is a weak argument to support the GPs' insistence you attend their meeting. In terms of virtue we could see another tension between you responding in tune with your holistic values and responsibility to the family against the values of the GPs who give greater value to the smooth running of their practice. As Friedson (1970) notes, the principal aim of the bureaucratic organisation is its own smooth running despite the rhetoric of patients first. Presumably, the GPs could easily debrief anything significant arising from the meeting at a later time?
Cathy: Yes, obviously from time to time people will miss the practice meeting for various reasons. I think they are just making a power play. I know they don't value the more relationship work with patients.
Chris: We can certainly see a conflict of values and claims to autonomy. There is also a communication breakdown linked to Brenda's admission to hospital. It's ultimately a power game and you fear the consequences of not conforming. One discourse of power relationships is to view nursing and caring as feminine struggling against a dominant patriarchal view characteristic of medicine and managerialism. The work of Gilligan might help you frame this idea. Gilligan (1982) showed how men and women differ in ethical priorities; women lean towards an ethic of caring and responsibility, whereas men lean towards an ethic of justice.

Let me draw this:

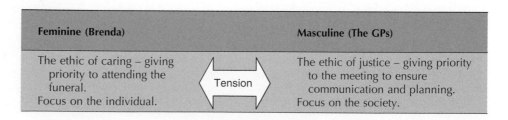

Feminine (Brenda)		Masculine (The GPs)
The ethic of caring – giving priority to attending the funeral. Focus on the individual.	Tension	The ethic of justice – giving priority to the meeting to ensure communication and planning. Focus on the society.

Both perspectives are important and need synthesis. I sense the 'team meeting' is a ritual of power flexing and control where the dominant voice of the doctors and power pattern of relationships with subordinates is reinforced. This requires subordinates to attend. Not attending the meeting to attend a funeral may seem an innocuous event in itself, yet from a power perspective, the decision is a symbolic challenge to the status quo. Your decision to attend a funeral undermines their patriarchal dominance. The power game is to diminish your autonomy and become a 'team player' – where they set the rules of the game.

Cathy: I don't like power games – why can't healthcare professionals collaborate in the patients' best interests?

Chris: You would think so. But it's a naïve perspective. The world is governed by power interests rather than what's necessarily best despite the rhetoric of valuing the 'patient's experience' as a primary measure of the quality of care. A kind of lip service where the reality doesn't measure up. Watson (1990, p. 62) notes that patriarchy presents a potent barrier to nursing's realisation of its holistic vision.

Cathy: Gilligan's feminist perspective is enlightening, especially when a couple of the GPs are actually women.

Chris: Reverby (1987) explored the way caring has been viewed as an extension of being a woman. She asserts that nurses' lack of power stems from this relationship between womanhood and caring and the subordinate relationship of nurses to doctors.

Cathy: I'm aware of the research by Lawler (1991) and James (1989) – who noted how caring in nursing is largely invisible, often devalued by nurses themselves, and seen as largely unskilled, being the natural extension of woman's social roles.

Chris: Yes, Lawler's research was entitled *Behind the Screens*, concerned with bodywork, whilst James's research was entitled 'Emotional Labour', concerned with emotional work. Perhaps then, it's not surprising that nurses have tended to delegate this work to unqualified staff, valuing instead more medical type tasks as they seek recognition and acceptance into the dominant class (Roberts 1983).

Cathy: As I mentioned, as a team leader I have less time to be with my patients and need to delegate more and more to junior staff including National Vocational Qualification (NVQ) health assistants whom I'm meant to supervise.

Chris: One of my PhD students[5] shared with me recently a similar experience whereby she had found it difficult to challenge the diagnosis of the doctor until she could appreciate the subordinate role she was taking, reinforcing the stereotype that doctors exert power over nurses (Daiski 2004) and her hesitancy in dealing with issues of authority and power in her everyday relationships. Yet the medical team was actually asking for her opinion, recognising her authority and specialist knowledge. She concluded that the incident had enabled her to see her relationships more clearly. The insight was literally empowering and shifted her perception of herself vis-à-vis the doctors she worked with.

Cathy: That's helpful to know that other nurses face similar situations. I wonder if I can become empowered to reframe my relationship with GPs – to touch my power. I feel it tingling as I speak!

Chris: Feel the power! I like it! Not easy work. Buckenham and McGrath (1983) highlight how nurses have been socialised into passive, subordinate and powerless perception of self *vis-à-vis* medicine; a perception that renders them incapable of fulfilling their self-perceived role of patient advocate. Old research but still holds water. It is natural for dominant professions such as medicine to reinforce subordinate behaviour in other healthcare professions, such as nursing (Oakley 1984). In other words doctors are always motivated to maintain the status quo and resist rivalry for power. Nurses rationalise their compliance with medical domination because of the need to be valued.

Cathy: I recognise the need to be valued by doctors, and yet it is satisfying whenever they make a positive comment, which is rare, I might add.

Chris: Chapman (1983) suggested that doctors reinforced nurses' subordination through humiliation techniques that become a normative pattern of relating. The aim of

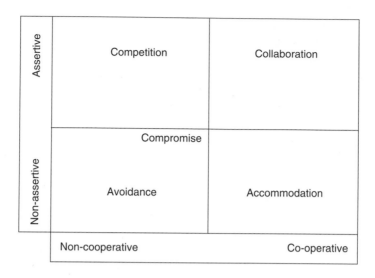

Accommodating is essentially a co-operative interaction but one in which the practitioner is not assertive, prepared to give up their own needs for the sake of maintaining harmonious relationships and need to be accepted by others – 'apologetic'.

Avoidance is characterised by negation of the issues and a rationalisation that attempts to challenge the behaviour of another are futile.

Collaboration involves an effort to seek effective problem solving – solve the issues towards a mutually satisfying conclusion – 'win–win' situation that is concerned with the needs self and others. Openly discuss issues surrounding conflict and attempt to find suitable means to resolve the conflict.

Competition is pursuing his or her own needs at the exclusion of others – usually through open confrontation (results in win–lose situations).

Compromise is realising that in conflict situation, every party cannot be satisfied – accepting at times.

Figure 18.2   The Thomas and Kilmann conflict mode instrument (http://www.kilmann.com/conflict.html).

the game is to keep nurses 'in their place'. Stein (1978) illuminated the nature of the doctor–nurse game whereby the nurse suggests to the doctor what to do in such a way that the doctor can claim credit for the idea. The point of the game is to ensure the doctor does not lose face. The game also reinforces the nurse's subordination. The game is also important for the doctor to play because he or she realises the significance of the nurse's knowledge. The pay-off for the nurse is the doctor's patronage. Stein argues that failure to play the game is 'hell to pay'.

Cathy: I did sense that sanction would be taken against me. It's a strange feeling that they would do that considering I work with them. It reminds me that relationships can be no more than a thin veneer when it comes to the power crunch.

Chris: Power within bureaucratic systems such as the NHS have a typical authoritative pattern to ensure a docile and competent workforce (Foucault 1979). What sort of relationship would you like with the GPs?

Cathy: A collaborative-type relationship where we value and respect each other. At the moment I don't think they respect nurses. It makes working difficult.

Chris: The Thomas and Kilmann (1974) 'conflict mode instrument' offers you a framework to consider the conflict management style you use and the style you would prefer to use (Figure 18.2). They identify five conflict management styles organised along two axes: assertive – the degree to which individuals satisfy their own concerns, and co-operation – the degree to which individuals attempt to the concerns of others. The five conflict modes are avoidance, accommodation, compromise, competition and collaboration. Looking at the styles, what mode of managing conflict do you tend to use?

Cathy: With the doctors I tend to be accommodating. I don't like conflict at the best of times so I guess I generally try to avoid it.

Chris: Cavanagh (1991), using the Thomas and Kilmann instrument, researched the conflict mode styles of nurses and nurse managers. He found that avoidance was the most common mode followed by accommodation, compromise, collaboration and then competition. I suspect nurses avoid competition because they fear they will lose . . . so you're not alone.

Cathy: Whew – that's some relief.

Chris: What style would you like to use?

Cathy: Compromise or collaboration.

Chris: If you want to be collaborative and you are accommodating or avoiding – how can you move from one to the other?

Cathy: I can't imagine that's possible. I would need to be more assertive, less fearful.

Chris: We can rehearse being assertive. We can also use this map with each experience you reflect on and plot your journey moving from avoidance/accommodation to collaboration. How does that sound?

Cathy: OK. I know it's something I have got to work on if I am ever going to feel confident working with the GPs.

Chris: Cathy, can you let go of fear that the GPs will punish you?

Cathy: No, not easily . . . it takes two to tango.

Chris: You did say you would assert going to the funeral if the situation arose again?

Cathy: Yes, that's true, but whether I could actually assert myself is another issue.

Chris: OK, let's look at yourself using another tool. Dickson constructed an assertiveness stereotype map comprising four stereotypes of women (see Figure 18.3). Who are you?

Cathy: That's easy. I'm Dulcie – the GPs walk all over me.

Chris: Who would you like to be?

Cathy: Selma. I could never be like Agnes, that isn't my personality. I can see the risk of being an Ivy, bitching and backbiting. I know people like this, even at the surgery, and know how destructive these people are.

Chris: Oppressed people often respond this way – projecting their oppression onto others. So Cathy, how do you move from being Dulcie to becoming Selma?

Cathy: I need to believe in myself more, be more assertive.

Chris: Cathy, the most vital point is to assert your right to be treated with respect and to assert your point of view. Dickson constructed a rights of women scale comprising 11 'rights' (Table 18.2). Score yourself out of 10 against each point. The higher the score, the greater your sense of self. You can re-score at later times to review your progress.

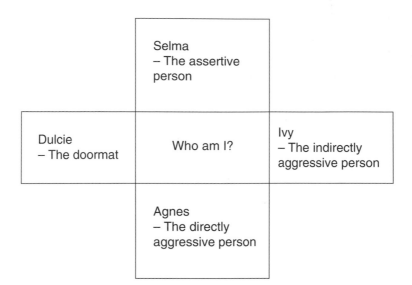

Figure 18.3   Four stereotypes of women.

Table 18.2   Rights of women scale (Dickson 1982)

Right	Score 1–10
• I have the right to state my own needs and set my own priorities as a person independent of any roles that I may assume in my life.	
• I have the right to be treated with respect as an intelligent, capable and equal human being.	
• I have the right to express my feelings.	
• I have the right to express my opinions.	
• I have the right o say 'yes' or 'no' for myself.	
• I have the right to make mistakes.	
• I have the right to change my mind.	
• I have the right to say I don't understand.	
• I have the right to ask for what I want.	
• I have the right to decline responsibility for other people.	
• I have the right to deal with others without being dependent on them for approval.	

Cathy: I'd rather not score myself – I know I won't score high. It makes me feel a bit inadequate – bit like beating myself up. I know I am a competent practitioner who gets on well enough with the GPs. I don't want to make a mountain out of a molehill and rock the boat. I'll soon get over this difficulty and move on.

Chris: Maybe the scale is a step too far. However, you do want to be more assertive. I devised the 'assertive action ladder' to guide practitioners towards more assertive action (Figure 18.4). You're not alone. Many practitioners, especially nurses, are not assertive. Indeed, the transactional culture of healthcare organisations may mitigate against being assertive. Better to know your place and keep your head down than raise it above the parapet and get it shot off. As one primary nurse once said to me, 'it doesn't pay to be assertive round here' (Johns 1989), suggesting that becoming assertive is not simply an individual effort but requires an

10	Treading the 'fine line' between pushing and yielding	
9	Playing the power game	
8	Staying in adult mode	
7	Being heard	
6	Just do it (JDI)	
5	Creating the optimum condition to assert self	
4	Making a good argument to assert self	
3	Authority to assert self	
2	Ethically right to assert self	
1	Feeling the need to assert self	

Figure 18.4 The assertive action ladder (adapted from Johns 2009a).

organisational effort to create a collaborative environment on the basis of shared vision.

Cathy: OK, lets look at this.

Note: I designed the assertive action ladder by analysing the pattern of becoming assertive with practitioners within guided reflection. It was apparent that nurses are not equipped to manage conflict positively leading to a huge wastage of energy and a low sense of self-esteem. It is true to say that the effective practitioner is an assertive practitioner and yet, in a culture where nurses are not expected to be assertive, this may itself cause conflict. The ladder has been adapted in light of reflection on its use in guided reflection although its basic tenets remains unchanged.

Up the assertiveness ladder Cathy quickly climbed rungs 1–3. She felt she now had the authority to assert herself although she remained cautious. At rung 4 she was flummoxed at how to make a good argument. Was there any evidence to support her perspective? She felt not and that her argument would be dismissed as sentimental nonsense. Some work to do on rung 4. Moving up to rung 5 I posed choice – to see the GPs as a group or as individuals? At a meeting or in the course of the day? Was one GP more sympathetic? The variables seemed endless. Rung 6 – can she carry it out? My guidance role was to infuse her with courage to act and deflate any sense of fear. At rung 7 I guided her through interaction skills based on John Heron's six-category intervention analysis (see Chapter 17), emphasising facilitative responses towards collaboration. At rung 8 I got Cathy to imagine the GPs response to her assertion. Possible tactics might include

- To deflect competition by staying focused on the issue rather than interpersonal stuff
- To confront the GPs with their caring values – it is often the organisation's Achilles heel to be revealed as uncaring – what I term as 'taking the moral high ground'
- To give the GPs behaviour back to them if they assert power over Cathy – 'asserting your power does not help solve the problem'
- To reduce their power by visualising them as bully boys trying to get their own way.

At rung 9 Cathy must manage her anxiety to stay in adult mode, especially the urge to flee into child mode to cope with the parental onslaught of Cathy being viewed as difficult and irresponsible (using a transactional analysis framework). The key is to keep the issue in focus rather than let it degenerate into competitive mode that she is ill-equipped to win. It is vital that Cathy is not fearful of sanction or loss of reward. Rung 10 is a heady sort of place – don't look down or you will topple off. The 'fine line' is the metaphorical line between of pushing an issue and yielding. Cathy may need to yield because the GPs are more powerful than her and refuse to accept her perspective.

As we ascended the ladder rung by rung, I felt a shift within Cathy, as if climbing the ladder was infusing her with a new confidence.

Cathy: Tell me about yielding.
Chris: Yielding is retreating with dignity holding collaborative intent, with one's integrity intact. Yielding is not being passive. It is being sensitive to energy flows and extending wisdom. 'Flow with the event rather than resist it, yet rooted with who you are' Jones and Jones (1996, p. 281). It is a strength, not a weakness. To fight when you cannot 'win' is to exhaust yourself and feel a failure. Some situations cannot be won.

Afterwards Cathy smiled: That was so helpful, maybe I can be more assertive than I imagined."

Chris: Only time will tell.

Hank's complaint

Karen was an associate nurse who contracted a guided reflection relationship with me as part of a project to investigate whether guided reflection facilitated more effective practice.[6] In one guided reflection session Karen revealed her dejection at a recent event at the hospital.

Karen: One night last week Hank complained to me about the actions of one of the night staff. He was very angry about it, so I wrote about his complaint in the notes, really to cover my own back because if something had happened because of that . . . if he had got worked up and had a heart attack. I didn't state who was involved or the nature of the incident. Christine (a night associate nurse) picked up what I had written in the notes and said that she felt 'very sad I had to write that, that some things were better said, not written'. She didn't deny the incident but criticised my documenting it.
Chris: The way you handled it?
Karen: Right. I reread my notes of the incident because I had written them in a hurry. I realised I had used a word that could have been replaced by a better one.
Chris: An antagonistic word?
Karen: Yes. I made a comment further on in the notes and replaced my initial note to make it clearer to people reading it. What got me was Christine criticising me about my way of documenting it when *The Nursing Times* goes on about 'whistle

blowing' and how complaints should be documented. I felt she was trying to cover for the person involved though she acknowledged that the event had happened.

Chris: And now?

Karen: I pointed it out to Leslie as he was the primary nurse. He said he would have a word with the person involved. I went home and worried about it all night, worried how she would take it, what she would say. So I need feedback.

Chris: I can sense your anxiety about this incident. What would you do differently if given the same situation again?

Karen: The only thing I could have done would have been to ring her and ask her to explain from her point of view.

Chris: Think of the response you might have got from doing that.

Karen: From my perspective, if it was me . . . I would have appreciated it.

Chris: And knowing the person involved?

Karen: I can't say . . . she could nearly be my grandmother.

Chris: How do you normally get on with her?

Karen: I see her in the evenings and nights when she works . . . but I don't have much to do with her. I suppose my relationship with her is superficial.

Chris: Do you think this action against Hank was out of character for her?

Karen: I think it was an exaggeration of her normal character.

Chris: You think?

Karen: I don't work with her. It's difficult to know how she is with other patients. The event itself was quite trivial, it's Hank's anger that got to me.

Chris: Do you think Hank's anger was reasonable?

Karen: I felt that at the time that if it had been me then I would have been upset and angry. She was inflicting her values on him, not respecting him.

Chris: I sense you feel you didn't handle Hank's complaint in the best way, although writing a report in the notes is the proper way of reporting patient distress. However, altering the notes might be construed as unprofessional, and perhaps should have been picked up by other staff. I know you were trying to damp down the conflict.

Karen: Yes I was. Discussing the situation at shift report would have been better but by then the night staff had departed. Reporting the incident to the primary nurse is good practice, and it is not unreasonable to have expected Leslie to deal with it – but he is a coward and conveniently forgets about it – or put another way he brushed it under the carpet. I could have reported it to the senior nurse, but that would have made it worse. I can imagine that they would have said I went running to mother and got them into trouble.

Chris: Reported it to the senior nurse was an option. What other options do you have? Think about what would have been the 'right' response – use ethical mapping.

Karen: Clearly Mandy was in the wrong – she abused a patient and that cannot be tolerated. She has no defence for this except to play down the incident or accuse Hank of lying. I know I should have been more mindful of the consequences of writing as I did in the notes. It wasn't the best way of reporting this. Altering the notes was not a good response as it looked as if I was trying to cover up my mistake. Leslie should have taken more responsibility. Everyone is so fearful of conflict. I do need to talk this through with the care assistant. If this isn't possible face to face then I could ring her at home.

Chris: Name the ethics involved.

Karen: Beneficence – acting for the patient's best interests and not doing harm. Perhaps I could have asked Hank if he wanted me to report the situation – I rather took that for granted. I also have a moral duty to care and expose situations of abuse.

Chris: Which you did. Do you still want Leslie to deal with it?

Karen: I never did in the first place, it was only because he had offered. Any tips for speaking with the care assistant?

Chris: OK, imagine I am her. The key factor is to keep the situation grounded in the situation rather than it becoming a secondary situation of interpersonal conflict, as indeed it has already become. Remember the supervision maxim: 'tough on the issues, soft on the person'. See taking action as an act of personal integrity as fearful as you are of its potential consequences of ostracism. Only time will tell.

We rehearsed what she might say to the care assistant.

In our next session, three weeks later . . .

Karen: I went home and phoned her!

Chris: Good for you. How did you feel when you picked up the receiver?

Karen: Terrified! She was angry but she didn't get as angry as she possibly could have done. I think she was also feeling guilty.

Chris: Have you learnt that it pays to belong to the harmonious team? If so, if a similar situation occurs, you will think twice before confronting it?

Karen: Remind me about the harmonious team.

Chris: The harmonious team is concerned with maintaining a facade of togetherness or teamwork. It does not talk openly about difficult feelings or issues between its members and seeks to protect itself from outside threat. Conflict is brushed under the carpet. As a consequence, conflict is inadequately resolved and continues to simmer under the apparent harmonious surface (Johns 1992). It undermines the ability of practitioners to collaborate in resolving conflict. It nurtures a perverse culture of being loyal to staff rather than to patients as you have discovered. As a consequence people become inauthentic and lose their integrity. What can you do about it?

Karen: I don't know. I'm really dejected and yet I can sense it's vital that I am not intimidated. If we can't raise issues because of fear of conflict then we all go about as if wearing masks. I can't simply sweep this under the carpet.

Chris: You haven't – you did phone her and refused to play the harmonious team game. Could you share this experience with your colleagues – to secure their support and assert the therapeutic team to offset this malignancy?

Karen: I felt like a chicken at the prospect of Leslie acting on my behalf. I'm now truly humbled. I didn't stop to think. I'm feeling very stupid. Why did Hank wait to see me?! He was probably just thinking about it when he saw me.

Chris: Perhaps he trusted you?

Karen: I like to think so. It's important patients can trust nurses to act for them as necessary.

Chris: How do you think Mandy (the care assistant) might be feeling now?

Karen: I hope she thinks I had the courage to ring her.

Chris: Be positive about this –your phone call to Mandy was an act of integrity. Her anger was her guilt. You enabled her to release that energy, yet she was also confronted with the fact that she did not act appropriately towards Hank. You can rationalise her anger in this way. It's imperative that you do not see yourself in the wrong.

Karen: I know . . . I hear what you say, but it's not easy.

Chris: I know but take strength. I am frustrated listening to you. If I was the senior nurse I would want to intercede and confront Mandy's behaviour. Summarise what insights you have gained.

Karen: It has reinforced my holistic values – the importance of listening to and working with patients like Hank. It involves a moral responsibility. I realise I do care about patients. I'm not good at conflict and felt intimidated. I need to develop a greater sense of poise so I am not so easily rattled by such issues. As a result, I feel I have grown through this experience – more grown up, more adult, less like a frightened panicky child. I must read about emotional intelligence and focus more on poise in future sessions. It has exposed the myth of collaborative relationships. The idea of the harmonious team is compelling- I can see it. My assertive and conflict management skills need developing – and yet I do feel more assertive. I also need to talk to Joyce (new senior nurse) – my hierarchical fears of punishment re-emerging.

As the text reveals, Karen was bruised in retaliation for breaking the norms of the harmonious team. The issue had twisted from being a patient-related issue to an interpersonal one where loyalty to the 'team' took precedence over loyalty to the patient. Karen's distress was the outcome of vilification – a reflection of the *force* of the harmonious team to regulate its members. Karen was motivated to limit the damage by accepting her villain role. As she noted, she was learning to play by the rules.

Yet despite Karen's distress, she said that she enjoyed going through the situation in supervision. She hadn't wanted to come to the follow-up session because she thought it was going to be too hard. She had a slight residual fear about retribution from the night staff, but at least the care assistant had gone on holiday for a month!

As her guide I urged Karen to act from a position of professional integrity – to respond ethically. Whilst we did not overtly use ethical mapping within the session, it is easy to perceive its capacity to reveal dilemmas and consider the perspectives of people involved in the situation and what would be the best response.

Clearly, patients cannot be abused. For that reason, I was pushing Karen against a power gradient that threatened her. To her great credit, she acted responsibly. My role was to help her lick her wounds and gather strength to tackle such issues more positively in the future. You might imagine how she might respond given the scenario again. Will her natural inclination to avoid conflict and conform to the harmonious team win the day or can she act on a newfound sense of integrity and loyalty to the patient?

Horizontal violence

Karen's experience reveals the phenomena of horizontal violence (Duffy 1995, McKenna *et al* 2003) – a toxic form of dealing with stress. The idea of *horizontal* stems from bureaucratic-hierarchical systems, whereby the subordinate person (the nurse) is unable to project her anger or frustration at her more powerful oppressors. She can only fire at those on her own level or below her. Yet, even on her own level, this violence is muted within the harmonious team, perhaps because people are motivated to be partially invisible, to keep their heads down to avoid criticism (Street 1992). Hence *harmonious* is a collusive strategy to contain the team's unresolved angst.

Conclusion

These three narratives of clinical supervision illustrate the value of ethical mapping as a practical tool for reflecting on what's best and appreciating factors that constrain acting for the best. Knowing what is best is not easily determined given the complexity of situations. It is a contestable space. It is not easy to push self against power gradients that are embedded in everyday practice that resist any pressure to shift.

The text illuminates the significance of guiding reflection or clinical supervision. However, in each case, I believe Michelle, Cathy and Karen would have benefitted from group supervision where peers may have added similar stories of ethical complexity and oppression by more powerful others.

Notes

1 This dialogue was recorded by Janet within a research project using clinical supervision as a model of clinical leadership (Johns 2003).
2 Janet refers to six-category intervention analysis (Heron 1975) that she had introduced to Michelle in previous sessions.
3 Cathy was in an individual-guided reflection relationship with me as an experimental delivery of an academic programme – being and becoming a reflective and effective practitioner in the practitioner's own work setting. The programme spanned 30 weeks. Usually this programme was delivered within the classroom in group-guided reflection.
4 See Figure 3.3.
5 Lou was a PhD student using narrative as a journey of self-inquiry and transformation towards realising her vision of practice as a spasticity nurse a lived reality. See 'From significance to insights' (Jarrett 2008, pp. 59–72) and 'Constructing the reflexive narrative' (Jarrett and Johns 2005, pp. 162–179).
6 This was an integral to my PhD study (Johns 1998a).

Chapter 19

Therapeutic journalling for patients

Therapeutic of journalling is a healing modality for people who suffer (DeSalvo 1999). Consider the patients you work with who have had a difficult time or have difficulty with expressing their feelings. Ask yourself, would keeping a journal benefit them? Writing is cathartic and healing – enabling the person to make sense and heal. Such stories also help others appreciate the author's experience, especially if the person is unable to express herself coherently.

Moira Vass

Moira wrote her story of living with motor neurone disease because she wanted her carers to understand what she was experiencing (Box 19.1). Writing gave her dying some purpose and enabled her to express her feelings of despair and anger. Moira was keen to publish her journal. I met with Moira to discuss this possibility in an earlier edition of this book.

My reflection

On 4 August, I arrive 10 minutes late. Moira is not there. Louise, the hospice day sister, says she has been delayed because her catheter had blocked. I sit with the group of patients and staff preparing for the day. Moira arrives. She is small and frail in her wheelchair. She has a piece of tissue coming out of her mouth that soaks up the excess secretions she can no longer control. She has her 'lite speaker' with her to communicate with me. I tell her who I am and clarify why we are meeting together – to consider her journal on living with motor neurone disease and ways it might be published. I had been strongly moved reading her journal.

Using her 'lite writer', Moira tells me about her experience this morning with her catheter being removed. The district nurse had asked Louise to replace it. Moira says it was awful. I sensed this and asked if it was embarrassing? Moira grimaces. She says she

Becoming a Reflective Practitioner, Fourth Edition. Christopher Johns.
© 2013 John Wiley & Sons, Ltd. Published 2013 by John Wiley & Sons, Ltd.

Box 19.1   Moira Vass – living with motor neurone disease

I have motor neurone disease (MND). This is a disease that relentlessly destroys the nerves that enable us to control all our movements, while leaving the intellect and senses unaffected. There is no cure for this disease. I was told the cause was unknown and it was terminal. However, there is a ray of hope – the drug Rilutek. This is not a cure, but has been shown in trials to extend survival in people with MND. Its cost is somewhere between £1000 and £2000 per patient per year, yet it gives the patient time and some hope. It slows down the paralysing effect. My attitude to Rilutek is if it does not cure then why take it? It only prolongs the agony and postpones the inevitable. The paralysis goes on unabated and death is by strangulation, a form of choking due to the fact that the intercostal muscles are affected and you cannot breath or cough. From day one I became slowly and deliberately useless and within 6 months I could no longer speak, eat, drink or walk unaided. Artificial ventilation via an endotracheal tube merely prolongs the suffering. Patients remain alert to the end and many need treatment to relieve their distress, as well as oxygen to assist breathing.

Living with feeding at home
MND affects the nerve endings and consequently affects the muscles in most of my body, but particularly all the muscles in my throat which means I cannot speak, eat, drink, or swallow. I was referred by my neurologist to a dietician as the time had come for me to be fed by tube. My reaction was disbelief, anger and a lot of tears. Then more tears.

By the time I came to see the nutritionist consultant, I had calmed down and accepted the fact that this was my only option if I wanted to go on living. The tube is attached to the gastrostomy. My reaction was despair. How can I live with this? The first thing that crossed my mind was no more baked or roast potatoes. No more predinner sherry, wine, all the joys of living. One of my favourite hobbies was cooking; adventurous cooking, dinner parties, BBQ with the family, like any normal person.

The first feed was only 200 mL. At 50 mL per hour. The feed type was 'Nutrison' and it was not a painful procedure. When the feed was finished this was followed by 60 mL. Syringe of water to flush out the tube and give you extra fluid and thereafter a water flush every 4 hours, totalling 240 mL per day to prevent me from getting dehydrated – feed at night and water during the day.

However, it did little to calm my anger. I just wanted to stop the whole business and go to God. I could not see myself living with a 'Kangaroo' pump and a plastic bag full of 1000 mL of 'Nutrison Energy Plus' to be given overnight. The idea of the night feed was to enable me to be free during the day apart from the water flushes.

I lay awake for the first three nights in hospital, my anger only getting worse. Anger that felt like someone pouring boiling oil over my body. On the third night, I reached down and closed the roller clamp. I forgot about the bleep sound from the pump, which brought two nurses to the pump who duly restarted the feed. They sat with me for a while and we had a chat. I was finding it impossible to come to terms with my new way of life, but I decided to take a more positive look at my feelings and especially the word ANGER. It struck me the word 'anger' is almost a cocktail of emotions:

A Aggressive, to myself and the staff – zero tolerance
N Negative thinking
G Grief, crying
E Emotions out of control
R Resentful – 'why me' syndrome

So I decided, for the sake of my family, my husband but especially my three grandchildren, to make an effort because they all thought the feeding pump was a great idea. I made up my mind to come to terms with tube feeding at home although the sight of the tube at my stomach brought back the anger.

On Saturday morning, 14 February 1998, I was found unconscious by Gordon, who was unable to rouse me. It was decided to admit me to the hospice. I have no recollection of the tragedy. I came round with my granddaughter Kerry, aged 16, crying, telling me to squeeze her hand if I could hear what she said: 'Please wake up Nan, we love you'. Twenty four hours later, I was awake to the reality of my condition. My living will meant they could not feed me if I went unconscious. As a result they were anxious to stat the feed but I said 'No, no, leave me be.' By the fourth day I gave in and the 'kangaroo' pump and plastic bag with the 1000 mL of food was back. I was back to square one – I had to give in for the sake of my family.

Once I had come to terms with home feeding I found it extremely easy to live with, and having the feed at night was more convenient. You are free during the day to do what you please and go where you like. It is very easy to take a water flush with you. It took about 6 weeks to establish a routine. I would set it up downstairs in the kitchen, sit back in my armchair and watch TV. The feed takes 10 hours to go through. When I am in bed, I make sure the tube is free and to that I attach the tube from the pump by holding it in place with sellotape on my thigh – so far it has never woken me up. If you can still eat anything that is a bonus.

The hospice
Following my admission to the hospice as an inpatient in February, I received wonderful care, especially as I spent 4 days on 'hunger strike'. To me, this was the only way out – to stop all treatments, drugs and feed. The staff respected my wishes, and while I was unconscious my living will (advanced directive) stated *no treatment*. When I regained consciousness I made the decision to continue cessation of all treatments. I found my family were devastated, and my three grandchildren cried and pleaded with me. On day 5, I came back to earth to the delight of everyone. The nursing care in the hospice was a special kind of nursing, but I would rather have had my rights and my way.

On discharge I was invited back 1 day per week as a day-care patient. On the first day this caused me unbelievable distress. They collected me in a hospice ambulance; there was the driver, a nurse and myself. As my husband waved goodbye I started to cry – another step down the MND road to death. Suddenly my anger exploded and I lost control, crying excessively and choking. The nurse told the driver to pull over to the side of the road until I had calmed down sufficiently. On arrival at the hospice I was taken into the quiet room, and there I remained for the rest of the day. With their special kind of care and continuous oxygen for 20 minutes, I calmed down enough and fell asleep again.

I have come to terms now with the hospice-type care for terminally ill patients. I am going into the hospice for a week of respite care – the last week of the world cup!

Car in the community
Learning to live with a progressive neurological condition, and in my case the advance has been rapid, has not been easy. Since my collapse in February on St. Valentine's Day, I am totally helpless and require 24-hour care. The equipment needed to assist in my care has built up gradually over a period of time. It takes one nurse to get me up in the morning, washed and dressed. I bring myself down on the chair lift. We found the easiest dress code for my needs consists of a silk top, slacks, knickers with pad, socks and sandals. What does break my heart is that I can no longer wear my size 12 outfits. Since the introduction of the tube feeding my waistline has increased to size 16. The position the night team leave me in bed has to be the right one for comfort as there I remain until morning. I can no longer move in bed or raise my head. I was provided with an air mattress to prevent pressure sores. My gratitude to the team. They always chat to me about nursing, clothes and fashion. I feel guilty that I need so much of their time. My particular hate was losing my independence and in particular my personal hygiene. This added to my despair and anger.

It is at times like this when I wish we had voluntary euthanasia. The patient should certainly have a say when and where to die. Life with MND is like a living hell on earth. Your whole body is dead. All I am left with is sight, smell, taste, hearing and sensation. Family gatherings and Sunday dinners have never been the same. I can take no part in family laughter and discussion. I take no part in the kitchen or food shopping. Anywhere I go I must take the suction machine, my talking machine, a large bunch of tissues and a carer familiar with my management. Controlling the saliva which flows from my mouth is not only depressing but also embarrassing. I fold the tissue into one inch widths, fourfold deep and roll the top end down into a narrow roll. I put about three rolls in the side of my mouth since I can no longer cough, but if I have an occasional sneeze. This prevents me from biting my tongue and my lip which is very painful. If I sneeze again within 5–10 minutes I hit the same spot. The surgery lent me a nebuliser to help remove very thick mucus.

Through Social Services I have obtained a wheelchair. I cried my heart out when it first arrived. Life in a wheelchair is a very different world. You feel so vulnerable and at risk. As the disease progresses, I find waking up in the morning a slow process. My friend, the practice nurse, suggested 10–20 minutes oxygen is supplied. Someone has to open my eyelids for me – usually Gordon. The only way I can sum up the sad journey is with a poem I have written. What more can I say!

My living hell on earth
I walk alone
Along this path
Leaving life's hope,
Sorrow, love and pain
Standing at my gate.

I speak no more
I sing no more
I eat no more
IN MY LIVING HELL.

Sometimes I wish
I could swallow,
But there's always
Something at my throat.

I drink no more
I kiss no more
I smile no more
IN MY LIVING HELL.

I see and hear
My world go by,
But reach out
I can not do.

My smiles have gone
I have no joy
I walk no more
To join my crowd
IN MY LIVING HELL.

I'm wheeled along
In my wheelchair
To a sea of knees
And a lot of pushchairs!

Some smiles I get
Some yawns and cries
Thank God they're not
IN MY LIVING HELL.

I tried to find
The peaceful way
But the road is closed
And I must stay.

Animal rights have a say
They can die
When they say;
Please God why can't I?
IN MY LIVING HELL.

could write so much more. I say she has written enough, that her message is powerful and will enable others to understand and learn.

I say to Moira that I understand she wants to publish whilst she is still alive. I ask her 'How long do you expect to live?' My pulse quickens asking this question yet Moira takes it in her stride. She says her GP refused to answer that question, but she expects to die soon. Of course, no one knows for certain, but do we as practitioners avoid such difficult questions and conversations? Does Moira's despair and obsession with euthanasia encourage us into avoidance tactics?

I understood Moira's need to write as a testament that her life and death were not without meaning. She had been a health visitor and teacher. She said she loved nursing and wanted to give something if it would help others to understand. Keeping a journal was a therapeutic act for her. It was cathartic, enabling her to pour out her feelings and helping her make sense of her despair in the face of her relentless physical deterioration towards death.

The catheter was yet another marker along this trajectory. She had become incontinent, and she is a proud woman. Another devastating blow as it took away what pride she had left. I asked her if there was anything that made her smile – the sun shining in the morning or a sparrow singing? In response she smiled. She said, 'I feel like the weather.' It was raining hard outside. She had shed many tears that morning. In her absence of words she drew the tear lines down her cheeks with her fingers. There was no way anybody could take away her despair. There was no way she could rationalise what was happening to her, yet focusing on something positive as her journal and the possibility to publish it did ameliorate her despair, as if the sun had come out for a moment. She was grateful to me. She joined her hands in thanks. I felt touched by this woman in this moment, privileged to sit with her and experience her dying. I was conscious that she, like other patients I had met and written about, were teaching me something profound along my own journey of realising myself as caring. When I left her, I sensed a lightness, a soft spring in my feet. Why was this? Perhaps I should have felt burdened with her despair. But no, on the contrary I had been lifted by the experience. I felt such a calmness and sense of humility. I felt that I had given Moira some warmth and light within her living hell. Moira nourished others, comforted and cared for those who would care for her. She did not want to be a burden but sensed the struggle her carers must feel caring for her. She had shared her story with her carers when perhaps they had not realised how she felt and had been insensitive to her plight. They were touched, and it changed their caring towards her. It had opened their eyes to what Moira was feeling inside. Moira died shortly afterwards. Moira's story offers deep insights into the way people respond to disability, terminal illness and face death. Her writing became her sanctuary, her space where she could scream out loud and communicate to others – so they knew and could understand. That was so important to Moira. Perhaps she sensed it was only too easy to see the demanding, complaining, depressed and angry woman rather than the suffering woman who deeply loved her grandchildren. Her writing made it easier for her and family to dwell together.

Therapeutic benefit

Telling the story may be more significant than just writing it. Smith and Liehr (1999) note that when individuals tell their personal health story to one who truly listens, a change in perspective takes place. Citing Campbell (1988), they state 'Self-discovery is embedded in story. Through story, persons search for clues or messages that potentiate understanding and the experience of being alive described as a "resonance within one's innermost being and reality"' (p. 5). Smith and Liehr did not ask their respondents to journal. They noted that peoples' stories are often disjointed, suggesting the difficulty people may have in expressing their thoughts and feelings. Hence writing may have help people to work through their feelings more coherently.

Smyth *et al* (1999) sampled 112 patients with asthma or rheumatoid arthritis (RA). They assigned them in random-controlled trial (RCT) groups to write either about the most stressful event of their lives or about neutral topics. Outcomes were evaluated at 2 weeks, 2 months and 4 months after writing. They reported that patients with mild to moderately severe asthma or RA who wrote about stressful life experiences had clinically relevant changes in health status at 4 months compared with those in the control group. These gains were beyond those attributable to the standard medical care that all participants were receiving. For the asthma patients, the primary outcome measure was forced expiratory volume in 1 second (FEV_1). An improvement is measured as 15% improvement in functioning. Evaluations of RA patients were made with a structured interview completed by the treating rheumatologist – rating diagnostic symptoms, global assessment of disease activity, symptom severity, distribution of pain, tenderness, swelling throughout the affected joints, presence and severity of deformities, assessment of daily living capacity and general psychosocial functioning. This was based on a categorical scale (asymptomatic/mild/moderate/severe/very severe). There was a 47% improvement (shift in rating) in experimental groups compared with 24% in control groups. Improvement was maintained in asthma patients whereas the change for RA patients was not evidenced until the 4-month period, suggesting that underlying physiological processes differ in different chronic processes. This study was the first of its kind with groups of patients, in contrast with earlier studies using healthy respondents. The study indicates that writing about illness experience does reduce physical symptoms.

Alexander (1998), in her role as writer-in-residence at a Hospice noted: 'Writing is no solution to pain or illness. It cannot cure or heal physical damage but it can help a person to feel whole again, a human being with a story to tell' (p. 178). Alexander's role was to help others to express themselves in words. Whether words can heal is an interesting challenge and the focus for her present study. Of course, this is no surprise, because it is the essence of art therapy (Mayo 1996, Tyler 1998).

Facilitating therapeutic writing

Given the known therapeutic value of reflective writing both for others, it might be a useful therapy to incorporate within clinical practice. How to do this? I might commence by helping the person find a still place inside themselves where they can be reflective (bringing the mind home). I might suggest writing in the afternoon, play some music, or have some complementary treatment beforehand.

When they are relaxed, I sit with the person and help them talk about their experience and then suggest writing about the experience – perhaps as a letter to someone they love and want them to understand. Perhaps start by writing down the strongest feeling specially if they have been resisting it. As such, writing the word down is both cathartic and confronting. I suggest they explore the feeling of thought they have written – why do I feel that way? The cues of the model for structured reflection (MSR) (Box 3.1) offer a pathway to facilitating reflection with the person. If the tone of the experience is negative, I might encourage the person to write something positive about their experience, either something happening now or from memory. The intention is to balance any negative thoughts or feelings with positive ones – to seek balance and harmony through writing.

And of course, to be available to the person to help them talk through the things they have written. In doing so, offer them guidance, courage, compassion and let them know they are not alone. Encouraging people to write is caring. It is empathic inquiry. It shows the person that you care about them and their experience. It is easing suffering.

Conclusion

Encouraging and listening to patient stories enable self-expression and healing, alongside similar activities such as art and music therapy. From a research perspective, reflective writing offers a privileged view into the life of others, enabling practitioners to really appreciate what it means to live with illness.

As Burkhardt and Nagai-Jacobson (2002, p. 296) note, 'In the process of telling and hearing stories, persons often come to new insights and deeper understandings of themselves because stories include not only events in our lives, but also the meanings and interpretations that define the significance of events for particular lives.'

Chapter 20

Nurse bully and the timid sheep: an adventure in storyboard

Storyboard offers an engaging visual approach to narrative that is both simple and effective. It is a technique developed in the 1930s from the Walt Disney Studio (Canemaker 2010).

In Figure 20.1a,b we set out a storyboard of Otter's experience of being bullied at work. The title of the storyboard doesn't mince with words. Getting to the point graphically is characteristic of storyboard. Otter is an artist and thinking visually is second nature for her.

The storyboard is constructed as a sequence of scenes around a central plot of Otter's perception of being bullied. Storyboard literally paints the picture. Whilst one scene prompts the next, the scenes can be rearranged. A brief commentary accompanies each scene. We feel it best to keep the words to a minimum, just enough to show and convey the intended messages.

The storyboard was conceived in two parts. The first part is Otter's tale of despair of being bullied. Bullying is an insidious and debilitating experience that is not easy for the victim to resist, possibly because the 'bully' has sensed that. Perhaps that is why Otter was singled out. The group of staff are caught up in a pattern of behaviour that no one can break free from.

In the second part of the storyboard, Otter was prompted by the model for structured reflection (MSR) cue – 'how might I respond differently, more effectively given the situation again?' This cue is the bridge between the two storyboards. As such, the first storyboard is mimetic, trying to accurately recall the situation, and the second storyboard is fiction. Whether Otter and the others could respond in this way and the imagined consequences are speculative and yet grounded in possibility. That is the nature of this MSR cue. The storyboard considers the cultural background to the experience, whereby others stand back too timid to act, as if they too might become victims. It also exposes the somewhat Machiavellian notion that another might benefit from Otter's bullying.

Becoming a Reflective Practitioner, Fourth Edition. Christopher Johns.
© 2013 John Wiley & Sons, Ltd. Published 2013 by John Wiley & Sons, Ltd.

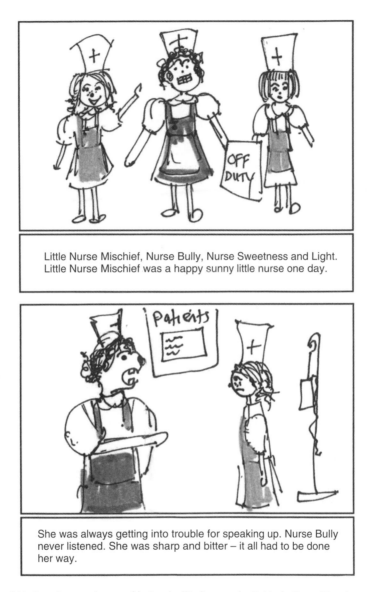

Figure 20.1 **(a and b)** Otter's experience of being bullied at work. © Linda Rose (Otter).

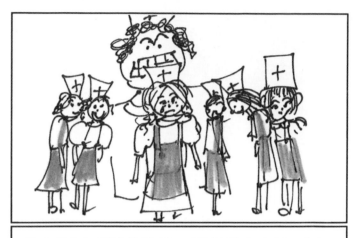

Nurse Bully humiliated Little Nurse Mischief in front of the whole team. Little Nurse Mischief soon lost her confidence and dreaded going to work.

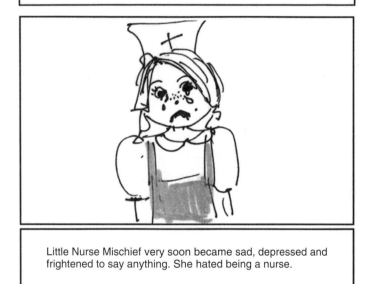

Little Nurse Mischief very soon became sad, depressed and frightened to say anything. She hated being a nurse.

Figure 20.1   *(Continued)*

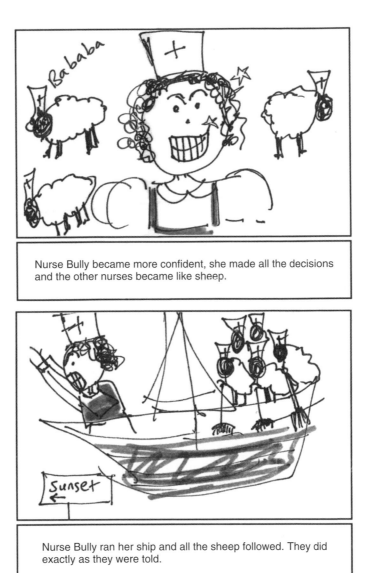

Nurse Bully became more confident, she made all the decisions and the other nurses became like sheep.

Nurse Bully ran her ship and all the sheep followed. They did exactly as they were told.

Figure 20.1 *(Continued)*

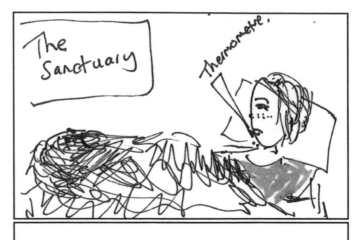

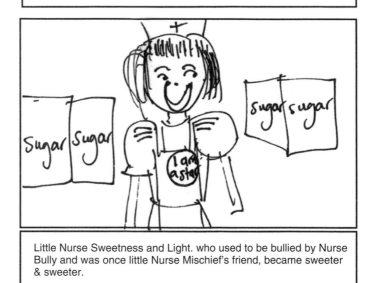

Figure 20.1 (*Continued*)

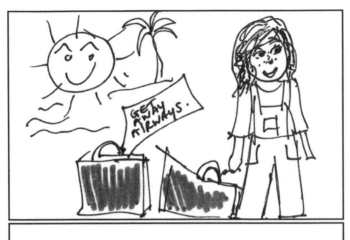

With no resolve, Little Nurse Mischief could see nothing was going to change for the better, it was sad... but she felt she had to leave.

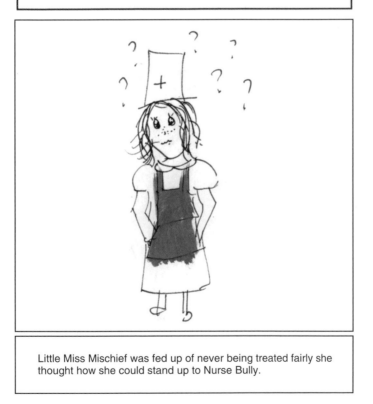

Little Miss Mischief was fed up of never being treated fairly she thought how she could stand up to Nurse Bully.

Figure 20.1   *(Continued)*

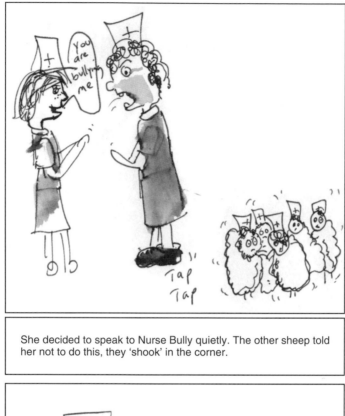

She decided to speak to Nurse Bully quietly. The other sheep told her not to do this, they 'shook' in the corner.

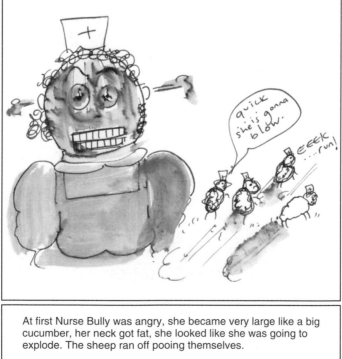

At first Nurse Bully was angry, she became very large like a big cucumber, her neck got fat, she looked like she was going to explode. The sheep ran off pooing themselves.

Figure 20.1 *(Continued)*

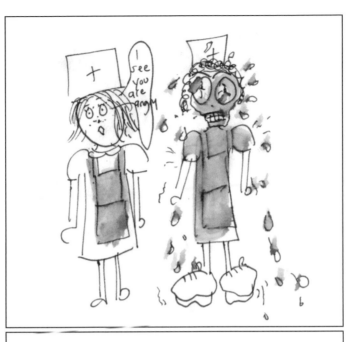

Little Nurse Mischief calmy said "I see you are angry..." after Nurse Bully had completely exploded leaving a trail of mess everywhere!

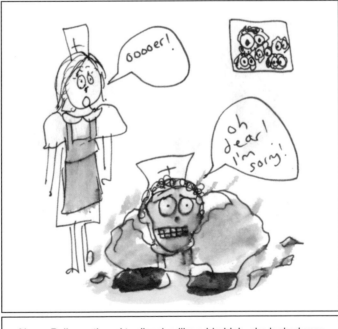

Nurse Bully continued to dissolve like a big blob, she looked very sad and said she was sorry she never listened and sorry she bullied me – the sheep hid nearby.

Figure 20.1 *(Continued)*

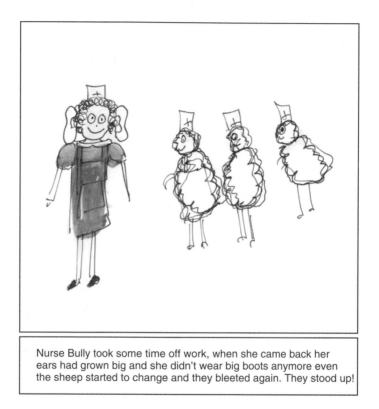

Nurse Bully took some time off work, when she came back her ears had grown big and she didn't wear big boots anymore even the sheep started to change and they bleeted again. They stood up!

Figure 20.1 *(Continued)*

I wonder if nurse bully realises she is a bully? I sense behind the scenes she is an anxious manager out of her depth looking for a soft target to vent her anxiety. Perhaps that is why Otter envisages her crumbling when confronted with her behaviour.

When we 'performed' this storyboard in the USA (July 2012), the audience response supported this interpretation. Indeed, they recognised the authenticity of the storyboard from their own experiences. The dialogue led into an exploration of how individuals and organisations can better resist bullying. It was agreed it should not be tolerated and yet recognising that its endemic nature made this difficult. It was a topic that organisations handled poorly and wanted to turn a blind eye too. The dialogue pursued these threads into deeper political and cultural aspects of organisation.

We minimally searched the literature for evidence to support bullying. We typed into Google – 'bullying in nursing'. Needless to say we got a significant number of hits. One example from NursingTimes.net: 'Healthcare commission chair Sir Ian Kennedy has called for renewed focus on nurse leadership and issued a warning about the "corrosive" nature of bullying in the National Health Service (NHS). Sir Ian said "bullying was one of the biggest untalked about problems in the delivery of good care to patients." '. He felt the problem was caused by the NHS's hierarchical culture and occurred across all staff groups. His comments follow last week's staff survey, in which 8% of respondents said they had experienced bullying, harassment or abuse from a manager or team leader and 12% said they had from colleagues.' (3 April 2009).

Turning to scholarly articles we find 16 papers written between 2000–2010. For example, Hutchinson *et al* (2006)'s 'Workplace Bullying in Nursing: Towards a More

Organisational Perspective'. Pursuing these papers we found links to 'whistleblowing', 'oppressed group behaviour' and 'horizontal violence', and so the paper trail continues. One thing leads to another into a complex and seemingly murky organisational and professional culture. What is clear is that bullying is big academic business besides a topic of significant distress for its victims. We also find advice on how to stop it.

Otter's advice to the workshop audience is 'do not worry about artistic skill. You can represent people as stick people or even thumb prints'. Of course, people do worry about artistic skill just as people unaccustomed to writing poetry worry about writing poetry. This type of response reminds us that people's imagination has been trimmed. They are uncomfortable with play, sensing that they will be publicly exposed and judged as not very good.

In the workshop, people quickly learn to play again and recover the lost imagination. Otter is good at that, at infusing this sense of play with her wild enthusiasm and conviction that everyone can succeed. We ran the workshop on consecutive days. On the first day Otter talked generally about storyboard and gave up some examples of her work.

On reflection, we felt it would be better to perform a whole storyboard to enable people to experience its power. As such, on the second day we performed the storyboard. This experience was further to prove to me (as if I needed it) that all reflective theory is better shown, not told, followed by dialogue where elements can be told as necessary. The performance creates the experience for reflection. The humour built into the storyboards is a vital ingredient as evidenced by audience reception, that even the darkest of topics can be infused with a humorous light emerged as significant. Humour facilitated audience engagement in ways we believe that verbal narratives may struggle with. Some people in the workshops thrived in the storyboard narrative milieu. Others not so much. Analysing this response supported our appreciation that some people are more visual and others are more verbal.

Conclusion

Storyboard offers a more visual representation of reflexive narrative. It opens a door to video and film narratives, media I have yet to explore in my own work and yet exciting to contemplate.

Chapter 21

Reflective prose poetry

Representing reflective learning or insights in narrative form can take diverse visual and verbal forms. Some of us have a natural leaning towards visual modes of expression and some of us lean towards verbal modes of expression. Indeed 'finding the right words' can be a frustrati ng and constraining force.

Wagner (1999) interviewed 18 nurses for their reflections of family impact on the dying experience. She reduced these experiences into a set of categories using fragments of the nurses' reflections to justify each category. In doing so, I felt she lost the meaning in these nurses' stories. However, she then reinterpreted the nurses' words into poetry – 'as a way of knowing subjectively and inter-subjectively the fullest meaning of the data' (p. 21). Her poetry reflects a deeper level of interpretation beyond cognition; in my mind it heals the story and makes it possible to connect with the experience because it is whole.

Prose poetry offers a powerful mode of verbal expression. Poetry transforms ideas into art – with the intent of revealing meaning. Everyone is a poet although you, the reader, may not realise that potential within you. Remember, limits exist only in the mind. Some of us have had our imaginations so trimmed that we believe poetic endeavour is beyond us. Practitioners often say that they do not know where their poetic words have come from. Many are astonished that they can write poetry, as if it is some untapped, latent potential within us all. Yet the latent artist lives within each of us . . . just needs to be woken up and injected with some spirit. On a one-day workshop I would have you writing poetry that you would never believe possible at the beginning of the workshop. Just let go and let the creative juices flow – easier said than done when the creative juices have dried up in the left brain world. Moving into poetic mode we stretch into the right brain moving beyond the confines of the left brain.

As I have suggested, writing story (reflections on experience) enables practitioners to move beyond normal use of language governed by cognitive processes. It opens a creative space.

Breaking down story into single lines further opens this space, and helps the practitioner to draw insights which can then be planted within the text as turning points. Language techniques such as litany, repeating phrases, imagery, analogy, signs and metaphors are utilised to hold and communicate meaning. These techniques all serve to enrich the text and invite the reader's engagement.

In prose poetry, there is no determination to rhyme or verse and yet it has a metre noticeable in the length of the lines that becomes evident when the poems are recited.

Becoming a Reflective Practitioner, Fourth Edition. Christopher Johns.
© 2013 John Wiley & Sons, Ltd. Published 2013 by John Wiley & Sons, Ltd.

Poetry is like taking a short cut to the unconscious, bypassing the cognitive realm. As such aesthetic expression balances the more cognitive approaches to reflection, a more holistic approach that draws on and uses all the senses and tap the deep pool of tacit knowing (Polanyi 1958).

I offer some examples of my own prose poetry in the following set of poems. I wrote them as spontaneous descriptions yet knowing I was going to transform them into prose poems. As such, the mode of prose poetry comes to shape my description. It is a short cut to gaining insight in much the same way as storyboard does for visual reflection as explored in the previous chapter.

The major plot of these prose poems is always the same – to ease the other's suffering and to enable the person's growth through their health–illness experience. This plot is my vision of practice. It is what I intend in my practice as a complementary therapist working in hospice.

The sub-plots or nuances reveal the multiple shades of easing suffering. In contrast with my longer narratives and performances, I try not to infuse with the prose poem with multiple messages. It is better to have one message to communicate, although inevitably it is garnished with signs to other aspects of easing suffering. As with all reflective reading, readers draw their own meanings.

The prose poems collectively reflect on my experiences with patients who resist my offer of therapy. They evoke the complex relationship between suffering and therapy.

> *Alfie Boundary*
> Despair ripples through him like a harsh wind,
> It blows and distorts his countenance.
> His face crumples to the inquiry;
> Heart failure has reduced him,
> Taken his vitality.
> In the hands of others now.
> His wife at her brother's funeral;
> 'I should be there' he cries.
> Tears fall,
> He has fallen.
> I move a chair close to his bed
> sit, move closer,
> as if moving into his suffering
> whereas before, standing, I was on the margin.
> Anxiety spills about going home,
> 'How will she cope?
> She doesn't know yet. . . .?'
> Words that drift off,
> Others spoken in the silence.
> Silence
> Lost for words
> How can such suffering be eased with words?
> He declines a therapy.
> Not in the right frame of mind
> as if healing needs a particular frame.
>
> *Naomi*
> 91 years old
> Never had a thing wrong

Until this.
This small lady looks up at me
Wearing delicate red lipstick
Such thin legs
The football stomach looks incongruous
The ascites being drained
Had her lungs done a while ago.
Ovarian cancer.
I sit
I am in no hurry
And now she can see my face more clearly
rather than my belly.
She tries to be rational
I've had a good life
The last 20 without my husband
Surrounded by a good family
She tries the brave face
But underneath her suffering ripples.
A nurse pops in to check the drainage tap
No sense she disturbs the flow
Naomi declines a therapy,
She has found a comfortable position
As if that position is precarious,
Takes my offered hand
And thanks me for my attention.

Dora Franke
Standing by her bedside
She murmurs 'I don't think I want a treatment thank you'
Her eyes search mine
'*How are you*' I inquire holding her eyes
from my six foot height
Space opens
She talks at length about her husband's
dying in the hospice 2 years ago.
'*How do you feel being here because of that?*'
'Ok, the care Don received was so good.'
As if she can now take comfort in her own care
She is 68
Breast, bowel, bone, and renal cancer spread through her
No pain.
The notes in the green file said she was depressed
Insinuation
Such labels stick
I would say more preoccupied, wistful
and a little fearful.
She knows what is happening to her
And seems ok about that
Perhaps working out old grief
As if preparing to join him.

Mrs Wells
'Good morning Mrs Wells'
banter style

She's been here four weeks now;
more grey, more subdued
Her breathing increasingly laboured
End stage lung disease
She says in her lugubrious way 'just waiting now'
Her husband sits by the window
He endures.
I stand
As if standing is my normal pose
In passing by
I ask how he is and he says 'ok'
What else can he say in this waiting room?
I won't ask you if you want a therapy
No need to burden you with the 'No' game
we learnt to play.
I say *'it's cold out there*
Just 2 degrees
Feel my hand'
She takes it and exclaims how cold it is
Her warmth transforming my cold
Caring is a mutual thing
And she smiles
I sense she has some peace
I am pleased I stopped by to dwell these few minutes.

Belinda
Unresponsive
At first I wondered if you had died
And then your chest moved slightly
Your family about you
Solemn faces
Searching mine
Who is this stranger at this time?
I have stepped into a death parlour
Perhaps I intrude into this room
tucked away as it is at the end of the long corridor
One can hardly be passing by.
I say who I am
dropping by to see if I could help in anyway?
My words spoken from the edge
No chair pulled up to join the throng
'No, they don't think so'
Caught up as they are in death's dance
Waiting for the music to play out its final notes.
They thank me.
'my compassion with you' I murmur
Such words felt right in the moment
As if some words need saying
To rectify the intrusion.

George Keeler
Few words spoken between tumultuous tears
His grief for Dandy who died last September

She had collapsed in the bathroom
A brain tumour
Dead in three days
Ripped away from him after 62 years of marriage.
Prostate cancer has spread through his bones
Now – he just wants to close his eyes and not wake up again
Nothing has meaning
Not even his great granddaughter expected soon
Grief obliterates any future.
I sit with him
Breaking the silence he says 'Drink'
I help him sip
His cup empty
'What do you like to drink?'
'Apple juice'
I fetch him cool apple juice from the fridge
I do not try to understand him
Or fix his despair with platitudes
That might more comfort me.
Alex James quotes a bereaved woman[1]
  'We were together forever.
  I can't quite believe it was 63 years.
  It has flitted by all too soon.
  I can't imagine going on without him.
  No amount of time would have been long enough for us.
  I wasn't ready for it yet
  and I want to slap those who keep saying
  he had a good innings.'
Words that help imagine George's suffering
It is enough to dwell with him
My presence a confrontation that life goes on
When he might prefer to be alone
Caught between worlds.
He says 'never mind' repeatedly.
Her picture on the table watches over him
Black and white
I say *'what message might she give you?'*
He sobs 'I don't know'
He calms as if she now holds his hand.

Frank Seymour
He puts aside the GWR illustrated text
A railway man of old
First the signals on the track
And then exams
Into the clerical office at Euston.
Railways his love
but spent the last 20 working years for Charles Forte
I do not ask why the job shift.
Me too an ex railway man
Building bridges and stations
With the Southern engineers
Connection
20 minutes in recollection

Then some talk of the cancer that grips you
and will take your life.
Matter of fact stuff
No emotional release
He doesn't think he needs a therapy.
Later I say to Wendy '*I had a talk with Frank.*'
She smiles 'He would like that, talking to a man.'
Therapy has many shades
Next Thursday
'*Hello Frank*'
Framed within the open door
'Chris . . . come in'
I hover as if in transition
'Sit down . . . chair over there. . . .
you can move that stuff off there'
I sit and sense the significance of sitting
Rather than stand as if passing by
With its insidious message 'I am busy'
or worse, 'you are an object'
Sitting is a commitment.
'I have time'
'I value our talk'.
I remind you about the job shift.
They wanted to relocate you to Derby
Your base at Harrow and Wealdstone
A small hut on the platform
No consultation
A fait accompli, seeing only the job and not the person
As if standing rather than sitting.
So you decided to quit
You had wanted to be a plateman
But your father, also a railwayman,
A defiant no . . . too dangerous.
So signals and telegraph it was.
You were envious of your friend
Who became a plateman.
Frank sucks in between his words
The nasal cannula and the green tube
A constant reminder as you wait
For the nursing home to be sorted.
You must sense I am restless
Thank me for dropping by and talking.
'*I guess you don't want any therapy?*' I say
'No, no thank you I'm happy as I am.'
Therapy is listening.
Stories are remembering, ordering, healing, connection
The piecing together of a life puzzle
So he can die intact.

Bernard Barker
He barks 'you've come at the wrong time'
A retort that reflects his discomfort
Waiting for a doctor to come to him
Problem with his eye

His anxiety spills
'I am too unwell' in response to my offer of a therapy later
I say '*I meet many people who are unwell.*'
A rue smile – 'good point'
He softens and sees I'm on his side
That he needn't fight me.
Alliance rather than adversarial[2]
No impasse.[3]
I say '*I'll find the doctor for you*'
He thanks me
Offers me his calloused hand.

Rita Pyke
Your green file lies on the table.
Opening I read you are 56.
breast cancer.
The mood word 'flat' grabs my attention.
'Flat' a word that conjures disturbance of the spirit
Insinuation
My curiosity aroused
Even at this late hour
The sky dark outside.
A visitor with you
Your dismissive NO
To my invitation for therapy
My poise disturbed
I was only trying to help!
Paradoxically I move closer
When perhaps I should bow my retreat
And apologise for the intrusion.
I draw attention to the fat robin
who flits across the lawn
Distraction
Saving face?
But you cannot see it
'*No matter*' I say
'*I'll leave you to your visitor*'
Caught on the hop
Like the robin
I exit uneasily.
Nothing flat about this force
Rarely am I thrown against the wall
Normal patterns twisted.

Mattingly (1998, p. 71) writes citing Sacks (1984, 1995), 'but sickness and tragedy have their own curious effects, not least of which is a sort of detachment, a leave taking of the body, a disinclination to care about anything, or a disowning of one's troublesome parts.'[4]

Rita, do these words fit the bill?
But then, what is the bill?
I cannot tune in and if I cannot tune in
how can I help you?
Perhaps I shouldn't try

> But to try is why I'm here?
> My dilemma
> I cannot expect relationship
> Or can I?
> Li argues,[5] relationship should be symbiotic niceness
> And Rita is not playing the game!
> Doesn't she know I am a miner
> to excavate the deep veins of her suffering?
> Yet I know my presence can put people 'on the spot',
> disturb their control
> when life is itself out of control.
> Intrusive
> 'unwelcome or uninvited and causing a disturbance or annoyance'[6]

Mattingly (1998, pp. 64–5] writes, 'therapist concern with a future strongly organises the meaning of the present and makes therapist vulnerable to disjuncture [contradiction] between what they have wished for and what actually unfolds.'[7]

> I feel the contradiction
> I who had put myself out to stay on
> Rebuffed unceremoniously!!
> I rationalize to pull myself free from anxiety
> It is, after all, isn't it, a reflection of her 'flatness'?
> But that would be to reduce her to a symptom
> When I seek humanness beyond the symbiotic niceness
> She doesn't play the 'nice' game I inadvertently fall into.
> My face slapped for such impertinence
> Wake up and read the road sign!
> Flat
> The tyranny of label[8]
> Rarely do I read notes first
> Preferring to find the person
> Than the patient wrapped up in labels;
> Flat – as if I might lift her
> Flat – a violation of her spirit
> as if someone has not understood.

Janet Younger (1995, pp. 53–4) writes, 'Suffering makes one a stranger . . . and the reaction of others is to turn away from this stranger who now lives in a world others may be reluctant to enter . . . but when by chance it is suddenly revealed in all its nakedness, people shiver and recoil.'[9]

> Recoil
> I hit the wall
> Can I bounce back?
> Two weeks pass
> The green file reveals Rita may now have brain mets
> A new 'label' to explain her 'unfriendly' behaviour
> To rationalise her 'disturbance';
> She lies on her bed alone
> Idly watching TV
> Wears red framed glasses
> A touch of colour to lift the 'flatness'

A slight smile of recognition
'*Hello Rita? I'm Chris the complementary therapist..*'
I pause as if to let the words sink in
'*Do you remember me?*'
No reply
'*How are you?*' I persist
'Bored, waiting'
Tentatively I inquire '*Waiting for what?*'
She does not answer.
Turns her head away
'*You have had some complementary therapy since being here?*'
Yes
'*Was it helpful?*'
Yes.
'*But not today?*'
No . . . but she is not unfriendly.
'*I'll let you rest*'
banal, but I need to have the last word.
I move away
A lingering trace of disquiet
I wanted to say more
But did not know how.
I mention this to a nurse
'Everyone finds her difficult,' she says
'You shouldn't take it personally.
She wasn't like this before.'
She suggests its Rita's problem rather than mine.
The dark side of nursing.[10]
But I disagree.
Randall and Downie (1999) note,

Those working in palliative care are strongly motivated to reduce 'suffering', but at the same time realise that our ability to do so is limited because we cannot personally meet the patient's needs. This does not mean that we will not do all in our power to alleviate this complex suffering, but rather acknowledge the limits of professional knowledge and skills, and explore the possibility of relieving distress by means of ordinary human contact informed by our knowledge.[11]

Another week passes
Her door partially open
She is in there
But I do not enter
My fear of intrusion
I know her resistance
the demand I impose
Simply by being there.
I stay outside
Held at bay.
Yet today might have been different?
Another week passes
Breath to bring myself present
Shake away the fear.
Rita is alone, lies on her bed

Viewing TV through her familiar red framed glasses
'I like your glasses. . .'
A slight smile of welcome.
I hover
Perhaps waiting to be invited to sit
Sitting cannot be assumed
'just passing by to say hello,
to let you know I am here today if you would like a therapy?'
'No'
I smile, *'That's fine as well.'*
She takes my offered hand and I am free.
But I am left wondering if
my persistence adds to her suffering.
Therapy like suffering is complex.
A week later
Her name no longer on the name board.

The poems are presented in a sequential pattern culminating with Rita Pyke. Unlike the other prose poems, this final poem was first written as a story. It was a difficult poem to write as I struggled to understand my emotional reaction to Rita. To help me, I drew on various literature to help frame the issues emerging. Perhaps most significant was the idea of 'symbiotic niceness' and that Rita refused to play this game. It was not an idea I was aware of and the realisation that I and other staff might play this game was disturbing. Failure to play this game by the patient results in labelling: 'she is the problem', and the therapeutic potential is subsequently diminished.

Using footnotes enables the reader to explore a relevant literature in relation to the issues I raise within the poems. In a public reading I invite the audience to dialogue with me, enabling me to link my experience within an informing literature.

Notes

1   James A (undated) *Living with Bereavement*. Right Way Books, Tadworth.
2   Mclaughlin AM and Carey JL (1993) The adversarial alliance: developing therapeutic relationships between families and the team in brain injury rehabilitation. *Brain Injury* 7(1): 45–51.
3   Ramos MC (1992) The nurse–patient relationship: theme and variations. *Journal of Advanced Nursing* 17: 498–506. (In this paper Ramos indicate that nurses have two impasses to therapeutic work – emotional and power).
4   Mattingly C (1998) *Healing Dramas and Clinical Plots*. Cambridge University Press, Cambridge.
5   Li S (2004) 'Symbiotic niceness': constructing a therapeutic relationship in psychosocial palliative care. *Social Science & Medicine* 58(12): 2571–58.
6   Compact Oxford English Dictionary (third edition) (2005) (C Soanes and S Hawker, Eds) Oxford University Press, Oxford, p. 533.
7   Mattingly C, op.cit.
8   Trexler JC (1995) Reformualtion of deviance and labeling theory for nursing. *IMAGE: Journal of Nursing Scholarship* 28(2): 131–135.
9   Younger J (1995) The alienation of the sufferer. *Advances in Nursing Science* 17(4): 53–72.
10 Corley MC and Goren S (1998) The dark side of nursing: impact of stigmatizing responses on patients. *Scholarly Inquiry for Nursing Practice: An International Journal* 12(2): 00–121.
11 Randall F and Downie RS (1999) *Palliative Care Ethics*, 2nd edition. Oxford University Press, Oxford.

Chapter 22
Through a glass darkly

Introduction

Moving narrative into performance is a logical development. However, performance, to be effective in engaging the audience, needs to be well crafted. I write narrative with a view to performance – what I term the *performance turn*. Performance opens up the sixth dialogical movement as a space to dialogue with an audience towards social action. As you can imagine, it is a more active engagement than reading narrative. I know that people tend to read narrative with their heads, although the storyteller's art can engage at a more visceral level. I also know that people tend to listen with a more subliminal awareness. In other words, performance is more gut or heartfelt than head felt. The writer's craft is to engage the audience, to draw the audience into the text as if they are living the experience for themselves.

Performance has a time span followed by appropriate dialogue time, with a 'processing' break in between. The processing break is vital, given the often emotional reaction to performance that requires some time to stand back from before engaging in dialogue.

The performance turn is influenced by the ideas of performance ethnography, in particular that performance is social action towards improving health care (Denzin 2003). The performance is a trigger to spur the audience to action.

Performance design

Performance may take many shapes. At its simplest level, it is no more than reading a narrative to an audience. The more crafted the narrative around its key turning points and insights, for the specific audience, the more effective it will be. To create dramatic ambience, I use movement, music, images and installation. However, it is important not to use such technique to embellish the performance. At times, too much 'going on' around the narrative is distracting for the audience and is ultimately counterproductive.

Giving voice

In some performance narratives, I represent the voice of others as empathic poems. In this way I 'give voice' to other people referred to in the narrative. It helps balance my

Becoming a Reflective Practitioner, Fourth Edition. Christopher Johns.
© 2013 John Wiley & Sons, Ltd. Published 2013 by John Wiley & Sons, Ltd.

own voice – that my voice is not privileged. Writing empathic poems opens a new dimension to performance. It adds an authenticity – that I have considered the voice of others. I first used the idea of 'giving voice' to others in 'Jane's Rap' (Groom and Johns 2002/2010, Johns and Marlin 2010) where I represented the voices of eight self-harm patients in an accident and emergency (A&E) department through empathic poems. These poems were composed by a third party as a response to the narrative. In various performances of Jane's Rap, I invited different people to read these poems within the performance. Initially I used one person, moving across eight chairs – where each chair represented the self-harm person.

In another performance, I worked with eight psychiatric nurses representing each self-harm patient. In another performance, I worked with university drama students (the educational impact of working with students in this way is developed in Chapter 8). I created the stage as a stark A&E department. In my performance of 'Anthea' I employed an actor to play Anthea for greater dramatic effect.[1]

In 'Climbing Walls' (Johns 2010b), I worked with a dancer and actor who moved around me as I read my narrative. This performance was professionally directed and performed on public stage.[2] My craft has benefited greatly working with performance teachers. Performance is much more than simply standing up and reading a narrative, as engaging as that might be.

In performances of 'My Mother's Death', I have performed with a musician – moving into an extemporised dialogue between my words and music. Conveying meaning without words is a medium I begin to explore, for example, using shapes and colours.

Through a glass darkly preamble

I have performed this text just once in Hiroshima at the Red Cross Hospital's Peace and caring conference in March 2012 to an audience of approximately 600. I performed it with Otter, my partner.

The narrative text concerns 1 day in my practice as a complementary therapist working within a hospice inpatient unit. My narrative is ongoing, constructed around its core plot to ease suffering. It is part of a larger reflexive narrative that plots my ability to ease suffering that stems back to 2000.[3]

Over the years I have come to know something about suffering and my ability to ease it.

There are many facets to easing suffering that are recurring threads that ripple through the narrative. Insights are subtle and ever deepening like the many different shades of colours. What is clear, at least to me, is that suffering is unique and uncertain. It can never be known outside the moment. As such, to know suffering is to tune into the suffering person's wavelength and move in rhythm with it.

The narrative is edited from the actual performance text, adjusting the syntax to make it more readable. Obviously, the music and images used as background cannot be shown or heard.

The performance commences with an artist painting a large enso. She then writes the word 'heiwa' (meaning peace in Japanese) inside the enso accompanied by the music of Pink Floyd's 'Obscured by Clouds' – a metaphor for the way clarity of mind is obscured by false ideas and creates conflict.

The music fades, leaving me sitting at my desk painting the enso as a prelude for reading my narrative. The narrative includes a number of empathic poems to represent voices of different people I engage with. In the performance these were read dramatically by the artist. I had asked if they might be read by Japanese nursing students, but this proved too difficult to arrange.

I have used extensive endnotes so as not to 'fill' the narrative with extraneous detail and references. Since this performance, I have altered small parts of the text as a consequence of performing it. My reading had simultaneous Japanese translation. The performance was followed by 30-minute audience dialogue.

Through a glass darkly

After a shift at the hospice, I write my reflections on the people I have worked with that day. I usually do this within 24 hours of the experience. Some reflections are just a few lines, whilst others, seemingly more significant, are developed into a more substantive form. One shift involved me working with six patients. A recurrent theme in my understanding of suffering was the idea of *waiting*, and how, as a therapist, I might ease the suffering of waiting.

Sitting here I paint ensos – zen circles of enlightenment. The circle expresses the totality of our being.[4] It is a spiritual practice. Alongside one enso I write, 'Everything that happens to you has the potential to deepen you.'[5]

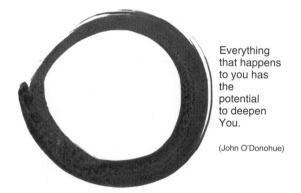

Everything that happens to you has the potential to deepen You.

(John O'Donohue)

These words reflect the essence of reflective practice that, by paying attention to our lived experiences, we can learn and gain insights that change us. By paying attention, I become increasingly mindful of myself within my practice, more mindful of my thinking, feeling and actions and any contradiction between my vision – of who I want to be and an understanding of my lived reality.[6] This creative tension is the learning potential of reflective practice.[7] It is the hermeneutic circle[8] – the constant play between the whole and its parts, resulting in an ever deeper understanding. Narrative opens a dialogical space for readers to consider its insights in terms of their own experiences. It is a trigger for social action towards creating a better, more peaceful world.

My vision as both a therapist and nurse is to help ease others' suffering and enable their growth. The idea of easing suffering is enshrined within the WHO definition of palliative care. Suffering is complex. It's nature is elusive despite conceptual attempts to 'know it'.[9] I have always appreciated Cassell's succinct description of suffering as distress brought about by an actual or impending threat to personal integrity.[10] It is sensed by tuning into to the patient's story. Yet, how easily suffering can be increased, rather than eased, by careless practitioners.

The idea of growth stems from the writing of Milton Mayeroff (1971, p. 1). He writes, 'To care for another person, in the most significant sense, is to help him grow and actualize himself.' Mayeroff identifies the major ingredients of caring: knowing, alternating rhythms, patience, honesty, trust, humility, hope and courage. He doesn't mention love? I wonder why?

Opening Rumi[11] I read:

> Love is longing and longing, the pain of being parted;
> No illness is rich enough for the distress of the heart
> A lover's lament surpasses all other cries of pain.

Rumi's (2006) poems offer beautiful perspectives on love and suffering. Reading these words I imagine the lament of patients and their relatives as they waited. I know that love is healing energy; it is the strange attractor that patterns healing. Healing is the return to wholeness that is so often fragmented by cancer.[12] I wonder, is it possible to really understand and case the lament that surpasses all other cries of pain?

As I move through the day from patient to patient, from family to family, I imagine moving through a series of six gates as transitional moments within my unfolding practice narrative.

My eyes scroll down the names of patients room by room. Familiar names mixed with new names. Much has changed since last week.

I walk along corridors where some doors stand open and others closed, behind which is a world of wonder and not-knowing, where curiosity, not certainty becomes the saving grace.[13] Perhaps 'a gate' would be a better descriptor than 'a door', for a gate opens to a path that the dying person and the family step along; a path risky for all of us.

The first gate

Before the closed door I pause to gather my breath to bring myself fully present to this moment. I knock and quietly enter. Jeannie Martin lies here. Last week you were so jolly. The room full of noise and laughter with memories of times past. You were quite a lass it seems. Planning the renewal of vows in the chapel. Something you had missed before in your life. Death had then seemed far away. Now, you seem at peace lying here. I say 'seem' because looks can be deceptive. Your agitation bludgeoned into submission with sedation. I wonder, What do you feel beneath the sedation blanket? Do you struggle? A question I have often asked myself in my struggle with this most pervasive and invidious practice. A question I challenge others about sedative practice.[14] How easy to slip into such practices as if by routine – as if we see the agitation as a symptom to subdue rather than the person. An old nutshell.

Words by Radbruch[15] come to mind:

> is the primary goal of sedation alleviation of intolerable suffering? If so, what level of consciousness should be achieved? Does the patient have to be unconscious or merely very sleepy but rousable? For longer periods, is sedation designed to be irreversible, or should trials of dose reduction be planned periodically to check the extent of the suffering and whether the patient wants to revise his (or her) decision on sedation? Sedation as a therapeutic option should be the last resort when other options are not available.

Words I have used before[16] as if practice is a merry-go-round where we collectively learn little. I do not know if the sedation was negotiated with Jeannie.

Murphy, your husband, sits alone by your side. His head bowed.

Waiting.

The waiting can be so hard. It is not easy for him to dwell by your side when you are caught in death's strong tide. I sense the loneliness of the dying journey.[17] My hand, briefly on his shoulder, my touch tries to convey sympathy.[18] Perhaps I should sit alongside and fill the room with reiki, and then perhaps the sedation could be put aside if we had the imagination or even the science.

Later, more family about, but no noise, no shout.

All is subdued in the afternoon light.

Your daughter says 'my feet are killing me'. Her knowing look my way. She knows we offer relatives therapy. My eye catch the full demand. 'A quickie then' I say. How many can I fit into any 1 day?

Now she can let go, if just for a moment, surrender into another's hands. My hands take the strain and then the longing is not so hard to bear. Blackwolf's mantra – 'Touch, the harmonic the grieving spirit craves.'[19]

Later, as I leave the hospice with the light fading fast, I pass Murphy who walks outside. His head slightly bowed. No doubt a cigarette or two smoked. Seeking relief from the strain, or so I imagine. My nod of recognition, soft eyes in the darkening light. No words passed. I feel uneasy passing him imbued by his sadness. Imbued – from the Latin *imbuere* – meaning 'moisten'[20], as if I have soaked up his tears.

I imagine his lament:

> Murphy's lament
> Round and round the garden
> Like a teddy bear
> One step two step
> Yet I stumble alone into the gathering darkness
> My children's noise deafens me
> Fine words fade like dew
> I am beyond words now
> Stumbling on
> No 'tickly under there'.

The second gate

In the room lies Rhona Hepworth. A sculptor's name. Her art reflective in the way it opens and shapes space.[21] I imagine you in your studio shaping imagination in the way I might sculpt energy and open healing spaces. Creating new patterns out of suffering.

Your brother makes his farewell. You say, 'Would you be bothered if I didn't wear my head scarf?'

Your head bald from the constant chemotherapy. Do you suggest that others recoil? I know women who do not like being seen bald.[22] Hair such an important statement, even in a hospice where you might imagine appearances would not be so important.

'No' I say.

You love reflexology, the way it helps you to relax. I imagine the strain of the remorseless toil of cancer and its treatments. The battle against the odds. Vain hope as you lose ground to its inexorable advance. The sense of fragmentation.[23] Death hovers but I hear you say 'not yet', 'not yet'. The towel held firm. Not yet thrown in. No surrender.

You say 'I am more at peace now' – as if you have sculpted your requiem. The material stuff stripped away. The mortal coil unwinding to reveal your soul.

You say 'I am going home tomorrow, the hospice bed is open if I should need it.' Reassuring words that ease the strain of uncertainty.

I listen as you unwind your story.

Rachel Remen[24] writes,

> Listening is the oldest and perhaps the most powerful tool of healing. It is often through the quality of our listening and not the wisdom of our words that we are able to effect the most profound changes in the people around us. When we listen, we offer with our attention an opportunity for wholeness. Our listening creates sanctuary for the homeless parts within the other person. That which has been denied, unloved, devalued by themselves and others. That which is hidden.

The hospice a sanctuary. But sometimes we listen to things but never hear them.[25]

I mix my oils; vetiver with lavender. Vetiver – the 'oil of tranquillity'.[26] Its deep earthy aroma pungent as if connecting you with the earth, that is, if you believe the books.[27]

My hands listening, sculpting, shaping energy into healing pattern in the quiet afternoon. Energy shifts, lifts.[28] No disturbance except just once, voices outside, a slight creak of the door as if someone not daunted by the 'do not disturb' sign, anxious to go about her business, had pressed down upon the handle.[29] Once again, I leave you asleep, careful not to wake you, as I clear away my stuff and wash my hands. Asleep, you look peaceful as if suffering had lifted from you.

I imagine your lament.

> Rhona's lament
> Alone but not alone
> In the middle of this circle that comforts and disturbs
> Like a dot that others move carefully around
> My precarious hold as I trip along the edge
> Too many nice people, too many words
> Thinking they can understand
> It's easier to be alone
> Yet I'm grateful for the space.
> Sorry if I'm abrupt.
> But I have to do this my way.

The third gate

Roland Baker, you were admitted yesterday.

Cancer in the pancreas and liver. 'Nothing to be done' you say, in response to my inquiry about treatment. Your words spoken with resignation. No trace of self-pity as if that is simply the way it is. Here for pain control. Pain in the hips and lower back disturb you. Your struggle to find a comfortable position. I will return later.

Some time later, Kay, your wife, sits at the end of the bed. We negotiate a reflexology for you as if you have become a spectator to your own dance. You acquiesce, but I sense an intolerance playing along the edge. Is it your wife's insistent anxiety? I do not ask but sense her longing, the pain of being parted. So many years married and now the end.

But first, to lift you in the bed. Women in dark blue tunics are called and come to lift you, straighten you out so I can work your feet. Your 6'2 frame extends beyond the bed's end. Overhanging feet. 'Size 13' your wife discloses. 'We'll need plenty of cream to cover those' I quip, in vain attempt at humour to soften the lament. Roland laughs, 'My brothers were all 6'6. My son too.'

Oils mixed. My hands along the soles of your feet. Listening for the tides coming in and going out, strengthening the tides that infuse the body with energy.[30]

Hands move across skin. But you are not comfortable on your back.

I pull you through so you lie on your side and work the feet as best I can.

You slip into sleep. Your wife too, sleeps. I imagine her tired with the caring strain. And when she wakes she exclaims, 'I slept', surprised, as if such moments are rare.

Reflex infuses the room and covers all in its calming blanket; shifts the energy, as molecules of lavender and grapefruit seduce the air with their fragrance, re-patterning the drama. And, for the moment, the longing seems easier.

I imagine Kay's lament.

> Kay's lament
>   I needed that sleep
>   I hope I didn't drool or worse, snore!
>   But I am so exhausted
>   Roland has had a great fall
>   and all the doctors and nurses can't put him back to together again
>   it's all in vain
>   and I don't know what to do
>   words no longer reassure
>   and now he snores and I sit here alone.

The fourth gate

Samuel Grey. Your name matches your pallor and beard. Your wife greets me as if we have met before. Have we? Ah yes, memories flood back. It was some months ago, a different room. Even then your breathing was compromised as the oesophageal cancer tightened its grip around the trachea. Then I had given you reiki. The relief it brought lifting the veil of suffering as it pressed heavy.

Mary, your wife, smiling, animated, hopeful that I can lift it again. Her smile a mask, a brave face in adversity to hide the pain of being parted. Hope mingles with despair even at this late hour as the light dims.

Trish, your daughter, the image of her mother. Your grandson plays with trucks on the floor absorbed in his play, seemingly oblivious to the unfolding drama. His name is Adam.

'I remember my dinky toys,' I say 'the pleasure they gave.'

You ask if I still have them.

'No,' I say.

Your wife quips they would be of value, especially if kept in their box. Mine were chipped and battered in the play. Long discarded with no thought of future value. Perhaps they still exist in some collectors haven?

I wonder, does such banter lighten the mood, quieten the lament, normalise my dwelling within the family so they feel less alone in this place of dying?

Perhaps I am an intrusion that forces social pleasantry when the blood churns inside? Dying *is* lonely, I cannot pretend otherwise.[31] As a healthcare worker I must always be mindful of positioning myself within the family and my manner, familiar, but not too familiar. Simultaneously tuning into the diverse wavelengths.[32]

Adam tidies his toys. Unusual for him, his mother says.

The family rise to go so you can have your therapy. 'Stay' I say. But they move away, perhaps needing space to stretch and gather. Mary aches for him. Out of sight her love turns to tears. The longing, the pain of being parted. A lover's lament surpasses all other cries of pain.

Reiki hands hold your brow and neck.

Reiki hands across your chest.

Reiki hands hold each foot.

Thirty minutes pass in reverent silence. Afterwards you say you can breath normally. Relief; relief against the stack of three concentrators that line the facing wall, relief against death's reaching tendrils. Your yellow eyes tell the story.

You say 'I am going now.'

And I imagine you crossing a bridge where the light illuminates the path.

You ask 'Are you here next week?'

'I am,' I say. And you say you hope to see me but you are not sure about that.

Heart strings pluck atonal notes, but then death is not a sweet melody I can pretend. Life is not a riddle to solve. It is a mystery to live.[33]

I imagine Adam's lament.

> Adam's lament
> Ring-a-ring o' roses
> A pocket full of posies
> A-tishoo! A-tishoo!
> We all fall down.
> Ring-a-ring o' roses
> A pocket full of posies
> A-tishoo! A-tishoo!
> We all fall down.

The fifth gate

Edith Ponting is hunched up on the bed, wrapped in a shawl.

'Hello dear' you say 'How are you?'

'I'm ok. And you?' I ask

'A little better today thank you.'

The TV control in her small hand. She is bothered by the intermittent loss of TV sound. The TV loud as if she might be hard of hearing.

'I'll contact the maintenance people,' I say

'Thank you dear.'

Last week you did not want my attention, but today you think it might be nice to have your feet massaged. You had it done last week.

'A woman did it,' you say. 'It was very nice.'

Edith is 82 years old. Her husband at home is 86.

'How is he?' I ask.

'Not so good . . . I look after him. My daughter three doors down holds the fort.'

Your face wrinkles, tears close to the surface. The pain of being parted. Your lament silent but I feel it like a cold wind.

Aromas of lavender and grapefruit delight you. In your undemonstrative way you say 'that's nice dear.' I smile and gently massage your feet. My hands move as if a healing dance.

'Did you like dancing?' I say

'Oh yes but my husband didn't.'

'Did you convert him?'

'No . . . he wasn't interested so I gave it up.'

The way women give way to men. Words drift into silence in the quiet afternoon. Some birdsong penetrates from outside. I ponder the cue – how do you see the future?[34] But I do not ask; it is enough to respond as I do.

We play out the game of symbiotic niceness.[35]

I imagine Edith's lament.

> Edith's lament
> No bother dear
> Every one is so nice here
> But the truth is I'm dying
> Dying of worry about hubby
> But I won't worry anyone
> Let's just have a cup of tea
> And everything will be better.
> Reminds me of an old nursery rhyme
> Polly put the kettle on
> Polly put the kettle on
> Polly put the kettle on
> We'll all have tea
> Sukey take it off again
> Sukey take it off again
> Sukey take it off again
> They've all gone away
> Me too soon.
> Never mind dear.

The sixth gate

Hettie Blake. We have met the past three Mondays. On no occasion did I give you a therapy. The first time we met your eyes lit up with possibility and then, suddenly, you were whisked away to the general hospital. An abscess found that needed draining.

The second time you looked tired, imbued by a sadness, surrounded by family who stood vigil. You had turned to look at me. Consternation in your look that pushed me away. I understood.

Now you lie comatose, life energy seeping away. Not many more hours for this world. Your sisters move about you, dignified with quiet lament. Your son, Tom, bending to the strain, like a reed that bows to the relentless rain. When will the rain stop?

Your sister urges him to have a therapy. My hands move to ease his strain.

'That's good,' he sighs.

Later, one sister plays the piano rallying the gathering troops. The hospice a nomadic camp. The lament ripples through the gathered host, muted in case of giving offence.

How hard the waiting, not knowing quite how to be. No apparent order in the drama. No discernible pattern. We fumble in the dark as the sun drops below the horizon and the evening draws its long shadows.

I imagine Hettie's lament.

> Hettie's lament
> Entombed in a tunnel of darkness
> A faint light one end fading slowly,
> the distant sound of muffled voices.
> Do they not hear my cry?
> No one comes for me
> I am alone.
> I feel as if I should fly
> But my wings are heavy.

I imagine Tom's lament.

> Tom's lament
> Mum, mum, you seem far away
> Can you hear me?
> Feel my hand hold yours
> It is so hard to sit here
> the strain pulls me down
> tears well
> and yet I hold them back
> released in the pulsing touch.
> I feel alone within this gathering crowd
> Words dry up
> Like a desert river in hottest summer
> With buzzards circling.

I pause from my journal. Turning over the words that reveal something of the drama of the day, I ask myself, 'Do I help ease the pain of being parted, the longing and longing of the distressed heart, and the lament that surpasses all other cries of pain?' Could I help ease this pain better?[36] Am I able to see things clearly for what they really are?[37] For sure, it is not easy to see through a glass darkly. And yet, I do know that Love *is* healing energy.

No question of it.

Michele Petrone, the artist who died of Hodgkin's disease, writes:

A serious illness does for your appetite for love what steroids do for your appetite for food. When feeling low and vulnerable, your appetite for love can become insatiable. Fortunately, love came tome from so many sources, some expected, others surprising. From my family and friends, of course, from my lover – well that goes without saying. The nurses and counsellors and even the cleaners gave so much love. It means so much to me even now. Some of the doctors also expressed love. Is a doctor a better doctor if he or she is loving? Undoubtedly. No question of it.[38]

No question of it. Love enters into dark places and showers them with beauty and light.[39] Perhaps compassion is an easier word than love; compassion is concern for the suffering of others from the latin 'compati – to suffer with',[40] a focused type of love, whereas love is more evocative, embarrassing, confrontational. Do we shrink from words like love because, as Okri writes, we live in fractured world where such words give offence?[41] Love is not a flowery thing. It is much deeper than that. Whilst dying could be peaceful it rarely is, either for those dying or those who watch and wait. But then, in a post-religious age there is little solace. Peace an illusion we grasp at. Love *is* solace.

John O'Donohue (1997) writes:

> . . . when love awakens in your life, in the night of your heart, it is like the dawn breaking within you. Where before there was anonymity, now there is intimacy; where before in your life was awkwardness, now there is a rhythm of grace and gracefulness; where before you were jagged, now you are elegant and in rhythm with yourself. When love awakens in your life, it is like a rebirth, a new beginning.[42]

The pain of being parted is love running through you. Easing suffering is tuning into this love and nourishing it rather than shrinking from it. To boldly go, so to speak, armed with sensitive compassion. Laments are expressions of love. Each patient and family's suffering is unique. I must be open to the possibilities of each moment, mindful of treading sensitively on such hallowed ground.

To ease suffering I must learn to tune into the other's suffering. To do this I must wipe away any preconceptions. My hands listening, learning in the stillness.

Becker[43] writes:

> We have to learn to feel, but it doesn't happen by being taught. I can't teach you anything about it; you have to learn it yourself on a one-on-one basis. Patients taught it to me from within themselves. I learned it within them by listening from within myself about how to work with the body physiology. I still don't know everything I'm supposed to feel, I'm still learning.

Reflective practice is being like Newton's Child, turning over pebbles, while great possibilities of wonder stretch out ahead of us into eternity.[44]

Notes

1. Performance of Anthea to an audience of GP trainees, North London Deanery (February 2012).
2. See Diedrich *et al* (2010) for a reflection on their involvement in 'Climbing Walls'.
3. This journal has been published in books and journal papers. In particular see: Johns C (2004) *Being Mindful, Easing Suffering*. Jessica Kingsley Publishing, London and Johns C (2006) *Engaging Reflection in Practice*. Blackwell Science, Oxford.
4. Seo AY (2007) *Enso: Zen Circles of Enlightenment*. Weatherhill, Boston, p. xi.
5. O'Donohue J (1997) *Anam Cara*. Bantam Press, p. 26.
6. Johns fundamentally defined reflective practice as paying attention to and working towards resolving the contradiction between what one's vision of what is desirable and one's actuality. Johns C (2009) *Becoming a Reflective Practitioner*, 3rd edition. Wiley-Blackwell, Oxford.
7. Senge described this as creative tension. See Senge P (1990) *The Fifth Discipline*. Century Business, New York.
8. I have designed an approach to reflexive narrative construction based on six dialogical movements within the hermeneutic circle – described as narrative as a journey of self-inquiry and transformation towards self-realisation (however that might be expressed). See Johns C (2010) *Guided Reflection: A Narrative Approach to Advancing Professional Practice*. Wiley-Blackwell, Oxford.

9   For example, Daneault S *et al* (2004) The nature of suffering and its relief in the terminally ill: a qualitative study. *Journal of Palliative Care* 20(1): 7–11.

10 Cassell EJ (1982) The nature of suffering and the goals of medicine. *New England Journal of Medicine* 306: 639–645.

11 Rumi – Words of paradise (selected and translated by Raficq Abdulla). Frances Lincoln Ltd, London, p. 4.

12 Colyer H (1996) Womens' experiences of living with cancer. *Journal of Advanced Nursing* 23: 496–501.

13 Wheatley M (1999) *Leadership and the New Science*, 2nd edition. Berrett-Kohler, San Francisco, p. 8

14 In a conversation with the hospice medical director, a recent audit of sedation revealed 81% died under sedation. She agreed that the practice of sedation had become routine rather than tailored to individual need.

15 Radbruch L (2002, p. 239) Reflections on the use of sedation in terminal care. *European Journal of Palliative Care* 9(6): 237–9.

16 Johns C (2005) *Being Mindful, Easing Suffering*. Jessica Kingsley Publishing, London.

17 Elias N (1985) *The Loneliness of the Dying*. Basil Blackwell, Oxford.

18 There is a considerable literature on 'touch'. I view it a as a primary mode of connection, although mindful that touch can be misconstrued or unwelcome. As O'Donohue states, 'touch brings presence home' (ibid., p. 101).

19 Jones, R and Jones G (1996) *Earth Dance Drum*. Commune-A-Key, Salt Lake City, p. 184.

20 *Compact Oxford English Dictionary*, p. 504.

21 http://www.barbarahepworth.org.uk/sculptures/

22 See 'Climbing Walls' in Johns C (2010) *Guided Reflection: A Narrative Approach to Advancing Professional Practice*. Wiley-Blackwell, Chichester (see chapter 4, pp. 1§64–177).

23 Colyer, H. (1996) Womens' experiences of living with cancer. *Journal of Advanced Nursing* 23: 496–501.

24 Remen R (1996) *Kitchen Table Wisdom; Stories That Heal*. Riverhead Books, New York, p. 220.

25 O'Donohue J (1997) *Anam Cara*. Bantam Press, London, p. 99.

26 Davis P (1999) *Aromatherapy: An A-Z*. The CW Daniel Co Ltd, Saffron Walden, p. 308.

27 I make this comment to reflect the weak evidence base for the efficacy of aromatherapy. I have no sense that either lavender or vetiver would have a beneficial effect, in the described situation, in easing suffering. However, the aroma in itself has a therapeutic benefit although I have no way of 'proving' that from any scientific perspective.

28 'lifts' – the way people use their energy to 'lift' people to a higher level of being. It would seem fundamental that all therapists and nurses tune into and develop this energy for 'lifting' their patients and colleagues. See Rael J (1993) *Being and Vibration*. Council Oak Books, Tulsa.

29 Disturbance – focus of a paper submitted for publication.

30 Becker R (1997) *Life in Motion*. Stillness Press, Portland, OR.

31 Elias N (1985) *The Loneliness of the Dying*. Basil Blackwell, Oxford.

32 Wavelength theory; see Johns C (2009) *Becoming a Reflective Practitioner*, 3rd edition Wiley-Blackwell, Oxford.

33 Osho (1994) *No Water No Moon: 10 Zen Teaching Stories for Everyday Life*. Element, Shaftesbury.

34 The question How do you view the future? is one of the Burford NDU Model: Caring in Practice cues that guide the way I 'see' patients from a holistic perspective. See Johns C (2009) *Becoming a Reflective Practitioner* (ibid.), p. 109–110.

35 Li S (2004) 'Symbiotic niceness': constructing a therapeutic relationship in psychosocial palliative care. *Social Science & Medicine* 58(12): 2571–258.
    Abstract – 'The concept of symbiotic niceness illustrates a mutually shared advantage in the nurse–patient relationship. This relationship is premised on the co-production of niceness through the doing of psychosocial care. This paper presents an account of "symbiotic niceness"

produced in palliative care nurses' talk. The data are collected from two hospices and one general hospital for the dying. The analysis of talk demonstrates how psychosocial care can be understood as the collaborative practice of "niceness" in the daily activities of participants, and how they collaboratively achieve reciprocal and therapeutic relevance for their talk. Participants co-engage in a "selling game". Through the activities of selling, a set of personal assets that constitute their personal curriculum vitae (CV) are revealed. It suggests that nurses' assets, when combined with patients' assets, function as marketable "products" to produce an impression of nice patients and professionals. This in turn leads to the production of an impression of "nice" organisations. Impression management is presented as a key strategy for the production of marketable niceness. Through the co-performance of niceness in talk, both nurses and patients are constructed as people who are somewhat charismatic, friendly, informal, understanding and concerned. This paper argues that underpinning the co-enactment of symbiotic niceness is the sharedness of patients' and nurses' experiences and a reciprocal notion of therapeutic help. It serves as a means of managing relations between palliative care nurses and dying patients. Symbiotic niceness thus represents a core component of professional and patient identity which works to maintain social orderliness as well as to advance personal, professional and organisational aspirations.'

36   This is my universal question – the raison d'etre of reflection – giving focus and meaning for my reflections.

37   Lather talks about false consciousness – suggesting that the reflective effort always involves this critical challenge to discern what factors influence the way I think, feel and respond within the situation – notably the tension between 'expectations from self' and 'expectations from others' how I should act. See Johns C (2009) *Becoming a Reflective Practitioner*, 3rd edition. Wuley-Blackwell, Oxford and Lather P (1986a) Research as praxis. *Harvard Educational Review* 56: 257–277.

38   Petrone M (2003) 'The emotional cancer journey'. MAP Foundation. I was fortunate to meet Michele in 2005 at the North Devon Hospice conference.

39   Jones R and Jones G (1996) *Earth Dance Drum*. Commune-A-Key Publishing, Salt Lake City, p. 66.

40   *Compact Oxford English Dictionary*, 3rd edition, 2005, p. 196.

41   Okri B (1997) *A Way of Being Free*. Phoenix House, London, p. 29.

42   O'Donohue J (1997) *Anam Cara*. Bantam Press, London, p. 26.

43   Becker R (1997), op. cit., p. 143.

44   Okri B (1997), op. cit., p. 28.

Appendix
Clinical supervision evaluation tool

This tool has been designed to enable you to reflect on the quality of your individual or group supervision. The information will facilitate giving feedback to your supervisor concerning the effectiveness of supervision.

How long have you been in supervision with your current supervisor?	
Is your supervisor (please circle)	Line manager Non-line manager within the organisation Outside the organisation
What is your grade?	
What is the grade/position of your supervisor?	
How frequently did you contract supervision?	Every . . . . days
How frequently (on average) do you actually have supervision?	Every . . . . days

Whilst completing the tool is perhaps time-consuming, please complete it carefully and honestly. *In particular please comment on your scores with specific examples.*

Mark along each scale the extent you agree with each statement:

5   most strongly agree
1   least agree

1	I felt safe to disclose my experiences.	5	4	3	2	1

Comment

2	It was easy to identify experiences to reflect on.	5	4	3	2	1

Comment

Becoming a Reflective Practitioner, Fourth Edition. Christopher Johns.
© 2013 John Wiley & Sons, Ltd. Published 2013 by John Wiley & Sons, Ltd.

3	I always came to each session prepared to share an experience.	5	4	3	2	1

Comment

4	I never cancelled sessions.	5	4	3	2	1

Comment

5	The balance of challenge and support was excellent (I didn't feel too threatened or comfortable).	5	4	3	2	1

Comment

6	Supervision has inspired me.	5	4	3	2	1

Comment

7	Supervision helped me clarify key issues and gain new insights into my practice.	5	4	3	2	1

Comment

8	I have become very reflective.	5	4	3	2	1

Comment

9	I have become more open and curious about my practice.	5	4	3	2	1

Comment

10	I felt I was being moulded into becoming a 'supervisor' clone.	5	4	3	2	1

Comment

11	I have become aware of the factors that influence the way I think, feel and respond within situations.	5	4	3	2	1

Comment

12	I am more aware/focused on my role responsibility, authority and autonomy.	5	4	3	2	1

Comment

| 13 | The input of theory was both relevant and substantial. | 5 | 4 | 3 | 2 | 1 |

Comment

| 14 | Work has become more meaningful and interesting. | 5 | 4 | 3 | 2 | 1 |

Comment

| 15 | Supervision picked me up when I felt overwhelmed. | 5 | 4 | 3 | 2 | 1 |

Comment

| 16 | Reflection has helped me to express my ideas, opinions and feelings. | 5 | 4 | 3 | 2 | 1 |

Comment

| 17 | Supervision enabled me to tackle issues that I might otherwise have avoided. | 5 | 4 | 3 | 2 | 1 |

Comment

| 18 | Supervision helped me deal with negative emotions (such as anger, failure, outrage, guilt, distress, resentment). | 5 | 4 | 3 | 2 | 1 |

Comment

| 19 | I am more in control of 'who I am'. | 5 | 4 | 3 | 2 | 1 |

Comment

| 20 | My supervisor really listened to me. | 5 | 4 | 3 | 2 | 1 |

Comment

| 21 | I was happy with my supervisor. | 5 | 4 | 3 | 2 | 1 |

Comment

| 22 | I never felt judged by my supervisor. | 5 | 4 | 3 | 2 | 1 |

Comment

| 23 | We constantly reviewed the way supervision has helped me to develop and sustain my practice. | 5 | 4 | 3 | 2 | 1 |

Comment

| 24 | We always commenced each session by reviewing the previous session. | 5 | 4 | 3 | 2 | 1 |

Comment

| 25 | Supervision sessions were never interrupted. | 5 | 4 | 3 | 2 | 1 |

Comment

| 26 | I always knew what I needed to do at the end of each session. | 5 | 4 | 3 | 2 | 1 |

Comment

| 27 | My supervisor always wanted 'to fix' the problem for me. | 5 | 4 | 3 | 2 | 1 |

Comment

| 28 | My supervisor was overly parental and patronising. | 5 | 4 | 3 | 2 | 1 |

Comment

| 29 | The environment for supervision was excellent. | 5 | 4 | 3 | 2 | 1 |

Comment

Use this space to make any further comment

Supervision evaluation tool /f – revised March 2002.

References

Alexander L (1998) Writing in hospices. In C Kaye and T Blee, Eds, *The Arts in Health Care: A Palette of Possibilities*. Jessica Kingsley, London.

Alfano G (1971) Healing or caretaking – which will it be? *Nursing Clinics of North America* 6(2): 273–80.

Aristotle (2004) *Nicomachean Ethics* [revised edition] [trans. J Thomson]. Penguin Books, London.

Armitage S (1990) Research utilisation in practice. *Nurse Education Today* 10: 10–5.

Ashworth P, Longmate M and Morrison P (1992) Patient participation: its meaning and significance in the context of caring. *Journal of Advanced Nursing* 17: 1430–9.

Atkins S and Murphy K (1993) Reflective practice. *Nursing Standard* 9(45): 31–7.

Atkinson RL, Atkinson RC and Smith E (1990) *Introduction to Psychology*. Harcourt Brace, New York.

Ausubel D (1967) *Learning Theory and Classroom Practice*. Ontario Institute for Studies in Education, Toronto, ON.

Autton N (1996) The use of touch in palliative care. *European Journal of Palliative Care* 3(3): 121–4.

Bailey J (1995) Reflective practice: implementing theory. *Nursing Standard* 9(46): 40–1.

Barker AM and Young C (1994) Transformational leadership: The feminist connection in post-modern organizations. *Holistic Nursing Practice* 9(1): 16–25.

Bass B (1985) *Leadership and Performance Beyond Expectations*. Free Press, New York.

Batehup L and Evans A (1992) A new strategy. *Nursing Times* 88(47): 40–1.

Batey M and Lewis F (1982) Clarifying autonomy and accountability in nursing service: part 1. *The Journal of Nursing Administration* 12(9): 13–8.

Beck CY (1997) *Everyday Zen*. Thorsons, London.

Becker R (1997) *Life in Motion*. Stillness Press, Portland, OR.

Begley A-M (1996) Literature and poetry: pleasure and practice. *International Journal of Nursing Practice* 2: 182–8.

Belenky MF, Clinchy BM, Goldberger NR and Tarule JM (1986) *Women's Ways of Knowing: The Development of Self, Voice, and Mind*. Basic Books, New York.

Benner P (1984) *From Novice to Expert*. Addison-Wesley, Menlo Park, CA.

Benner P (2003) Clinical reasoning: articulating experiential learning in nursing practice. In L Basford and O Slevin, Eds, *Theory and Practice of Nursing: An Integrated Approach to Caring Practice*. Nelson Thornes, Cheltenham.

Benner P and Wrubel J (1989) *The Primacy of Caring*. Addison-Wesley, Menlo Park, CA.

Benner P, Tanner C and Chesla C (1996) *Expertise in Nursing Practice: Caring, Clinical Judgement, and Ethics*. Springer, New York.

Benjamin M and Curtis J (1986) *Ethics in Nursing*, 2nd edition. Oxford University Press, New York.

Berne E (1961) *Transactional Analysis in Psychotherapy. The Classic Guide to Its Principles*. Grove Press, New York.

Biley F (1992) Some determinants that affect patient participation in decision-making about nursing care. *Journal of Advanced Nursing* 17: 414–21.

Biley F and Wright S (1997) Towards a defence of nursing routine and ritual. *Journal of Clinical Nursing* 6(2): 115–9.

Blackford J (2003) Cultural frameworks of nursing practice: exposing an exclusionary healthcare culture. *Nursing Inquiry* 10(4): 236–2424.

Bochner A and Ellis C (2002) *Ethnographically Speaking: Autoethnography, Literature, and Aesthetics*. AltaMira Press, Walnut Creek, CA.

Bohm D (1996) *On Dialogue*, N Lee, Ed. Routledge, London.

Bolton S (2000) Who cares? Offering emotion work as a 'gift' in the nursing labour process. *Journal of Advanced Nursing* 32: 580–6.

Boud D, Keogh R and Walker D (1985) Promoting reflection in learning: a model. In D Boud R Keogh and D Walker, Eds, *Reflection: Turning Experience into Learning*. Kogan Page, London.

Boyd E and Fales A (1983) Reflective learning: key to learning from experience. *Journal of Humanistic Psychology* 23(2): 99–117.

Brodersen L (2001) Creatively capturing care: poetry and knowledge in nursing. *International Journal for Human Caring* 6(1): 33–41.

Brookfield S (1995) *Becoming a Critically Reflective Teacher*. Josey-Bass, San Francisco, CA.

Brooks S (2004) Becoming a transformational leader. Unpublished Masters in Leadership dissertation, University of Bedfordshire.

Bruner J (1986) *Actual Minds, Possible Worlds*. Harvard University Press, Cambridge, MA.

Bruner J (1994) The remembered self. In U Neisser and R Fivush, Eds, *The Remembering Self: Construction and Accuracy in the Self Narrative*. Cambridge University Press, New York.

Bruner J (1996) *The Culture of Education*. Harvard University Press, Cambridge, MA.

Buckenham J and McGrath G (1983) *The Social Reality of Nursing*. Adis, Sydney, NSW.

Bulman C (2004) An introduction to reflection. In C Bulman and S Schultz, Eds, *Reflective Practice in Nursing*, 3rd edition. Blackwell Publishing, Oxford.

Burkhardt M and Nagai-Jacobson M (2002) *Spirituality: Living Our Connectedness*. Farrar, Straus and Giroux, New York.

Burnard P (1995) Nurse educators' perceptions of reflection and reflective practice. A report of a descriptive study. *Journal of Advanced Nursing* 21: 1167–74.

Burnard P and Morrison P (1991) Nurses' interpersonal skills: a study of nurses' perceptions. *Nurse Education Today* 1: 24–9.

Burns J (1978) *Leadership*. Harper Row, New York.

Burrows D (1995) The nurse teacher's role in the promotion of reflective practice. *Nurse Education Today* 15: 346–50.

Burton A (2000) Reflection: nursing's practice and education panacea? *Journal of Advanced Nursing* 31(5): 1009–17.

Bush T (2003) Communicating with patients who have dementia. *Nursing Times* 99(48): 42–5.

Butler S and Rosenblum B (1991) *Cancer in Two Voices*. The Women's Press, London.

Butterfield P (1990) Thinking upstream: nurturing a conceptual understanding of the societal context of health behaviour. *Advances in Nursing Science* 12(2): 1–8.

Callahan S (1988) The role of emotion in ethical decision making. Hastings centre Report June/July 9–14.

Callanan M and Kelley P (1992) *Final Gifts: Understanding the Special Awareness, Needs, and Communication of the Dying*. Bantam, New York.

Cameron D *et al* (2008) Expressing voice and developing practical wisdom on social justice through art. In C Delmar and C Johns, Eds, *The Good, the Wise, and the Right Clinical Nursing Practice*. Aalborg Hospital, Arhus University Hospital, Denmark, pp. 59–72.

Campbell J (1988) *The Power of Myth*. Doubleday, New York.

Canemaker J (2010) *Paper Dreams, the Art and Artists of Disney Storyboards*. Hyperion Press, New York.

Carmack B (1997) Balancing engagement and detachment in care-giving. *Image: The Journal of Nursing Scholarship* 29(2): 139–43.

Carper B (1978) Fundamental patterns of knowing in nursing. *Advances in Nursing Science* 1(1): 13–23.

Carson J (2008) *Spider Speculations: A Physics and Biophysics of Storytelling*. Theatre Communications Group, New York.

Casement P (1985) *On Learning from the Patient*. Routledge, London.

Cassell EJ (1982) The nature of suffering and the goals of medicine. *New England Journal of Medicine* 306: 639–45.

Cavanagh S (1991) The conflict management style of staff nurses and nurse managers. *Journal of Advanced Nursing* 16: 1254–60.

Chang OS (2001) The conceptual structure of physical touch in caring. *Journal of Advanced Nursing* 33(6): 820–7.

Chapman G (1983) Ritual and rational action in hospitals. *Journal of Advanced Nursing* 8: 13–20.

Charmaz K (1983) Loss of self: a fundamental form of suffering in the chronically ill. *Sociology of Health & Illness* 5(2): 168–95.

Cherniss G (1980) *Professional Burn-Out in Human Service Organisations*. Praeger, New York.

Cioffi J (1997) Heuristics, servants to intuition, in clinical decision making. *Journal of Advanced Nursing* 26: 203–8.

Cixous H (1996) Sorties: out and point: attacks'ways out/ forays. In H Cixous and C Clement, Eds, *The Newly Born Woman*. Tauris, London.

Clarke M (1986) Action and reflection: practice and theory in nursing. *Journal of Advanced Nursing* 11: 3–11.

Clough P (2000) Comments on setting criteria for experimental writing. *Qualitative Inquiry* 6: 278–91.

Cochran L and Laub L (1994) *Becoming an Agent: Patterns and Dynamics for Shaping Your Life*. State University of New York Press, Albany, NY.

Colyer H (1996) Womens' experiences of living with cancer. *Journal of Advanced Nursing* 23: 496–501.

Cooper M (1991) Principle-oriented ethics and the ethic of care: a creative tension. *Advances in Nursing Science* 14(2): 22–31.

Cope M (2001) *Lead Yourself. Be Where Others Would Follow*. Pearson Education Ltd, Harlow.

Corley MC and Goren S (1998) The dark side of nursing: impact of stigmatizing responses on patients. Scholarly Inquiry for Nursing Practice. *An International Journal* 12(2): 00–121.

Costello E (1983) Everyday I write a book. Punch the Clock-F-Beat (UK) Columbia Records.

Cotton A (2001) Private thoughts in public spheres: issues in reflection and reflective practices in nursing. *Journal of Advanced Nursing* 36(4): 512–9.

Cowling WR (2000) Healing as appreciating wholeness. *Advances in Nursing Science* 22(3): 16–32.

Cox M (1988) *Structuring the Therapeutic Process: Compromise with Chaos* [revised edition]. Jessica Kingsley Publications. London.

Cox H, Hickson P and Taylor B (1991) Exploring reflection: knowing and constructing practice. In G Gray and R Pratt, Eds, *Towards a Discipline of Nursing*. Churchill Livingstone, Melbourne, VIC, pp. 373–90.

Daiski I (2004) Changing nurses' disempowering relationship patterns. *Journal of Advanced Nursing* 48(1): 43–50.

Daneault S *et al* (2004) The nature of suffering and its relief in the terminally ill: a qualitative study. *Journal of Palliative Care* 20(1): 7–11.

Davidhizar R and Giger J (1997) When touch is not the best approach. *Journal of Clinical Nursing* 6(3): 203–6.

Davis P (1999) *Aromatherapy A-Z*. C.W. Daniel & Co., Saffron Walden.

Davis-Floyd R (2001) The technocratic, humanistic and holistic paradigms of childbirth. *International Journal of Gynaecology and Obstetrics* 75(1): 5–23.

Day C (1993) Reflection: a necessary but not sufficient condition for professional development. *British Educational Research Journal* 19(1): 83–93.

De Hennezel M (1998) *Intimate Death* [trans C Janeway]. Warner Books, London.

De La Cuesta C (1983) The nursing process: from development to implementation. *Journal of Advanced Nursing* 8: 365–71.

Delmar C and Johns C, Eds (2008) *The Good, the Wise and the Right Clinical Nursing Practice*. Aalborg Hospital, Arhus University Hospital, Denmark.

Denzin N (2003) *Performance Ethnography*. Sage, Thousand Oaks, CA.

Department of Health (1996) *Clinical Audit in the NHS*. HMSO, London.

Department of Health (2007) *Maternity Matters: Choice, Access and Continuity of Care in a Safe Service*. HMSO, London.

Department of Health (2008) *High Quality Care for all*. HMSO, London.

Department of Health & Social Security (DHSS) (1972) *Report of the Committee on Nursing* [Chairperson, Professor Asa Briggs] HMSO, London.

Department of Health & Social Security (DHSS) (1986) Neighbourhod nursing – a focus for care [The Cumberlege Report] HMSO, London.

DeSalvo L (1999) *Writing as a Way of Healing: How Telling Our Stories Transform Our Lives*. The Women's Press, London.

Deutsch M (1971) Towards an understanding of conflict. *International Journal of Group Tensions* 1: 42–54.

Dewey J (1933) *How We Think*. J.C. Heath, Boston.

Dickson A (1982) *A Women in Your Own Right*. Quartet Books, London.

Downe S (2004) *Normal Childbirth Evidence and Debate*. Churchill Livingstone, London.

Dreyfus H and Dreyfus S (1986) *Mind over Machine*. Free Press, New York.

Druskat V and Wolff S (2001) Building the emotional intelligence of groups. *Harvard Business Review* 79: 81–90.

Duffy E (1995, April) Horizontal violence: a conundrum for nursing. *Collegian: Journal of the Royal College of Nursing Australia* 2(2): 5–17.

Dunham J and Klafehn K (1990) Transformational leadership and the nurse executive. *Journal of Advanced Nursing* 20(4): 28–33.

Dyer I (1995) Preventing the ITU syndrome or how not to torture an ITU patient (part 2). *Intensive and Critical Care Nursing* 11(4): 223–32.

Edwards S (1998) An anthropological interpretation of nurses' and patients' perceptions of the use of space and touch. *Journal of Advanced Nursing* 28: 809–17.

Eifried S, Riley-Giomariso O and Voight G (2000) Learning to care amid suffering: how art and narrative give voice to the student experience. *International Journal for Human Caring* 5(2): 42–51.

Eliade M (1991) Images and symbols (P. Mairet, trans). In C Delmar and C Johns, Eds, *The Good, the Wise, and the Right Clinical Nursing Practice*. Aalborg Hospital, Arhus University Hospital, Aalborg.

Elias N (1985) *The Loneliness of the Dying*. Bssil Blackwell, Oxford.

Elliot G (1876/1996) *Daniel Deronda*. Wordsworths Editions, London.

Ellis C (2004) *The Ethnographic I: A Methodological Novel about Autoethnography*. AltMira Press, Walnut Creek, CA.

Estabrooks C and Morse J (1992) Toward a theory of touch: the touching process and acquiring a touching style. *Journal of Advanced Nursing* 17: 448–56.

Evans D (2002) The effectiveness of music as an intervention for hospital patients: a systematic review. *Journal of Advanced Nursing* 37(1): 8–18.

Farrar M (1992) How much do they want to know? *Professional Nurse* 7(9): 606–10.

Faugier J and Butterworth T (undated) *Clinical Supervision: A Position Paper*. School of Nursing Studies, University of Manchester, Manchester, UK.

Fay B (1987) *Critical Social Science*. Polity Press, Cambridge, UK.

Feil N (1993) *The Validation Breakthrough: Simple Techniques for Communicating with People with 'Alzheimer's-Type Dementia'*. Health Profession's Press, Baltimore, MD.

Ferruci P (1982) *What We May Be*. St. Martin's Press, New York.

Fordham M (2008) Building bridges in homelessness, mindful of phronesis in nursing practice. In C Delmar and C Johns, Eds, *The Good, the Wise, and the Right Clinical Nursing Practice*. Aalborg Hospital, Arhus University Hospital, Denmark, pp. 73–92.

Fordham M (2010) Falling through the net and the spider's web: two metaphoric moments along my journey. In C Johns, Ed., *Guised Reflection: A Narrative Approach to Advancing Professional Practice*, 2nd edition. Wiley-Blackwell, Oxford, pp. 145–63.

Fordham M (2012) Doctoral thesis. Unpublished PhD thesis. University of Bedfordshire.

Foucault M (1979) *Discipline and Punish: The Birth of the Prison* [trans. A Sheridan]. Vintage/Random House, New York.

Frank A (2002a) Relations of caring: demoralization and remoralization in the clinic. *International Journal of Human Caring* 6(2): 13–9.

Frank A (2002b) *At the Will of the Body: Reflections on Illness*. Mariner Books, Boston.

Fredriksson L (1999) Modes of relating in a caring conversation: a research synthesis on presence, touch and listening. *Journal of Advanced Nursing* 30(5): 1167–76.

Freire P (1972) *Pedagogy of the Oppressed*. Penguin Books, London.

French J and Raven B (1968) The bases of social power. In D Cartwright and A Zander, Eds, *Group Dynamics*. Row Peterson, Evanston, IL, pp. 150–67.

Friedson E (1970) *Professional Dominance*. Aldine Atherton, Chicago.

Gadamer H-G (1975) *Truth & Method*. Seabury Press, New York.

Gadow S (1980) Existential advocacy. In S Spickler and S Gadow, Eds, *Nursing: Image and Ideals*. Springer, New York, pp. 79–101.

Garland D (2004) Is the use of water in labour an option for women following a previous LSCS? *Midwifery Digest* 14(1): 63–7.

Garland D (2006) Is waterbirth a 'safe and realistic' option for women following a previous caesarean section? *Midwifery Digest* 16(2): 217–20.

Garside P (1999) The learning organisation: a necessary setting for improving care? *Quality in Health Care* 8: 211.

Gaydos H (2008) Collage: an aesthetic process for creating phronesis in nursing. In C Delmar and C Johns, Eds, *The Good, the Wise, and the Right Clinical Nursing Practice*. Aalborg Hospital, Arhus University Hospital, Denmark, pp. 163–78.

Gibbs G (1988) *Learning by Doing: A Guide to Teaching and Learning Methods*. Further Education Unit, Oxford Polytechnic, now Oxford Brookes University, UK.

Gilbert T (2001) Reflective practice and clinical supervision: meticulous rituals of the confessional. *Journal of Advanced Nursing* 36(2): 199–205.

Gilligan C (1982) *In a Different Voice*. Harvard University Press, Cambridge, MA.

Goldstein J (2002) *One Dharma*. Rider, London.

Goleman D (1996) *Emotional Intelligence: Why It Can Matter More Than IQ*. Bloomsbury Publishing, London.

Goleman D, Boyatzis R and McKee A (2002) *Primal Leadership: Learning to Lead with Emotional Intelligence*. Harvard Business School Press, Boston, MA.

Gray G and Forsstrom S (1991) Generating theory from practice: the reflective technique. In G Gray and R Pratt, Eds, *Towards a Discipline of Nursing*. Churchill Livingstone, Melbourne, VIC, pp. 355–72.

Green A (1996) An explorative study of patients' memory of their stay in an acute intensive therapy unit. *Intensive and Critical Care Nursing* 12(3): 131–7.

Greene M (1988) *The Dialectic of Freedom*. Teachers College Press, Columbia University, New York.

Greenleaf R (1975) *Servant Leadership*. Paulist Press, New York

Groom J and Johns C (2002/2010) Working with deliberate self-harm patients in A&E. In C Johns, Ed., *Guided Reflection: Advancing Practice*. Blackwell Publishing, Oxford, pp. 169–85.

Habermas J (1984) *Theory of Communicative Action. Vol. 1: Reason and the Rationalisation of Society*. Beacon Press, Boston, and Basil Blackwell, Oxford, in association with Polity Press, Cambridge.

Hall C (2003) Nurse shortage in the NHS is near crisis point. *Daily Telegraph*, 29 April.

Hall L (1964) Nursing – what is it? *Canadian Nurse* 60(2): 150–4.

Halldórsdóttir S (1991) Five basic modes of being with another. In D Gaut and M Leininger, Eds, *Caring: The Compassionate Healer*. National league for Nursing, New York.

Halligan A and Donaldson LJ (2001) Implementing clinical governance: turning vision into reality. *British Medical Journal* 322(7299): 1413–7.

Hansen F (2008) Phronesis and eros – the existential dimension of phronesis and clinical supervision for nurses. In C Delmar and C Johns, Eds, *The Good, the Wise, and the Right Clinical Nursing Practice*. Aalborg Hospital, Arhus University Hospital, Denmark, pp. 27–58.

Hawkins P and Shohet R (1989) *Supervision for the Helping Professions*. Open University Press, Buckingham.

Heath H and Freshwater D (2000) Clinical supervision as an emancipatory process: avoiding inappropriate intent. *Journal of Advanced Nursing* 32: 1298–306.

Heron J (1975) *Six-Category Intervention Analysis*. Human Potential Resource Group, University of Surrey, Guildford.

Hewitt-Taylor J (2004) Challenging the balance of power: patient empowerment. *Nursing Standard* 18(22): 33–7.

Hickman P and Holmes C (1994) Nursing the post-modern body: a touching case. *Nursing Inquiry* 1: 3–14.

Holly ML (1989) Reflective writing and the spirit of inquiry. *Cambridge Journal of Education* 19(1): 71–80.

Hooks B (1994) *Teaching to Transgress: Education as the Practice of Freedom*. Routledge, New York.

Howse E and Bailey J (1992) Resistance to documentation – a nursing research issue. *International Journal of Nursing Studies* 29(4): 371–80.

Hunt J (1981) Indicators for nursing practice: the use of research findings. *Journal of Advanced Nursing* 6: 189–94.

Hutchinson M, Vickers M, Jackson D and Wilkes L (2006) Workplace bullying in nursing: towards a more critical organisational perspective. *Nursing Inquiry* 13(2): 118–26.

Isaacs W (1993) Taking flight: dialogue, collective thinking, and organizational learning. Centre for Organizational Learning's Dialogue Project. MIT.

James A (undated) *Living with Bereavement*. Right Way Books, Tadworth.

James N (1989) Emotional labour: skill and work in the social regulation of feelings. *Sociological Review* 37(1): 15–42.

Jarrett L (2008) From significance to insights. In C Delmar and C Johns, Eds, *The Good, the Wise, and the Right Clinical Nursing Practice*. Aalborg Hospital, Arhus University Hospital, Denmark, pp. 59–72.

Jarrett L (2009) Being and becoming a nurse specialist in spasticity management. Unpublished PhD thesis, City University, London.

Jarrett L and Johns C (2005) Constructing the reflexive narrative. In C Johns and D Freshwater, Eds, *Transforming Nursing through Reflective Practice*, 2nd edition. Blackwell Publishing, Oxford.

Jaworski J (1998) *Synchronicity: The Inner Path of Leadership*. Berrett-Koehler Publishers, San Francisco.

Jewell S (1994) Patient participation: what does it mean? *Journal of Advanced Nursing* 19: 433–8.

Johns C (1989) *The impact of introducing primary nursing on the culture of a community hospital.* Master of Nursing dissertation, University of Wales College of Medicine, Cardiff.

Johns C (1992) Ownership and the harmonious team: barriers to developing the therapeutic nursing team in primary nursing. *Journal of Clinical Nursing* 1: 89–94.

Johns C (1993) Professional supervision. *Journal of Nursing Management* 1(1): 9–18.

Johns C, Ed. (1994) *The Burford NDU Model: Caring in Practice.* Blackwell Publishing, Oxford.

Johns C (1995) Framing learning through reflection within Carper's fundamental ways of knowing. *Journal of Advanced Nursing* 22: 226–34.

Johns C (1996a) The benefits of a reflective model of nursing. *Nursing Times* 92(27): 39–41.

Johns C (1996b) Visualising and realizing caring in practice through guided reflection. *Journal of Advanced Nursing* 24(6): 1135–43.

Johns C (1996c) Using a reflective model of nursing and guided reflection. *Nursing Standard* 11(2): 34–8.

Johns C (1998a) *Becoming a reflective practitioner through guided reflection.* Unpublished PhD thesis. The Open University.

Johns C (1998b) Caring through a reflective lens: giving meaning to being a reflective practitioner. *Nursing Inquiry* 5: 18–24.

Johns C (1999) Unravelling the dilemmas of everyday nursing practice. *Nursing Ethics* 6: 287–98.

Johns C (2000) Working with Alice: a reflection. *Complementary Therapies in Nursing & Midwifery* 6: 199–203.

Johns C (2001a) Depending on the intent and emphasis of the supervisor, clinical supervision can be a different experience. *Journal of Nursing Management* 9: 139–45.

Johns C (2001b) The caring dance. *Complementary Therapies in Nursing & Midwifery* 7(1): 8–12.

Johns C (2003) Clinical supervision as a model for clinical leadership. *Journal of Nursing Management* 11: 25–34.

Johns C (2004) *Being Mindful, Easing Suffering: Reflections on Palliative Care.* Jessica Kingsley, London.

Johns C (2005) Balancing the winds. *Reflective Practice* 5(3): 67–84.

Johns C (2006) *Engaging Reflection in Practice.* Blackwell Publishing, Oxford.

Johns C (2008) Passing people by (why being a mindful practitioner matters). *Journal of Holistic Healthcare* 5(2): 37–42.

Johns C (2009a) *Becoming a Reflective Practitioner*, 3rd edition. Wiley-Blackwell, Oxford.

Johns C (2009b) Reflections on my mother dying: a story of caring shame. *Journal of Holistic Nursing* 27(2): 136–40.

Johns C, Ed. (2010a) *Guided Reflection: A Narrative Approach to Advancing Practice*, 2nd edition. Wiley-Blackwell, Oxford.

Johns C (2010b) Climbing walls. In C Johns, Ed., *Guided Reflection: A Narrative Approach to Advancing Practice*. Wiley-Blackwell, Oxford.

Johns C (2012 in press) Becoming a reflective leader. Unpublished.

Johns C and Freshwater D, Eds (2005) *Transforming Nursing through Reflective Practice*, 2nd edition. Blackwell Publishing, Oxford.

Johns C and Hardy H (2005) Voice as a metaphor for transformation through reflection. In C Johns and D Freshwater, Eds, *Transforming Nursing through Reflective Practice*, 2nd edition. Blackwell Publishing, Oxford, pp. 85–98.

Johns C and Marlin C (2010) Feminist slant. In C Johns, Ed., *Guided Reflection: A Narrative Approach to Advancing Practice*. Wiley-Blackwell, Oxford.

Johns C and McCormack B (1998) Unfolding the conditions where the transformative potential of guided reflection (clinical supervision) might flourish or flounder. In C Johns and D Freshwater, Eds, *Transforming Nursing through Reflective Practice*. Blackwell publishing, Oxford.

Johnson D (1974) Development of theory: a requisite for nursing as a primary health profession. *Nursing Research* 23(5): 373–7.

Johnson M and Webb C (1995) Rediscovering unpopular patients: the concept of social judgment. *Journal of Advanced Nursing* 21: 466–75.

Joiner A and Johns C (2010) Awakenings. In C Johns, Ed., *Guided Reflection: A Narrative Approach to Advancing Professional Practice*. Wiley-Blackwell, Oxford.

Jones R and Jones G (1996) *Earth Dance Drum*. Commune-E-Key, Salt Lake City, UT.

Jourard S (1971) *The Transparent Self*. Van Nostrand, Newark, NJ.

Kabat-Zinn J (1994) *Wherever You Go, There You Are*. Hyperion, New York.

Kelly M and May D (19182) Good and bad patients: a review of the literature and theoretical critique. *Journal of Advanced Nursing* 7: 147–56.

Kermode F (1966) *The Sense of An Ending*. Oxford university Press, New York.

Kieffer C (1984) Citizen empowerment: a developmental perspective. *Prevention in Human Services* 84(3): 9–36.

Kikuchi J (1992) Nursing questions that science cannot answer. In J Kikuchi and H Simmons, Eds, *Philosophic Inquiry in Nursing*. Sage, Newberry Park, CA.

King L and Appleton J (1997) Intuition: a critical review of the research and rhetoric. *Journal of Advanced Nursing* 26: 194–202.

Kitson A (1989) *A Framework for Quality: A Patient-Centred Approach to Quality Assurance in Health Care*. Scutari Press, Middlesex.

Klakovich M (1994) Connective leadership for the 21st century: a historical perspective and future directions. *Advanced in Nursing Science* 16(4): 42–54.

Knopf M (1994) Treatment options for early stage breast cancer. *MEDSURG Nursing* 3: 249–57.

Kopp P (2000) Overcoming difficulties in communicating with other professionals. *Nursing Times* 96(28): 47–9.

Kübler-Ross E (1969) *On Death an Dying*. Tavistock, London.

Lather P (1986a) Research as praxis. *Harvard Educational Review* 56(3): 257–77.

Lather P (1986b) Issues of validity in open ideological research: between a rock and a hard place. *Interchange* 17(4): 63–84.

Latimer J (1995) The nursing process re-examined: enrolment and translation. *Journal of Advanced Nursing* 22: 213–20.

Lawler J (1991) *Behind the Screens: Nursing, Semiology and the Problems of the Body*. Churchill Livingstone, Melbourne, VIC.

Lawrence M (1995) The unconscious experience. *American Journal of Critical Care* 4(3): 227–32.

Lee SC (1994) *The Circle Is Sacred: A Medicine Book for Women*. Council Oak Books, Tulsa, OK.

Leigh K (2001) Communicating with unconscious patients. *Nursing Times* 97(48): 35–6.

Levine M (1986) *Who Dies? An Investigation of Conscious Living and Conscious Dying*. Gateway Books, Bath.

Li S (2004) Symbiotic niceness': constructing a therapeutic relationship in psychosocial palliative care. *Social Science & Medicine* 58(12): 2571–83.

Lieberman A (1989) *Staff Development in Culture Building, Curriculum and Teaching: The Next 50 Years*. Teachers' College Press, Columbia University, New York.

Lliffe S and Drennan V (2001) *Primary Care and Dementia*. Jessica Kingsley, London.

Logstrup KE (1997) *The Ethical Demand*. University of Notre Dame Press, Notre Dame.

Lorde A (1980) *The Cancer Journals*. Spinsters Ink, Argyle.

Lunghi M (2004) Playing the endgame: reflections on waiting. *International Journal of Palliative Nursing* 10(8): 374–7.

Mackintosh C (1998) Reflection: a flawed strategy for the nursing profession. *Nurse Education Today* 18: 553–7.

Macleod M (1994) 'It's the little things that count': the hidden complexity of everyday clinical nursing practice. *Journal of Clinical Nursing* 3(6): 361–8.

Maddex E (2002) Shedding the armour: my leadership journey. Unpublished MSc Leadership in Health Care Dissertation. University of Bedfordshire.

Madison S (1999) Performing theory/embodied writing. *Text and Performance Quarterly* 19(2): 107–24.

Madrid M (1990) The participating process of human field patterning in an acute care environment. In E Barrett, Ed., *Visions of Martha Rogers's Science-Based Nursing*. National League for Nursing, New York.

Manjusvara (2005) *Writing Your Way*. Windhorse, Birmingham.

Margolis H (1993) *Paradigm and Barriers: How Habits of Mind Govern Scientific Beliefs*. University of Chicago Press, Chicago, IL.

Maslach C (1976) Burned -out. *Human Behaviour* 5: 16–22.

Maslow A (1968) *Towards a Psychology of Being*. Van Nostrand, Princeton, NJ.

Mattingly C (1998) *Healing Dramas and Clinical Ploys: The Narrative Structure of Experience*. Cambridge University Press, Cambridge, UK.

Mayeroff M (1971) *On Caring*. Harper Perennial, New York.

Mayo S (1996) Symbol, metaphor and story: the function of group art therapy in palliative care. *Palliative Medicine* 10: 209–16.

McCaffrey R (2002) Music listening as a nursing intervention: a symphony of practice. *Holistic Nursing Practice* 16(3): 70–7.

McElroy A, Corben V and McLeish K (1995) Developing care plan documentation: an action research project. *Journal of Nursing Management* 3: 193–9.

McKenna B, Smith N, Poole S and Coverdale J (2003) Horizontal violence: experiences of Registered Nurses in their first year of practice. *Journal of Advanced Nursing* 42(1): 90–96 91.

Mclaughlin AM and Carey JL (1993) The adversarial alliance: developing therapeutic relationships between families and the team in brain injury rehabilitation. *Brian Injury* 7(1): 45–51.

McNeely R (1983) Organizational patterns and work satisfaction in a comprehensive human service agency: an empirical test. *Human Relations* 36(10): 957–72.

McNiff S (1992) *Art as Medicine: Creating a Therapy of the Imagination*. Shambhala, Boston.

McSherry W (1996) Raising the spirit. *Nursing Times* 92(3): 48–9.

Menzies-Lyth I (1988) A case study in the functioning of social systems as a defence against anxiety. In I Menzies-Lyth, Ed., *Containing Anxiety in Institutions: Selected Essays*. Free Association Books, London.

Mezirow J (1981) A critical theory of adult learning and education. *Adult Education* 32(1): 3–24.

Miller L (2002) Effective communication with older people. *Nursing Standard* 17(9): 45–50, 53, 55.

Milne AA (1926) *Winnie-the-Pooh*. Methuen, London.

Moon J (2002) *Reflection in Learning and Professional Development: Theory and Practice*. Routledge, London.

Moore T (1992) *Care of the Soul*. HarperCollins, New York.

Morgan R and Johns C (2005) The beast and the star: resolving contradictions within everyday practice. In C Johns and D Freshwater, Eds, *Transforming Nursing through Reflective Practice*. Blackwell Publishing, Oxford, pp. 114–28.

Morse J (1991) Negotiating commitment and involvement in the nurse-patient relationship. *Journal of Advanced Nursing* 16: 552–8.

Morse J and Dobernect B (1995) Delineating the concept of hope. *Image: The Journal of Nursing Scholarship* 27: 277–85.

Morse J, Bottorff J, Anderson G, O'Brien B and Solberg S (1992) Beyond empathy: expanding expressions of caring. *Journal of Advanced Nursing* 17: 809–21.

Mott V (2000) The development of professional expertise in the workplace. *New Directions for Adult and Continuing Education* 86: 23–31.

Munhall P (1993) 'Unknowing': towards another pattern of knowing in nursing. *Nursing Outlook* 41(3): 125–8.

Mycek S (1999, April) Teetering on the edge of chaos. *Trustee: The Journal for Hospital Governing Boards* 10–3.

National Health Service Management Executive (NHSME) (1993) *A Vision for the Future*. Department of Health, London.

National Institute for Health and Clinical Excellence (NICE) (2004) *Clinical Guidelines. Caesarian Section.*

Nehring V and Geach B (1973) Why they don't complain: patient's evaluation of their care. *Nursing Outlook* 21(5): 317–21.

Newman M (1994) *Health as Expanded Consciousness*. National League for Nursing, New York.

Newman M (1999) The rhythm of relating in a paradigm of wholeness. *Image: The Journal of Nursing Scholarship* 31(3): 227–30.

Nicholson D (2009) Implementing the next stage review visions: the quality and productivity challenge. Memo to all chief executives of Primary health care Trusts in England, all chief executives of NHS Trusts in England, and all chief executives of NHS Foundation Trusts in England [Gateway reference 12396] Department of Health.

Nicklin P (1987) Violence to the spirit. *Senior Nurse* 6(5): 10–2.

Northouse L *et al* (1995) Emotional distress reported by women and husbands prior to breast biopsy. *Nursing Research* 44: 196–201.

Novelestsky-Rosenthal H and Solomon K (2001) Reflections on the use of Johns' model of structured reflection in nurse-practitioner education. *International Journal for Human Caring* 5(2): 21–6.

Nowlen P (1988) *A New Approach to Continuing Education for Business and the Professions*. MacMillan, Old Tappen, NJ.

Nursing and Midwifery Council (NMC) (2002) *Midwives Rules and Standards*. Portland Place, London.

Nunes Tucker A, Price A and Diedrich A (2010) *Guided Reflection: A Narrative Approach to Advancing Practice*, C Johns, Ed. Wiley-Blackwell, Oxford.

Oakley A (1984) The importance of being a nurse. *Nursing Times* 83(50): 24–7.

Ochs L (2001) This nurse suggests asking before you touch. *RN* 64(4): 10.

O'Donohue J (1997) *Anam Cara: Spiritual Wisdom from the Celtic World*. Bantam Press, London.

Okri B (1997) *A Way of Being Free*. Phoenix House, London.

Osho (1994) *No Water No Moon: 10 Zen Teaching Stories for Everyday Life*. Element, Shaftesbury.

Ottaway R (1978) A change strategy to implement new norms, new styles and new environment in the work organization. *Personnel Review* 5(1): 13–8.

Paramananda (2001) *A Deeper Beauty: Buddhist Reflections on Everyday Life*. Windhorse, Birmingham.

Parker M (2002) Aesthetic ways in day-to-day nursing. In D Freshwater, Ed., *Therapeutic Nursing*. Sage, London.

Parker R (1990) Nurses' stories: the search a relational ethic of care. *Advances in Nursing Science* 13(1): 31–40.

Parsons T (1952) *The Social System*. Routledge and Kegan Paul, London.

Pearson A (1983) *The Clinical Nursing Unit*. Heinemann Medical Books, London.

Pederson C (1993) Presence as a nursing intervention with hospitalized children. *Maternal-child Journal* 3: 75–81.

Pennebaker J (1989) Confession, inhibition and disease. *Advances in Experimental Social Psychology* 22: 211–44.

Pennebaker J, Colder M and Sharp L (1990) Accelarting the coping process. *Journal of Personality and Social Psychology* 58: 528–37.

Pennebaker J, Mayne T and Francis M (1997) Linguistic predictors of adaptive bereavement. *Journal of Personality and Social Psychology* 72: 863–71.

Perrella L (2004) *Artists' Journals and Sketchbooks: Exploring and Creating Personal Pages*. Quarry Books, Gloucester, MA.

Petrone M (2003) The emotional cancer journey. MAP Foundation.

Picard C, Sickul C and Natale S (1999) Healing reflections: the transformative mirror. *International Journal for Human Caring* 2(2): 40–7.

Pike A (1991) Moral outrage and moral discourse in nurse-physician collaboration. *Journal of Professional Nursing* 7(6): 351–63.

Pinar W (1981) Whole, bright, deep with understanding: issues in qualaitative research and auto-biographical method. *Journal of Curriculum Studies* 13: 173–88.

Pink D (2005) *A Whole New Mind: Moving from Information Age to the Conceptual Age*. Riverhead Books, New York. Penguin 74) Zen and the art of motorcycle maintenence.

Pirsig R (1974) *Zen and the Art of Motorcycle Maintenance: An Enquiry into Values*. Vintage, London.

Pitkin WB (1932) *Life Begins at Forty*. McGraw-Hill Book, New York.

Plath S (1975) *Letters Home*. Harper & Row, New York.

Platzer H, Blake D and Ashford D (2000) Barriers to learning from reflection; a study of the use of groupwork with post-registration nurses. *Journal of Advanced Nursing* 31(5): 1001–8.

Podurgiel M (1990) The unconscious experience: a pilot study. *Journal of Neuroscience Nursing* 22(1): 52–3.

Polanyi M (1958) *Personal Knowledge: Towards a Post Critical Philosophy*. Routledge and Kegan Paul, London.

Polkingthorne D (1996) Transformative narratives: from victimic to agentic life plots. *The American Journal of Occupational Therapy* 50(4): 299–305.

Prigogine L and Stengers L (1984) *Order Out of Chaos*. Bantam, New York.

Proctor B (1988) *Supervision: A Working Alliance*. (videotape training manual). Alexa Publications, St Leonards-on-Sea.

Puzan E (2003) The unbearable whiteness of being (in nursing). *Nursing Inquiry* 10(3): 193–200.

Quinn J (1992) Holding sacred space: the nurse as healing environment. *Holistic Nursing Practice* 6(4): 26–35.

Quinn J (1997) Healing: a model for an integrated health care system. *Advanced Practice Nurse Quarterly* 3(1): 1–7.

Radbruch L (2002) Reflections on the use of sedation in terminal care. *European Journal of Palliative Care* 9(6): 237–9, 239.

Rael J (1993) *Being and Vibration*. Council Oak Books, Tulsa, OK.

Ramos M (1992) The nurse-patient relationship: themes and variations. *Journal of Advanced Nursing* 17: 496–506.

Randall F and Downie RS (1999) *Palliative Care Ethics*, 2nd edition. Oxford University Press, Oxford.

Rao MT (1993) *Coping with Communication Challenges in Alzheimer's Disease*. Singular Publishing, San Diego, CA.

Rawnsley M (1990) Of human bonding: the context of nursing as caring. *Advances in Nursing Science* 13: 41–8.

Ray M (1989) The theory of bureaucratic caring for nursing practice in the organizational culture. *Nursing Administrative Quarterly* 13(2): 31–42.

Read S (1983) Once is enough: causal reasoning from a single instance. *Journal of Personality and Social Psychology* 45(2): 323–34.

Reisetter K and Thomas B (1986) Nursing care of the dying: its relationship to selected nurse characteristics. *International Journal of Nursing Studies* 23: 39–50.

Remen R (1996) *Kitchen Table Wisdom*. Riverhead Books, New York.

Reverby S (1987) A caring dilemma: womanhood and nursing in historical perspective. *Nursing Research* 36(1): 5–11.

Richardson L (2000) Evaluating ethnography. *Qualitative Inquiry* 6: 253–5.

Rinpoche S (1992) *The Tibetan Book of Living and Dying*. Rider, London.

Roach S (1992) *The Human Act of Caring*. Canadian Hospital Association Press, Ottawa, ON.

Roberts S (1983) Oppressed group behaviour: implications for nursing. *Advances in Nursing Science* 5(4): 21–30.

Robinson D and McKenna H (1998) Loss: an analysis of a concept of particular interest to nursing. *Journal of Advanced Nursing* 27(4): 779–84.

Robinson S Thorne S (1986) Relatives as interference. *Journal of Advanced Nursing* 9: 597–602.

Rodgers J (2001) *Bald in the Land of Big Hair*. HarperCollins Publishers, New York.

Rogers A *et al* (2000) 'All the services were excellent. It is when the human element comes in that things go wrong': dissatisfaction with hospital care in the last year of life. *Journal of Advanced Nursing* 31(40): 768–74.

Rogers C (1969) *Freedom to Learn: A View of What Education Might Be*. Merrill, Columbus, OH.

Rolfe G and Gardner L (2006) 'Do not ask who I am . . .': confession, emancipation and (self)-management through reflection. *Journal of Nursing Management* 14: 593–600.

Roper N, Logan W and Tierney A (1980) *The Elements of Nursing*. Churchill Livingstone, Edinburgh.

Rosenberg L (1998) *Breath by Breath*. Shambhala, Boston.

Rowe H (1996) Multidisciplinary teamwork – myth or reality? *Journal of Nursing Management* 4: 93–101.

Rumi (2006) *Words of Paradise* [trans. R Abdulla]. Frances Lincoln Ltd, London, p. 4.

Russell F (1999) An exploratory study of patient perception, memories, and experiences of an intensive care unit. *Journal of Advanced Nursing* 29(4): 783–91.

Sacks O (1976) *Awakenings*. Pelican books, London.

Sacks O (1984) *A Leg to Stand On*. Summit Books, New York.

Sacks O (1995) *An Anthropologist on Mars*. Alfred Knopf, New York.

Salovey P and Mayer JD (1990) Emotional intelligence. *Imagination, Cognition, and Personality* 9: 185–211.

Sangharakshita (1998) *Know Your Mind*. Windhorse, Birmingham.

Sangharakshita (1999) *The Bodhisattva Ideal*. Windhorse, Birmingham.

Saunders C (1975) The care of the dying patient and his family. Documentation in Medical Ethics, No. 5. Published by the London Medical Group.

Schön D (1983) *The Reflective Practitioner*. Avebury, Aldershot.

Schön D (1987) *Educating the Reflective Practitioner*. Jossey-Bass, San Francisco, CA.

Schuster JP (1994) Transforming your leadership style. *Association Management* 46(1): 39–42.

Seedhouse D (1988) *Ethics: The Heart of Health Care*. Wiley, Chichester.

Senge P (1990) *The Art and Practice of the Learning Organisation*. Century Business, London. The Fifth Discipline.

Seo AY (2007) *Ensō: Zen Circles of Enlightenment*. Weatherhill, Boston.

Sinha L and Scherera K (1987) Ask the patient. *Nursing Times* 83(45): 40–2.

Sisson R (1990) Effects of auditory stimuli on comatose patients with head injury. *Heart and Lung* 4: 373–8.

Sloan G and Watson H (2001) John Heron's six-category intervention analysis: towards understanding interpersonal relations and progressing the delivery of clinical supervision for mental health nursing in the United Kingdom. *Journal of Advanced Nursing* 36(2): 206–14.

Smith A and Jack K (2005) Reflective: a meaningful task for students. *Nursing Standard* 19(26): 33–7.

Smith M and Liehr P (1999) Attentively embracing story: a middle range theory with practie and research implications. *Scholarly Inquiry for Nursing Practice* 13(3): 3–27.

Smuts J (1927) *Holism and Evolution*. Macmillan, London.

Smyth J, Stone A, Hurewitz A and Kaell A (1999) Effects of writing about stressful experiences on symptom reduction in patients with asthma or rheumatoid arthritis. *Journal of the American Medical Association* 281: 1304–9.

Smyth WJ (1987) *A Rationale for Teachers' Critical Pedagogy*. Deakin University Press, Melbourne, VIC.

Soanes C and Hawker S, Eds (2005) *Compact Oxford English Dictionary*, 3rd edition. Oxford University Press, Oxford.

Soffarelli D and Brown D (1998) The need for nursing leadership in uncertain times. *Journal of Nursing Management* 6: 201–7.

Steier F, Ed. (1991) *Research and Reflexivity*. Sage Publications, London.

Stein L (1978) The doctor-nurse game. In R Dingwall and J McIntosh, Eds, *Readings in the Sociology of Nursing*. Churchill Livingstone, Edinburgh, pp. 108–17.

Stein L (1988) The doctor-nurse game 10 years on . . .

Stewart I and Joines V (1987) *TA Today: A New Introduction to Transactional Analysis*. Russell Press, Nottingham.

Stockwell F (1972) *The Unpopular Patient*. Royal College of Nursing, London.

Street A (1992) *Inside Nursing: A Critical Ethnography of Clinical Nursing*. State University of New York Press, Albany.

Street A (1995) *Nursing Replay*. Churchill Livingstone, Melbourne, VIC.

Strummer J and Jones M (1978) White man in Hammersmith Palais. Nineden Ltd (PRS). Sony Music Entertainment (UK) Ltd.

Subhuti (1985/2001) *The Buddhist Vision: A Path to Fulfilment*. Windhorse, Birmingham.

Sumner J (2001) Caring in nursing: a different interpretation. *Journal of Advanced Nursing* 35(60): 926–32.

Susuki S (1999) *Zen Mind, Beginners Mind* [revised edition]. Weatherhill, New York.

Sutherland L (1994) Caring as mutul empowerment: working with the BNDU model at Burford. In C Johns, Ed., *The Burford NDU Model: Caring in Practice*. Blackwell Science, Oxford.

Talton C (1995) Complementary therapies: touch-of-all-kinds is therapeutic. *RN* 58(2): 61–4.

Tann S (1993) Eliciting student teachers' personal theories. In J Calderwood and P Gates, Eds, *Conceptualizing Reflection in Teacher Development*. The Falmer Press, London.

Taylor B (1992) From helper to human: a reconceptualisation of the nurse as a person. *Journal of Advanced Nursing* 17: 1042–9.

Taylor D and Singer E (1983) *New Organisation from Old*. IPM Management Publications, London.

Thomas K and Kilmann R (1974) *Thomas Kilmann Conflict Mode Instrument*. Xicom, Toledo.

Torbert WR (1978) Educating toward shared purpose, self direction and quality work. The theory and practice of liberating structure. *Journal of Higher Education* 49(2): 109–35.

Tosch P (1988) Patients' recollections of their post-traumatic coma. *Journal of Neuroscience Nursing* 20(4): 223–8.

Trexler JC (1995) Reformualtion of deviance and labeling theory for nursing. *Image: The Journal of Nursing Scholarship* 28(2): 131–5.

Trihn M (1991) *When the Moon Waxes Red: Representation, Gender and Cultural Politics*. Routledge, New York.

Trnobranski P (1994) Nurse-patient dialogue: assumption or reality? *Journal of Advanced Nursing* 19: 733–7.

Tschudin V (1993) *Ethics in Nursing*, 2nd edition. Butterworth Heinemann, Oxford.

Tuffnell M and Crickmay C (2004) *A Widening Field*. Dance Books, Alton.

Turton P (1989) Touch me, feel me, heal me. *Nursing Times* 85(19): 42–4.

Tversky A and Kahneman D (1974) Judgement under uncertainty: heuristics and biases. *Science* 185: 1124–31.

Tyler J (1998) Nonverbal communication and the use of art in the care of the dying. *Palliative Medicine* 12: 123–6.

Tzu L (1999) *Tao Te Ching* [trans S Mitchell]. Frances Lincoln, London.

UKCC (1987) *Advisory Paper: Confidentiality – An Elaboration of Clause 9*. UKCC, London.

UKCC (1996) *Positional Statement on Clinical Supervision*. UKCC, London.

Vachon M (1988) Battle fatigue in hospice/palliative care. In A Gilmore and S Gilmore, Eds, *A Safer Death*. Plenum Publishing, New York.

Van Manen M (1990) *Researching Lived Experience*. State University of New York Press, New York.

Vaught-Alexander K (1994) The personal journal for nurses: writing for delivery and healing. In D Gaut and A Boykin, Eds, *Caring as Healing: Renewal through Hope*. National League for Nursing Press, New York.

Visinstainer M (1986) The nature of knowledge and theory in nursing. *Image: The Journal of Nursing Scholarship* 18: 32–8.

Wagner L (1999) Within the circle of death: transpersonal poetic reflections on nurses' stories about the quality of the dying process. *International Journal for Human Caring* 3(2): 21–30.

Wainwright P (2000) Towards an aesthetics of nursing. *Journal of Advanced Nursing* 32(3): 750–5.

Wall TD, Bolden RI and Borril CS (1997) Minor psychiatric disturbance in NHS trust staff. *British Journal of Psychiatry* 171: 519–23.

Ward K (1988) Not just the patient in bed three. *Nursing Times* 84(78): 39–50.

Waterworth D (1995) Exploring the value of clinical Nursing practice: the practitioner's perspective. *Journal of Advanced Nursing* 22: 13–7.

Waterworth S and Luker K (1990) Reluctant collaborators: do patients want to be involved in decisions involving care? *Journal of Advanced Nursing* 15: 971–6.

Watson J (1988) *Nursing: Human Science and Human Care. A Theory of Nursing*. National league for Nursing, New York.

Watson J (1990) The moral failure of the hierarchy. *Nursing Outlook* 38(2): 62–6.

Weinsheimer J (1985) *Gadamer's Hermeneutics: A Reading of Truth and Method*. Yale University press, New Haven.

Wheatley M and Kellner-Rogers M (1996) *A Simpler Way*. Berrett-Koehler Publishers, San Francisco, CA.

Wheatley MJ (1999) *Leadership and the New Science. Discovering Order in a Chaotic World*. Berrett- Koehler, San Francisco, CA.

White A (1993) The nursing process: a constraint on expert practice. *Journal of Nursing Management* 1: 245–52.

White J (1995) Patterns of knowing: review, critique and update. *Advanced in Nursing Science* 17(4): 73–86.

Whittemore R (1999) Natural science and nursing science: where do the horizons fuse? *Journal of Advanced Nursing* 30(5): 1027–33.

Wilber K (1991) *Grace and Grit*. Newleaf, Dublin.

Wilber K (1998) *The Eye of Spirit: An Integral Vision for a World Gone Slightly Mad*. Shambhala, Boston.

Wilkinson J (1988) Moral distress in nursing practice: experience and effect. *Nursing Forum* 23(1): 16–29.

Winterson J (2001) *The Powerbook*. Vintage, London.

Winterson J (2005) *Lighthousekeeping*. Harcourt, Orlando, FL.

Woodward V and Webb C (2001) Women's anxieties surrounding breast disorders: a systematic review of the literature. *Journal of Advanced Nursing* 33(1): 29–41.

Woolf V (1945) *A Room of One's Own*. Penguin Books, London.

Wuest J (1997) Illuminating environmental influences on women's caring. *Journal of Advanced Nursing* 26(1): 49–58.

Younger J (1995) The alienation of the sufferer. *Advances in Nursing Science* 17(4): 53–72.

Index

Page numbers in **bold** refer to tables, those in *italics* refer to figures

Becoming a Reflective Practitioner, Fourth Edition. Christopher Johns.
© 2013 John Wiley & Sons, Ltd. Published 2013 by John Wiley & Sons, Ltd.